T0254306

CREATE AN ENVIRONMENTAL PROTECTION

and

CANCER PREVENTION RESEARCH INSTITUTE AND CARRY OUT CANCER PREVENTION SYSTEM ENGINEERING

Open a new era of cancer prevention research and cancer prevention system engineering in the 21st century

How to conquer cancer? How to prevent cancer?
How to scientifically prevent pollution and pollution?
How to scientifically prevent cancer and control cancer?

(Part II of Prevention)

Authors: Xu Ze (China); Xu Jie (China) ; Bin Wu (America)
Translators: Bin Wu ; Lily Xu ; Zihao Xu
Editors: Bin Wu ; Lily Xu
Illustrators : Lily Xu ; Bin Wu

authorHOUSE®

AuthorHouse™
1663 Liberty Drive
Bloomington, IN 47403
www.authorhouse.com
Phone: 1 (800) 839-8640

© 2019 Xu Ze, Xu Jie, Bin Wu. All rights reserved.

No part of this book may be reproduced, stored in a retrieval system, or transmitted
by any means without the written permission of the author.

Published by AuthorHouse 09/27/2019

ISBN: 978-1-7283-2777-8 (sc)
ISBN: 978-1-7283-2776-1 (e)

Library of Congress Control Number: 2019914361

Print information available on the last page.

Any people depicted in stock imagery provided by Getty Images are models,
and such images are being used for illustrative purposes only.
Certain stock imagery © Getty Images.

This book is printed on acid-free paper.

Because of the dynamic nature of the Internet, any web addresses or links contained in this book may have changed
since publication and may no longer be valid. The views expressed in this work are solely those of the author and do not
necessarily reflect the views of the publisher, and the publisher hereby disclaims any responsibility for them.

Create an environmental protection and cancer prevention research institute and carry out cancer prevention system engineering

Open a new era of cancer prevention research and cancer prevention system engineering in the 21st century

How to conquer cancer? How to prevent cancer?

How **to scientifically** prevent pollution and pollution?

How **to scientifically** prevent cancer and control cancer?

(Part II of Prevention)

Authors: Xu Ze (China); Xu Jie (China) ; Bin Wu (America)

Translators: Bin Wu ; Lily Xu ; Zihao Xu

Editors: Bin Wu ; Lily Xu

Illustrators : Lily Xu ; Bin Wu

XZ-C proposes to create an environmental protection and cancer prevention research institute and carry out cancer prevention system engineering

—— Open a new era of cancer prevention research and cancer prevention system engineering in the 21st century

XZ-C proposes:

Dawning A type cancer prevention plan

Dawning B type cancer prevention plan

Dawning D-type cancer prevention plan

Combined with winning three major pollution battles,

scientific pollution prevention and pollution control

scientific cancer prevention, anti-cancer

Scientific research ideas and suggestions for how to fight well and win the three major pollution battles

(Part II)

TO THE READS

First, I deeply appreciate that you spend your precious time to open this book to read and you are willing to understand our innovation method how to prevent cancer and how to cure cancer and how to control cancer. Time is life.

Medicine is fascinating; Technology dramatically develops. Along with the recognition and understanding of the disease etiology and pathology and pathogenesis and pathophysiology, many disease can be prevented before it occurs and can be cured or controlled such as the common disease cancer and cardiovascular disease, others etc. Dr. Xu Ze did the detail and throughout cancer basic and clinical research and clinical verification about many clinical phenomenon such as how cancer metastasis and where the weak point is and why so many cancer patients had thrombosis and how to stop the disease process. During the experiment processes, he found that cancer occurrence and metastasis are closely **relate to immune function and** how cancer metastasis in our body and where the week line is so that how to stop cancer metastasis during the week point. The great achievements are the effective medications which only kill the cancer cell without killing the normal cell and so far there are no significant side effect after the patient take for the long term period and plus many innovated concept and way to prevent and to treat the cancer. Prevention is the key to conquer cancer. The work of cancer treatment and prevention should start at the same time and at the same attention and at the same level.

Reflection and review can improve and can promote the innovation such as in 1916 it was discovered that the incidence of breast carcinoma on mice could be reduced after removal of the ovary, indicating ovarian hormone may lead to breast ; 1932 the artificial hormone was injected to induce the breast carcinoma of mice, which implied that breast cancer is closed to hormone; in 1941, the hormone dependence of prostatic carcinoma was proven, physical castration therapy and estrogen chemical castration therapy could reduce tumor load of the metastatic prostatic carcinoma while the androgen injected could promote the metastasis, which implied the issue of prostate is closely related to hormone. All of these scientific researches can save thousands of the patient life.

It is a great passion to this modern medicine and as a medical profession and a doctor can help the patient and can save the life. Let us keep working hard to do good things for our world.

Bin Wu and Lily Xu

09-11-2019

In Timonium, MD in USA

CONTENTS

Note:

1. XZ-C is Xu Ze-China (Xu Ze - China), because science is borderless, but scientists are national and intellectual property.

2. Cancer is a disaster for all mankind. It must evoke the struggle of the people all over the world. Therefore, 15 of these series are exclusively in English and distributed worldwide.

WHAT THINGS ARE IN THIS BOOK?

XZ-C proposes to conquer cancer and to launch the general attack on cancer, and that it must establish the research institute of the environmental protection and cancer prevention and it must carry out cancer prevention system engineering. Open a new era of cancer prevention research and cancer prevention system engineering in the 21st century

While human being is in the search for the cause and condition of cancer, the most prominent thing is that it was found that more than 90% of cancers are caused by or closely related to environmental factors.

The Cancer Prevention Research Institute should conduct cancer prevention research, look for carcinogenic factors, detect damage to humans caused by carcinogens or carcinogenic factors, track the source of carcinogens or carcinogenic factors and study preventive measures of how to reduce or stop these carcinogens.

How to overcome cancer? How to prevent cancer?

XZ-C proposes:

Established the Research Institute of Environmental Protection and Health Prevention Cancer to carry out cancer prevention system engineering and establish a high-level laboratory

XZ-C proposes:

Dawning A type cancer prevention plan

Dawning B type cancer prevention plan

Dawning D-type cancer prevention plan

Because cancer patients cover the whole world, the pollution of industrial and agricultural wastewater, waste residue and waste gas also covers the whole world. Therefore, it is imperative that the global effort be made to conquer cancer and launch the general attack on cancer, or we must globally attack the cancer to attack the general attack, and put cancer prevention, cancer control, cancer treatment at the same level and the same attention and at the same time, especially cancer prevention is the top priority, study these sources of pollution, try to stop at the source, and strive to block the safety risks of cancer in the bud status.

How to fight well and win three major pollution battles?

XZ-C proposed: What is the source of pollution? To solve or to release the bell, you need to ring the bell.

How to <u>scientifically</u> prevent pollution and to treat pollution? How to <u>scientifically</u> prevent cancer and to control cancer?

<u>1.   How to scientifically prevent pollution and to treat pollution?</u>

XZ-C proposes that scientific thinking, scientific research, scientific analysis, and scientific discussion should be conducted:

a. What is the content of pollution? What contents are there? What are the ingredients? What contents are they included in? What are the chemical ingredients?

It should be used for chemical composition detection, analysis, trace element analysis, qualitative and quantitative.

b. Does this ingredient have any effect on human health? What is the damage? Whether is there a carcinogen or not?

c. What is the source of pollution? Why did it happen? Can it be tried to stop at the source? In scientific and research design, how is it avoided?

d. How to stop the pollution at the source?

It is to block at the source of the business.

XZ-C proposed that it is necessary to ring the bell in order to solve the bell, that is, it is to set up a special scientific research team within the enterprise to study and solve it.

Professor Xu Ze proposed to strive to study as much as possible before the product leaves the factory in order not to produce social pollution.

2. How does it try to stop the pollution at the source? How to prevent it at the source within the company in order to reduce pollution society?

To solve the bell, it needs to ring the bell. Industry is the main body of atmospheric pollutant emissions, energy production and consumption are the main sources of air pollutant emissions in China. Special scientific research groups for air pollutants should be established within the enterprise to study the composition analysis of atmospheric pollutants and their emission pathways, and to strive to conduct the research of pollution prevention and pollution control and pollution treatment before the product leaves the factory, and avoid social pollution as much as possible (such as airplanes, trains, cars, thermal power...)

In the route of emission of atmospheric pollutants, it can be purified.

Professor Xu Ze proposed how to overcome cancer and how to prevent cancer by I see

Situation analysis: (1)

- How to prevent cancer? Cancer incidence is rising

Situation analysis: (2)

- Cancer incidence is related to the environment

1). Why does the increase in cancer incidence have a relationship with the environment?

2). The cause of cancer is related to the carcinogenic factors of the external environment and the internal environment.

3). If we have a deeper understanding of the causes of cancer, then we can come up with more valuable suggestions in the future:

How should it prevent cancer-causing factors, how to monitor which carcinogenic factors, and which to eliminate cancer-causing factors, so that we can stay away from cancer and prevent cancer?

Situation analysis: (3)

--- Prevention should be based on improving the carcinogenic factors of external factors (external environment) and internal factors (internal environment)

Professor Xu Ze proposed:

The establishment of an innovative cancer prevention research institute and an innovative cancer prevention system project is an unprecedented and it must be practiced in person to seek health and well-being for mankind.

XZ-C proposed the general design of cancer prevention and cancer prevention system engineering.

Situation analysis: (4)

- **It should set up the Environmental and Cancer Research Group**

It is to monitor environmental pollution-causing factors and data, to research and develop the measures of cancer prevention and cancer control, and to research and develop the method of interventions.

a, from clothing, food, shelter and walking to prevent cancer

b, from the big environment of life to prevent cancer

c, from the small living environment to prevent cancer

d, from life behavior, life hobbies, and living habits to prevent cancer

Under the guidance of Xi Jinping's characteristic socialism in the new era, it strives to open a new situation in scientific research work in the new era, and overcome the scientific research work of cancer, we should make great strides forward, and strives to follow the path of independent innovation with Chinese characteristics and adhere to the road of independent innovation of "Chinese-style anti-cancer" with the combination of Chinese and Western medicine.

Innovation -

It walked out of the road of Immune regulation and control of treatment of cancer with "Chinese-style anti-cancer" of the combination of Chinese and Western medicine while we have accumulated 30 years of the basic and clinical research on anti-cancer and anti-cancer metastasis. We have accumulated clinical application experience more than 12,000 cases in 20 years which can be pushed to the country and can go to the world, can be connected to the "A Belt and A Road" to bring Chinese medicine to the world and to make "Chinese-style anti-cancer" and immune regulation and control of treatment of cancer with the combination of Chinese and Western medicine that not only develops and enriches the content of immunotherapy of cancer, but also brings China's medical modernization into line with international standards and is at the forefront of the world.

A BRIEF INTRODUCTION TO THE FIRST AUTHOR

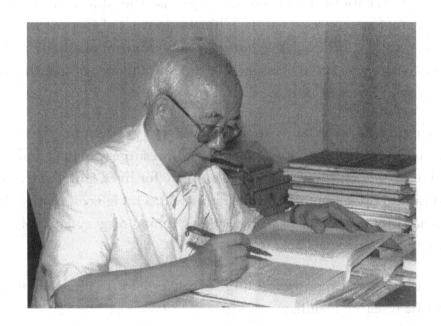

Xu Ze, male, was born in October 1933 in Leping City, Jiangxi Province, graduated from Tongji Medical College in 1956. He has served as the director of surgery, professor, chief physician, master's and doctoral supervisor of Hubei Affiliated Hospital of Hubei College of Traditional Chinese Medicine, director of the Experimental Surgery Research Institute of Hubei College of Traditional Chinese Medicine, director of the Department of Abdominal Oncology Surgery, and director of the Anticancer Metastasis and Recurrence Research Office. He has served as the executive director of the Wuhan Branch of the Chinese Medical Association, the vice chairman of the Wuhan Microcirculation Society, and the honorary president of the Wuhan Anticancer Research Association, member of the Standing Committee of the General Association of Hubei Branch of the Chinese Medical Association, member of the Hubei Provincial Schistosomiasis Research Committee, member of the Hubei Provincial Senior Health Technology Review Committee, member of the Hubei Provincial Academic Committee of the Academic Degree Committee, and member of the Academic Committee of Hubei College of Traditional Chinese Medicine, member of the Expert Group of China Medical and Health Science and Technology Appraisal and Evaluation of the Department of Science and Technology of the Ministry of Health, member of the scientific and technical peer review expert group of the Higher Education Institute, member of the Spleen Surgery Group of the Chinese Medical Association Surgical Society, senior editor of the China Series Magazine, and member of the National Natural Science Foundation of China, schistosomiasis advisory committee of Ministry of Health, academic member of the International Liver Disease Research Collaboration Center, member of the International Federation of Surgeons. The editorial board of the first, second, third and fourth sessions of the Chinese Journal of Experimental Surgery, the first, second and third executive editors of the Journal of Abdominal Surgery. He has made outstanding contributions to medicine and enjoys special government allowances from the State Council.

He engages in surgical work for more than 50 years, is proficient in the theory of this profession, and has rich clinical experience in radical surgery of lung and esophageal cancer in thoracic surgery and abdominal surgery for liver, gallbladder, pancreatic cancer and radical operation of gastrointestinal cancer. He is especially effective in the treatment of refractory ascites surgery and tumor surgery and spleen surgery for cirrhotic portal hypertension.

He has been engaged in experimental surgical research for 15 years and has achieved many scientific research results:

One is the experimental research and clinical application of the self-made Z-Cl abdominal cavity-venous bypass device for the treatment of refractory ascites in cirrhosis of the Hubei Provincial Science and Technology Commission. In 1982, the Hubei Provincial Science and Technology Commission presided over the identification of the domestic advanced level, won the second prize of Hubei Provincial Government Science and Technology Achievements, and won the first prize of scientific and technological achievements of Hubei Provincial Health Department. It is promoted and applied in 38 hospitals in 12 provinces and cities nationwide. After the results were published in English and German, they received letters from medical research institutions in Spain, France, Italy, Belgium, Japan and other countries. In 1983, he attended a conference on parasites in China and Japan and went to Australia in 1990 to present a thesis at the International Conference on Liver Disease Research. The other is the National Natural Science Foundation:

"Experimental study on the pathophysiology and pathogenesis of pulmonary schistosomiasis by experimental methods" was identified as an international advanced level under the auspices of the Provincial Health Department in 1986, which received the second prize for scientific and technological achievements of the Hubei Provincial Government.

In 1985, he made a petition to more than 3,000 patients with postoperative thoracic and abdominal cancer. He found that most patients relapsed or metastasized within 2 to 3 years.

Therefore, clinical basic research to prevent recurrence and metastasis must be carried out. In 1987, he began experimental tumor research, performed cancer cell migration, established a tumor animal model, and carried out a series of experimental tumor research:

To explore the mechanism and regularity of cancer recurrence and metastasis;

To explore the relationship between tumors and immune organs and immune organs and tumors;

From experimental tumor research it was found:

The progression of the tumor causes progressive atrophy of the thymus, impaired proliferation of thymocytes, and decreased immune function.

From a series of experimental studies, it has been found that thymus atrophy and low immune function may be one of the causes and pathogenesis of cancer, and should be treated with "protection of Thymus and Increase of Immune function".

More than 200 kinds of Chinese herbal medicines in the literature that may have anti-cancer and anti-cancer effects were screened in a rigorous scientific and repeated tumor-bearing animal model in vivo. After looking for a large number of natural medicines, 48 kinds of traditional Chinese medicines with anti-cancer invasion, metastasis and recurrence were screened out. Based on this, XZ-C immunomodulatory anticancer traditional Chinese medicine preparation was developed and invented. XZ-C1-10 was applied to clinical practice on the basis of successful animal experiments.

XZ-C immunomodulation anticancer Chinese medicine has been clinically proven in clinical cases over the past 20 years, and its curative effect is remarkable.

He has been teaching for 50 years and has trained many young doctors, 10 master students and 2 doctoral students. He published 126 research papers and participated in the compilation of eight medical monographs such as Hepatopathy Treatment, Hepatobiliary and Pancreatic Surgery, and Abdominal Surgery. In 2001, he published the monograph "New Understanding and New Model of Cancer Treatment", published by Hubei Science and Technology Press, Xu Ze, and issued by Xinhua Bookstore nationwide. In 2006, he published the monograph "New Concepts and New Methods for Cancer Metastasis Treatment", published by People's Military Medical Press, Xu Ze, and issued by Xinhua Bookstore nationwide. This book was awarded the "Three Hundreds" original book by the State Press and Publication Administration. In April 2007, the General Administration of Press and Publication of the People's Republic of China issued the "Three One Hundred" Original Publishing Engineering Certificate: "The New Concept and New Method of Cancer Metastasis Treatment" was selected into the first "Three Ones" of the General Administration of Press and Publication. This book is issued for the original book publishing project.

In this book, Xu Ze (XU ZE) published the basic research and clinical research of the new concept and new method of cancer metastasis treatment. The new findings of a series of experimental research and the theoretical innovation of clinical research are original innovations:

Xu Ze (XU ZE) first discovered and proposed the following five clinically applied oncology theoretical innovations in the world: theoretical innovation content:

1. Three manifestations of cancer in the human body; theoretical innovations;

2. The "two points and one line" theory of the whole process of cancer development; theoretical innovation content;

3. cancer transfer treatment "three steps"; theoretical innovation content;

4. Open up the third field of human anti-cancer metastasis treatment; theoretical innovation;

5. The animal laboratory of XU ZE has the following new findings:

In this book, Xu Ze published the basic research and clinical research of the new concept and new method of cancer metastasis treatment. The new findings of a series of experimental research and the theoretical innovation of clinical research are original innovations: Xu Ze first discovered and proposed the following five clinically applied oncology theoretical innovations in the world: theoretical innovation content:

1. Three manifestations of cancer in the human body; theoretical innovations;

2. The "two points and one line" theory of the whole process of cancer development; theoretical innovation content;

3. cancer transfer treatment "three steps"; theoretical innovation content;

4. Open up the third field of human anti-cancer metastasis treatment; theoretical innovation;

5. The new concept, new model of XU ZE cancer therapy.

The animal laboratory of XU ZE has the following new findings:

It was found:

1, Excision of the thymus (Thymus) can produce a cancer animal model; experimental findings;

2, the use of immunosuppressive drugs, so that the decline in immunity, is conducive to the production of cancer animal models; experimental findings;

3, As the cancer progresses, the thymus undergoes progressive atrophy; experimental findings;

4, cancer metastasis is related to immunity, immune function is low, may promote tumor metastasis; experimental findings

5, the rats inoculated, the thymus progressive atrophy, not inoculated, the thymus does not shrink, grow to the size of the fingertips, the thymus no longer shrinks; experimental findings;

6, the tumor will inhibit Thymu (Th) and caused the immune organs to shrink. Therefore, we speculate that solid tumors may produce a factor that is not yet known to inhibit Th(thymus), and is called "cancer suppressor factor."

A BRIEF INTRODUCTION TO THE SECOND AUTHOR

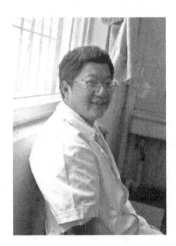

Xu Jie, male, graduated from Hubei College of Traditional Chinese Medicine in 1992, graduated from Hubei Medical University in 1996, Department of Clinical Medicine. Now He is chief physician in Hubei University of Traditional Chinese Medicine Hospital and Hubei Provincial Hospital of Surgery, engaged in experimental surgical tumor research and general surgery, urology clinical work.

Since 1992, he has been involved in the experimental tumor research of the Institute of Experimental Surgery of Hubei College of Traditional Chinese Medicine. He has carried out cancer cell transplantation and established a tumor animal model. He has carried out a series of experimental tumor research: exploring the mechanism of recurrence and metastasis of cancer and in vivo screening experiment of more than 200 kinds of Chinese herbal medicine in vivo tumor model of tumor inhibition s from a large number of natural medicine to find out, screening out of 48 kinds of anti-cancer invasion, metastasis, relapse traditional Chinese medicine

He participates in clinical validation and followed up for XZ - C immunoregulatory Chinese herbal medicine and completes the experimental research and clinical verification, data collection, collection and summary of this book.

A BRIEF INTRODUCTION TO THE THIRD AUTHOR AND THE MAIN TRANSLATOR AND ONE OF THE EDITORS

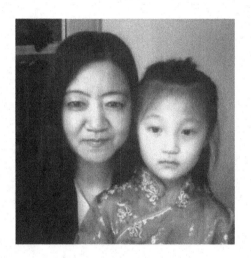

Bin Wu, MD, Ph.D., graduated from College of Yunyang of Tongji University of Medical Sciences for her MD degree; Studied her Master degree and her Ph. D degree in Sun Yat-Sen University of Medical Sciences. After she receive her Ph.D., she worked as a Post-doctoral Follews in the Johns Hopkins Medical School and University of Maryland Medical School. She passed all of her USMLE tests and is going to do her residency training in America. She dedicated herself to oncology ·clinical and research. Her goal is to conquer cancer, which she believes this great contribution to our health. She has a daughter, named Lily Xu who drew all of the pictures in this book.

A BRIEF INTRODUCTION TO THE ILLUSTRATOR AND THE ADVISOR

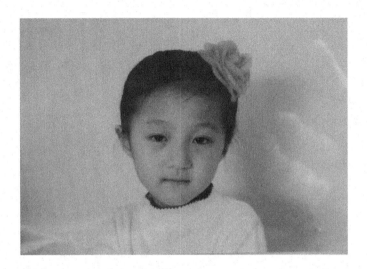

Lily Xu was born on November 17th 2006 and had an art presented in the Walter Art Museum in Baltimore at the age of 6; she got the fourth place trophy in the ES Double Digits or 24 and 24 games in the Baltimore County in Maryland; she got the first trophy in the BCPS STEM FAIR PHYSICS in Baltimore County; when she was in the sixth grade, she passed the advanced Math for 7th grade(which means the 8th grade math) test and moved the 8th grade math class and now she takes high school Math class; she loves the reading and the writing and she finished many seires of books and in 2019 summary she start to do volunteer job in the publish libarary. She got $6000 scholarship award for the Peabody music program in the Johns Hopkins University. She edits all of my books for the publishing and drew all of the pictures in this book. In 2018 and 2019 she was chosen into Baltimore county Middle school Honor Band. In 2018 the robotic team which she attended for years got designing-award from the Baltimore county so that this robotic team came to Maryland State for the Robotic contest in 2019. On January 19th, 2019 she got the Robotic designing award in Maryland. She edits all of my books for the publishing and drew all of the pictures in this book. In 2019 she was chosen by Baltimore County for one duel and one ensemble to play Clarion.

ACKNOWLEDGEMENTS

First, thank for everyone who takes time to open these series of books.

Second, this book is for all of people who concern human being health. We are deep grateful to all of people who like our new ways to improve our human being health. I appreciate to anyone who encourages me to continue working on my career. I thanks for any good word which is encouraging me.

Sometime life is extremely difficult for me and I faced the *traumatically family disaster,* however I keep working very hard day and night because I love to help the patients to live fear-free of disease and to help the patients to have happy and healthy live so that they can serve others.

My daughter Lily Xu gives me many smart and creative ideas while we were finishing this book. Lily Xu drew all of the pictures such as the Thymus etc. **The characteristics of she loves the challenge** and her judgment always encourages me to continue working hard to move on.

I would like to express our sincere gratitude to the following:

1. All of Authorhouse staffs

2. Dr. Xu Ze's family and Dr. Xu Jie's family

3. Mrs. Bo Wu's family and Mrs. Tao Wu's famly

4. I deeply thank my only daughter Lily Xu, for her help with me and for her understanding me and for her update knowledge and for her loving learning.

Bin Wu, M.D., Ph.D

09-11-2019 in Timonium, Maryland in USA

THE MAIN TOPICS

A. The outline of conquering cancer

Under the guidance of Xi Jinping's new era of socialism with Chinese characteristics, we should strive to open up a new phase of scientific research in the new era, and the scientific research work to overcome cancer should be advanced. We will strive to follow the path of independent innovation with Chinese characteristics and adhere to the road of independent innovation of Chinese and Western medicine combined with "Chinese-style anti-cancer". China will contribute more to the world's wisdom, China's programs, and China's forces to overcome cancer research, so that the sun of humanity's destiny will shine in the world.

XZ-C proposes to create an environmental protection and cancer prevention research institute and carry out cancer prevention systems engineering and open 21st Century Cancer Research

How to overcome cancer? How to conquer cancer and launch the general attack of cancer?

How to prevent cancer by I see? How to do cancer prevention research by I see?

How to scientifically prevent pollution and treat pollution?

How to scientifically prevent cancer and control cancer?

The purpose of the research work of conquering cancer is to make people's health and to keep away from cancer, and is also a great pioneering work or great initiative for future generations to seek health and welfare.

— *To establish an overall framework for the fight against cancer or for conquering cancer, to create the multidisciplinary of conquering cancer and the science city of the scientific research base of the cancer-related research of conquering cancer, which is the only way to conquering cancer*

— *Proposed the overall design, plan, plan, blueprint and implementation rules of Science City*

---- *Equivalent to designing an overall framework for Chinese characteristics to overcome cancer*

----- *The following is the outline which was proposed by XZ-C of about the implementation of how to overcome cancer:*

The main project to implement the outline of how to overcome cancer is:

The structural work:

Overcoming cancer and launching the general attack of cancer, focusing on prevention, control, and treatment together and at the same attention and at the same level.

Creating multidisciplinary and the scientific research base of cancer-related research---- - Science City

Two-wing project:

A wing - how to overcome cancer? How to prevent cancer?

----- - to reduce the incidence of cancer

B wing - how to overcome cancer? How to treat cancer?

---- - to improve cancer cure rate

Aims:

A: *Reduce the incidence of cancer*

B: *Improve cancer cure rate, prolong patient survival, and improve patient quality of life*

If it can be to implement and realize the overall design of cancer, planning blueprints, it is possible to overcome cancer.

How to implement, how to achieve this general guideline, programs, plans, blueprints to overcome cancer?

It should set up the cancer research team to "conquer cancer and launch the general attack of the cancer"

It is to invite famous experts, professors, academic leaders or leading scientists, entrepreneurs, leaders, and volunteers who support "overcome cancer and launch the general attack on cancer" who are invited to work together to make an unprecedented event in human history, "to overcome cancer and to launch the general attack of cancer," and "create a science city that conquers cancer, for the benefit of mankind.

The preparation for setting up:

"The first science city of the scientific research base in the country to overcome cancer"

"The world's first science city of the scientific research base to conquer cancer"

B. The detail of the Table of Contents

Table of Contents

A late scientific research report was 25 years late. The design was put forward during the "Eighth Five-Year Plan" and the plan was completed and the scientific research report was presented after 35 years.

The reason for being late is my acute myocardial infarction, and then there is the resting or recovery time for a long time, then slowly move forward.

A late scientific research report

1. The source background and experience of scientific research topics

(1) The source background and the course of completion of scientific research topics (the tortuous course)

(2) Some experiences (Annex 1)

1. Briefly describe the scientific research process of my anti-cancer research

(1) The first stage

(2) The second stage

(3) The third stage

(4) The fourth stage

2. Briefly describe the academic thinking and scientific research thinking of my scientific research process

(1) The first stage (1985-1999)

From the follow-up results it is found:

New findings from animal experiments:

Innovative thinking, changing concepts, and proposing new models and new understandings of cancer treatment

(2) The second stage (after 2001)

Targeting the research goals and the "targets" of cancer treatment to **anti-metastasis**, pointing out that the key to cancer treatment is anti-metastasis

(3) The third stage (after 2006)

The research focuses on the prevention and treatment of the whole process of cancer occurrence and development.

Closely combined with clinical practice, it proposes reform and innovation, research and development in response to the problems and drawbacks of current clinical traditional therapy.

Recognizing that the prevention and treatment strategies for cancer must move forward, the way out for cancer treatment is "three early", and the way out for cancer is prevention.

Put the research focus for the research on prevention and treatment of the whole process of cancer occurrence and development. Closely integrated with clinical practice, in response to the problems and drawbacks of current clinical traditional therapies, it proposes reform and innovation, research and development. Recognizing that the prevention and treatment strategies for cancer must move forward, the way out for cancer treatment is "three early", and the way out for cancer is prevention.

(4) The fourth stage (2011 -)

Now it is the fourth stage of scientific research, which is being carried out and proceeded. The research work is step by step, and the research goal or "target" is positioned to reduce the incidence of cancer, improve the cure rate and prolong the survival period. Professor Xu Ze (XZ-C) proposed an initiative to create the Environmental Protection and Cancer Research Institute and carry out cancer prevention system engineering to reduce the incidence of cancer.

XZ-C proposes to carry out "to overcome conquer and launch the general attack of cancer – cancer prevention, cancer control, cancer treatment at the same attention and at the same level and at the same time"

3. The formation process of the new theory concept of cancer treatment

(1) From the follow-up to the establishment of experimental surgical laboratory

(2) New findings

(3) Animal experimental research on finding new anticancer and anti-metastatic drugs in natural medicine

(4) Clinical verification work

4. The Scientific Research routes and research methods for new theories and new methods of related-cancer treatment

(1) Scientific Research route

(2) Research methods

(3) Academic value and academic status

(4) Dawning or Shuguang scientific research spirit

5. The tasks, missions, opportunities and challenges of anti-cancer research

(1) Research on anti-cancer metastasis is a current urgent need

1). It must know the current problems

2). It must know the problems in the current treatment

(2) Conducting anti-cancer metastasis research is the need for the development of oncology

(3) What to do and how to do it

6. The Research of Reform and Development on cancer treatment

7. What research work have we carried out? What scientific research achievements and scientific and technological innovation series have been made?

Briefly describe scientific research results, scientific thinking, academic thinking, theoretical innovation, and scientific dedication of anti-cancer research.

In the past 30 years, we have made scientific research achievements and scientific technology innovation series in the field of cancer research direction as conquering cancer.

In this series of "Monographs", the following 30 academic arguments are presented for the first time in the world, all of which are original papers, internationally pioneered, and internationally leading, and have reached the forefront of the world.

8. XZ-C put forward four major scientific contributions, all of which were first proposed internationally, all of which are international leaders.

9. What research work have we carried out?

In order to conquer cancer, a series of scientific research plans, overall design, scheme, projects, blueprints, master plans, overall framework and implementation details or rules are proposed.

"XZ-C proposes a scientific research plan to conquer cancer and launch the general attack of cancer"

(1). It is first proposed at the international level:

"Necessity and Feasibility of Overcoming cancer and launching the General Attack of Cancer"

-- The overall strategic reform of cancer treatment shifts the focus of treatment into prevention and treatment of cancer at the same attention and at the same time and at the same level.

(2) It is first proposed at the international level:

"Preparing for the establishment hospital with cancer prevention and treatment during the whole process of cancer occurrence and development"

—— The global demonstration of the prevention and treatment hospital

(3) It is first proposed at the international level:

"The report of the general attack design for conquering cancer and the basic design and feasibility of building the Science City for conquering cancer"

-It is equivalent to designing an overall framework for conquering cancer design with Chinese characteristics

(4). It is first proposed at the international level:

"The report of the necessity and feasibility which in the construction of a well-off society, it is recommended that "taking a ride to scientific research" to carry out scientific research on cancer prevention and tumors prevention and treatment work"

These four scientific research projects are all proposed for the first time in the world, and are the first in the world. The international leader has opened up a new field of anti-cancer research.

11. How to overcome cancer? How to treat cancer?

XZ-C first proposed in the world: Dawning or Shuguang C-type plan No.1-6

Dawning C-type plan No. 1:

"Conquering cancer and launching the general attack of cancer"

Dawning C-type plan No. 2:

"Creating a full-scale prevention and treatment hospital"

Dawning C-type plan No. 3:

"Building a scientific research base and the science city of conquering cancer"

Dawning or Shuguang C-type plan No. 4:

"Building the multidisciplinary and cancer research group"

Dawning C-type plan No. 5:

"The vaccine is human hope and immunological prevention"

Dawning C-type plan No. 6:

"The prospect of immunomodulatory drugs is gratifying"

12. How to overcome cancer? How to prevent cancer?

The XZ-C first proposed internationally:

Create "Innovative Environmental Protection and Cancer Prevention Research Institute" and carry out cancer prevention system engineering

XZ-C proposes:

Dawning A type cancer prevention plan

Dawning B type cancer prevention plan

Dawning D-type cancer prevention plan

Macro, micro, ultra-micro

13. The scientific research ideas or thinking path of how to fight well and win the three major pollution battles

XZ-C proposes:

How to scientifically prevent pollution and treat pollution?

How to scientifically prevent cancer and control cancer?

How to scientifically design, scheme, plan, scientific thinking, scientific and technological innovation, and win the three major pollution battles by I see (1), (2), (3), (4)

14. The scientific research thought or ideas and words or suggestions of how to fight well or lay a good and win the three major pollution battles

(1) XZ-C proposes:

Advising the World Health Organization:

1). It should promote scientific research ethics, medicine is benevolence, setting up ethics is the first

The scientific Research ethics:

products, achievements, patents, and technologies should have ethical standards

Standard:

the bottom line should not be harmful to human health

Basic ethics:

All products, achievements, patents, technology, goods and people are harmless and do not harm people's health, especially for children, and must not contain carcinogens.

All products, goods, and technology should have ethical standards.

2). It is recommended that all countries, provinces and states should establish anti-cancer research institutes (or institutions) to carry out anti-cancer system projects and carry out anti-cancer projects for their own country, province, state and city (because of various countries, provinces and states) There are a large number of cancer patients in each city)

3). Countries should establish anti-cancer regulations and carry out comprehensively (some should be legislated)

4). implementation of prevention-oriented policy: the way to cure cancer in the "three early", the way out of cancer prevention.

(2) XZ-C proposes:

To the World Health Organization and the United Nations:

1). XZ-C proposes:

It should save the mother river of the world.

2). XZ-C proposal:

"To solve the bell, you need to ring the bell" (all products: airplane, train, car...) should be harmless to human health, no complications, no sequelae, no harm to people's health, especially the three major pollution, can not contain cancer The product should be designed to avoid and remove when designing. When the product leaves the factory, it should be monitored by product ethical standards.

Research ethics:

It should be based on the standard of not damaging human health, especially the carcinogens.

Basic ethics:

All products, achievements, patents, goods and people are harmless and do not harm people's health, especially for children, and must not contain carcinogens.

3). XZ-C proposes an initiative:

The "Innovative Environmental Protection and Cancer Prevention Research Institute" should be established and the cancer prevention system project should be carried out.

—— Open a new era of cancer prevention research and cancer prevention system engineering in the 21ˢᵗ century.

Resolutely fight and win the three major pollution battles, scientific pollution prevention, pollution control, scientific management of smog, scientific cancer prevention, cancer control, this is a great initiative for the benefit of the country and the people, but it is also for the research work of cancer prevention, anti-cancer, and conquering cancer to create good opportunities. Conquering cancer is at the forefront of science and a worldwide problem. Cancer is a human disaster. The whole world and the people all over the world are eager to hope that one day they can overcome cancer and benefit mankind.

15. Adhere to walk the road of cancer prevention and cancer control innovation in a well-off society with Chinese characteristics

(1) At the same time as building a well-off society, it is recommended to carry out scientific research of cancer prevention and cancer control and work for cancer prevention and treatment.

(2) Following the scientific development concept and adhering to the innovative road of anti-cancer and anti-metastasis with Chinese characteristics

(3) Energy conservation, emission reduction, pollution prevention, pollution treatment, a well-off society, stay away from cancer

16. Building a resource-saving and environment-friendly society, which has great correlation with cancer prevention and cancer control.

17. The cancer prevention scientific research work cannot walk slowly and it should run ahead, save the wounded

18. **XZ-C proposed: it should promote scientific research ethics, medicine is benevolence, setting up the ethics it the first**

19. **The past and future of oncology development**

Prospects for cancer treatment, predictive assessment

20. **How to overcome cancer?**

XZ-C proposes that cancer is a disaster for all mankind. It is necessary for the people of the world to work together and China and the United States will jointly tackle the problem.

"Cancer moon shot" (US) and "Dawning C-type plan" (China) - march together and head to the science hall of conquering cancer

Why do you want to move forward together? What are you together? The advantages analysis and complementary advantages for China and the United States itself each

- For the past 100 years, the history record of the "Conquering Cancer" program has been raised or proposed internationally.

- Doing or Be an unprecedented event for the benefit of mankind

- Dawning C plan

- Situation analysis: (1), (2), (3), (4)

Our advantage is:

1. Traditional Chinese medicine, anti-cancer traditional Chinese medicine, immune regulation and control traditional Chinese medicine, activating blood circulation and removing blood stasis anti-cancer thrombus suppository Chinese medicine, Ruanjian Sanjie anti-small nodule Chinese medicine, heat-clearing and detoxifying to improve the micro-environment of cancer cells;

2. Combination of Chinese and Western medicine, combined with innovation

The advantages of the United States are:

Modern medicine, advanced diagnosis and treatment technology, targeted medicine

XZ-C believes that:

We should give full play to China's advantages and potentials. We should increase efforts to develop and explore the advantages of Chinese herbal medicine. Traditional Chinese medicine can improve symptoms, improve physical fitness, increase immunity, and prolong survival. (The lesions generally do not shrink, but they can survive with tumors and live for a long time.) can be used as an adjuvant treatment for surgery.

21. Pathfinding and footprint

- cause

- navigate

- Footprint (scientific footprint)

- Shuguang research spirit

- Thinking in the morning

22. Guide to read

23. Guide to act or to walk

24. Attachment (1—)

Note:

1. XZ-C is Xu Ze-China (Xu Ze - China), because science is borderless, but scientists are national and intellectual property.

2. Cancer is a disaster for all mankind. It must evoke the struggle of the people all over the world. Therefore, 15 of these series are exclusively in English and distributed worldwide.

FOREWORD (1)

The scientific research projects to overcome cancer, which are internationally the key scientific research, is the frontier of science.

This is to conquer cancer and to launch the total attack to cancer and to create the Science City of conquering cancer.

The overall design, planning, and blueprint of XZ-C's scientific research plan for cancer is the scientific thinking and theoretical innovation and experimental basis for conquering cancer. It is the overall strategic reform and development of cancer treatment in China. It is the result of my 60 years of experience in medical work and 30 years of scientific research, scientific and technological innovation, scientific thinking and scientific wisdom to overcome cancer. It is planned to set up a test area in the Huangjiahu University City of Wuhan City. The research project will be implemented by experts and professors of the research team.

The research plan to overcome cancer is a key scientific research in the world and a frontier of science.

On January 12, 2016, US President Barack Obama proposed the National Cancer Program to "conquer cancer" in his State of the Union address, and named the Cancer Moon Shot, which was implemented by Vice President Biden. The specific plan is unknown.

Cancer is a disaster for all mankind. It must fight with the world. The people of the world work together to gather wisdom and advance together to overcome cancer.

The disaster of cancer covers the whole world. People all over the world are eager to hope to overcome cancer one day. It is hoped that the state, government, experts, scholars, scientists and entrepreneurs can find out anti-cancer measures to keep people away from cancer.

According to the "2015 China Cancer Statistics" report published by the National Cancer Center and the National Cancer Registry, in 2015, the number of new cancer cases in China was about 4.292 million, and the number of deaths was about 2.814 million. Continued to increase, cancer has become the "number one killer" threatening human health, bringing great challenges to cancer prevention and control in China and the world, and also causing enormous economic burden on society.

The way out for cancer treatment is "three early", and the way out for cancer is prevention. Coping with this challenge through a combination of cancer prevention, early diagnosis and early treatment can reduce the economic loss of cancer to a certain extent and save people's lives.

Therefore, XZ-C proposed to carry out the initiative of "conquering cancer, launching a general attack - prevention, control, and treatment."

It is to put forward a new concept of XZ-C cancer treatment after summary collection and agglutination wisdom, which is the book "Walked out of the new way of immune regulation and control with the combination of Chinese and Western medicine for cancer treatment."

XZ-C proposed: "Creating an Research Institute Environmental Protection and Cancer prevention" and carrying out cancer prevention system engineering and project.

—— Open a new era of cancer prevention research and cancer prevention system engineering in the 21st century

FOREWORD (2)

<u>**The real record of scientific thinking from "clinical to experiment, then experiment to clinical"**</u>

In 1985, I conducted a petition with more than 3,000 patients who underwent radical surgery for various cancers. It was found that most patients had recurrence and metastasis 2 to 3 years after surgery, and some even metastasized several months after surgery. This made me realize that although the operation is successful, the long-term efficacy is not satisfactory. Postoperative recurrence and metastasis are the key factors affecting the long-term efficacy of the operation. It also reminds us that prevention and treatment of postoperative recurrence and metastasis is the key to prolonging postoperative survival. Therefore, basic research must be carried out, and **without breakthroughs in basic research, clinical efficacy is difficult to improve.** So we established the Institute of Experimental Surgery and spent a total of 24 years conducting a series of experimental research and clinical validation work from the following three aspects.

First

Explore the mechanisms of cancer onset, invasion and recurrence and metastasis, and carry out experimental research on effective measures to regulate and to control cancer invasion, recurrence and metastasis.

We have been conducting a full-scale clinical research work in the laboratory for 4 years, which is a basic clinical study.

The selection of the research project is a clinically raised question, in order to explain these clinical problems or solve these clinical problems through experimental research.

Second

The experimental study of looking for the new drug of anti-cancer, anti-metastatic, anti-recurrence for cancer from natural medicine.

The existing anticancer drugs kill both cancer cells and normal cells, and have large adverse reactions. We used anti-tumor experiments in cancer-bearing mice to find new drugs that inhibit cancer cells without affecting normal cells. We spent a full three years to conduct the tumor-inhibiting screening experiment in cancer-bearing animals for 200 kinds of Chinese herbal medicines used in traditional anti-cancer agents and anti-cancer agents reported in various places one by one.

RESULTS:

48 kinds of traditional Chinese medicines with good anti-tumor effect and good ascending effect were screened out, and the traditional Chinese medicine Huangla Teng ethyl acetate extract (TG) which can inhibit the new microvessels was found out.

Third,

Clinical validation work

Through the above four years to explore the basic experimental research of recurrence and metastasis mechanism, and after three years of experimental research screening from natural drugs, we have identified a batch of $XZ\text{-}C_{1\text{-}10}$ immunomodulatory anticancer Chinese medicine, and then passed the clinical verification of more than 12,000 patients with advanced or postoperative metastatic cancer in 20 years.

Through the clinical validation of more than 12,000 patients with advanced or postoperative metastatic cancer in 20 years, the use of XZ-C immunomodulation of anticancer traditional Chinese medicine has achieved good results, which can improve the quality of life of patients, improve the symptoms of patients, and significantly prolong the survival of patients.

Through the review, analysis, reflection and experience of my clinical practice cases for more than 50 years, combined with the results and findings of my own experimental research on tumor-bearing animals for more than 10 years. In January 2001, Hubei Science and Technology Press published "New Understanding and New Model of Cancer Treatment". In January 2006, the People's Military Medical Publishing House published "New Concepts and New Methods for Cancer Metastasis Treatment". The latter also won the "Three One Hundred" Original Book Awards issued by the General Administration of Press and Publication of the People's Republic of China in April 2007.

This book is a true record of the author's research thinking from experiment to clinical, and then from clinical to experimental. The summary of experimental research and clinical verification data has been raised to the theoretical essence, and new discoveries and new understandings have been proposed, such as clinical practical oncology theory, cancer treatment, research development and reform, and these clinical practical innovation **theories can be used to guide Clinical treatment work**.

The theoretical application of clinical application is because all clinical treatment, medication, and diagnosis must have a reasonable theoretical basis. More than 50 years of clinical tumor surgery practice has made me deeply understand that because the etiology, pathogenesis and pathophysiology of tumors are not well understood, "oncology" has become one of the most backward developments in medical science.

In the past 7 years, a series of clinical basic experimental research and basic problems have been explored on more than 6,000 tumor-bearing animal models. In vivo anti-tumor experiment 200 kinds of Chinese herbal medicines were screened in a tumor-bearing animal model. These are all done by my several graduate students. "Exploring the effect of spleen on tumor growth and the experimental study on the anti-cancer effect of Jianpi Yiqi Decoction" was completed by Master Zhu Siping; "Experimental study on the combined transplantation of fetal liver, spleen and thymus cells for the treatment of malignant tumors by immunoreconstruction" was completed by Dr. Zou Shaomin; "Experimental study on the anti-tumor effect of Fuzheng Peiben on S180 mice" was completed by Master Li Zhengxun; "Experimental study on the inhibitory effect of ethyl acetate extract (TG) on the neovascularization of transplanted tumors in mice" was completed by Master Liu.

The subjects of the master's and doctoral students are the sub-topics of my total research project, and they are the basic issues closely related to clinical practice. The graduate students have carried out and completed a lot of hard and meticulous experimental research work, contributing to the development of cancer prevention, anti-cancer and experimental oncology medicine.

-The book covers experimental research and clinically validated cases, as well as new concepts, new theories, and new models of cancer treatment that have risen to theory. **Some insights were first proposed for originality.** In the spirit of "Hundred Flowers Blossom", we will update our thinking and change our concepts to enlighten our thinking and further develop and innovate. Due to the rapid development of oncology medicine, and involving many disciplines such as molecular biology, molecular immunology, genetic engineering, etc., there are a wide range of knowledge. If there are errors or omissions in the book, please ask colleagues, experts and readers for your advice.

FOREWORD (3)

The experimental surgery is a key to open the medical restricted area, the laboratory is the key condition

Experimental surgery is extremely important in the development of medicine. It is a key to opening the medical exclusion zone. Many diseases are controlled by many animal experiments. The stability results which are gained and made are applied to the clinic, which promotes the development of the medical cause.

Developing science, technological innovation, and laboratories are key conditions. I deeply understand the importance of the laboratory. I am the first batch of college students in the post-liberation college entrance examination. I have not studied further for schooling or training or studied abroad. However, I have achieved many international achievements. The key is that I have a good laboratory. In the 1960s, I participated in the open heart surgery laboratory for cardiopulmonary bypass. In the 1980s, I established a laboratory for cirrhosis ascites. In the 1990s, I established the Institute of Experimental Surgery to focus on cancer. My animal laboratory has good equipment conditions, including animal experiments such as mice, rats, Dutch pigs, rabbits, dogs, and monkeys. There is a better sterilized operating room, which can be used for chest and abdomen major surgery and animal postoperative observation room. . It can bring various designs and ideas to achieve results or conclusions through the experiments.

Therefore, the laboratory is the key condition, and the key is to build a good equipment laboratory.

There should be a dual task on the shoulders of university teachers. One is to do a good job of teaching; the other is to develop science.

University teachers should have good laboratories for scientific research, follow the scientific development concept, base on known science, explore unknown science, face the future science, emerging disciplines, marginal disciplines, interdisciplinary, face the frontiers of science, strive for innovation, advance, which for the scientific hall, it adds bricks and tiles.

In summary, experimental research and basic research are very important. Without experimental research and breakthroughs in basic research, clinical efficacy is difficult to improve, and it is difficult to propose new understandings, new concepts, and new theoretical insights. Among them, the experiment is the key. I have a good laboratory. I am the director of the Institute of Experimental Surgery and the director of clinical surgery. The experimental research, basic research and clinical verification are convenient for overall planning.

Basic research in medicine is very important for achieving progress in combating diseases. Experimental oncology is the basic science of cancer prevention research and has promoted the continuous development of cancer research in China.

Our Institute of Experimental Surgery conducted a series of experimental studies to explore the mechanisms of cancer onset, invasion and recurrence and metastasis. We have been conducting laboratory research for a full 4 years in the laboratory. From experimental tumor research it was found:

Thymus atrophy and the decline of immune function may be the cause of tumor, one of the pathogenesis. And how to prevent thymus atrophy? How to regulate and to control the reduction of immune function? How to promote immunity? How to "protect Thymus and to increase immune function "?

Immune regulation should be carried out, and it should embark on a new path of conquering cancer with China characteristics of the combination of Chinese and Western medicine at the molecular level.

Facing the future of medicine, we will look forward to the future. After 20 years of hard work, we will practice the scientific development concept and face the frontier of science, striving for innovation and progress. To overcome cancer, it must be from the clinical, through experimental research, to the clinical, to solve the actual problems of patients; it must seek truth from facts, use facts, speak with data; it must constantly self-transcend, self-advance; in scientific research it should emancipate the mind an break away the traditional old ideas and it is to base the foot on independent innovation and original innovation; our research route for decades is to find problems → ask questions → study problems → solve problems or explain problems, the road walked out just like this, step by step, difficult trek, we hope Stepping out of an innovative road of anti-cancer and anti-metastasis with Chinese characteristics and independent intellectual property rights.

Our research model for oncology is based on patients, discovering and asking questions from clinical work, conducting in-depth basic research on animal experiments, and then turning basic research results into clinical applications to improve the overall level of medical care and ultimately benefit patients.

FOREWORD (4)

The review, analysis and reflection from clinical practice cases

I am a clinical surgeon. Why do you do research or study cancer? This is due to the results of a petition to a group of cancer patients after surgery.

In 1985, I made a petition to more than 3,000 postoperative patients with chest and abdominal cancer whom I performed the operation on. The results from the petitions: It was found that the most patients have recurrence or metastasis 2 to 3 years after surgery, and some even relapsed and metastasized several months and one year after surgery.

From the follow-up results, it was found that postoperative recurrence and metastasis were the key factors affecting the long-term efficacy of surgery.

Therefore, it also raised an important question for us:

That is, clinicians must pay attention to and study the prevention and treatment of postoperative recurrence and metastasis, so as to improve the long-term efficacy after operation. Therefore, it is necessary to conduct an experimental study of the clinical basis of recurrence and metastasis. Without a breakthrough in basic research, clinical efficacy is difficult to improve.

So we established the Experimental Surgery Laboratory (later established the Experimental Surgery Research Institute of Hubei College of Traditional Chinese Medicine in 1991, the research direction is to overcome cancer).

We have studied from the following two aspects: one is animal experimental research, and the other is clinical research. Based on the success of animal experiments, it is applied in clinical practice for clinical validation. After 28 years of hard work and hard effort, a series of experimental research and clinical verification work were carried out, and a series of scientific and technological innovation research results were obtained.

Through experimental research and clinical medical practice cases, combined with the review, analysis, evaluation and self-reflection of traditional medical practice cases for half a century,

the positive and negative experiences and lessons of the successes and failures of clinical medical cases in the past 60 years was summarized and there are the following new findings, new thinking, new understanding, and new treatment concepts.

The new findings in anti-cancer and anti-cancer metastasis research

First, the new discoveries

1. The things were found from **the results of follow-up**

(1) Postoperative recurrence and metastasis are the key factors affecting the long-term efficacy of surgery.

(2) Clinicians must pay attention to and study the prevention and treatment measures for postoperative recurrence and metastasis.

2. The things was found From **the experimental tumor research**:

(1) Our laboratory removes the thymus (Thymus: TH) from mice, which can be used to create a model of cancer-bearing animals. Injection of immunosuppressive agents can also contribute to the establishment of cancer-bearing animal models. The research conclusions prove that: The occurrence and development of cancer are obviously related to the thymus and its function of the host immune organs.

(2) When we explored the effect of tumor on the immune organs of the body, we found that the thymus was progressively atrophied (600 mice bearing cancer model mice) as the cancer progressed. The host thymus is acute progressive atrophy after inoculation of cancer cells.

3. Through the review and analysis, evaluation and reflection of clinical practice cases of postoperative adjuvant chemotherapy cases, it was found that there are problems:

(1) Some patients with postoperative adjuvant chemotherapy failed to prevent recurrence;

(2) Some patients did not prevent metastasis after adjuvant chemotherapy;

(3) Some patients have chemotherapy that promotes immune failure.

4. Analysis and reflection from clinical practice cases on why postoperative chemotherapy failed to prevent cancer recurrence and metastasis

Analyze and reflect from the role of chemotherapeutic drugs in the cancer cell cycle; analyze and reflect on the inhibition of the overall immune function by chemotherapeutic drugs; analyze and reflect from the drug resistance of chemotherapeutic drugs:

(1) There are some important misunderstandings in current chemotherapy:

(2) There are several major contradictions in current chemotherapy.

5. Through the review, analysis, evaluation and reflection of clinical medical practice cases, the following problems are found:

"Analysis, evaluation and questioning of systemic intravenous chemotherapy for solid tumors";

"A Century Review, Analysis and Review of the Three Major Therapies for Cancer Tradition";

"Chemotherapy needs further research and improvement."

Second, update thinking, update understanding

Through 7 years of experimental observation of cancer-bearing animals and 6 years of diagnosis and treatment of more than 6,000 cases in specialist outpatient clinics, review, analysis, evaluation and self-reflection, it was to summarize the experience and lessons of both positive and negative aspects of success and failure, and consider why traditional therapy does not significantly reduce mortality, why not control recurrence and metastasis? What is the problem with the traditional concept of traditional therapy. It has gradually made me realize that there may still be some problems with the current traditional cancer therapy, such as:

1. Traditional chemotherapy inhibits immune function and inhibits bone marrow hematopoietic function;

2. Traditional intravenous chemotherapy for intermittent treatment, intermittent treatment can not be treated. The intermittent cancer cells continue to proliferate and divide;

3. The traditional therapy damages the host, because the chemotherapy cell poison is a "double-edged sword", which kills both cancer cells and normal cells;

4. The traditional therapy goal only focuses on chemotherapy can kill cancer cells, but ignores the host's own resistance to cancer, because the occurrence and development of tumors depends on the level of host immune function and the biological characteristics of the tumor itself, that is, decided Both the biological characteristics of the tumor cells and the host's influence on the constraints are both dominant, and if the two are balanced, they are controlled, and if the two are unbalanced, the progress is made. Traditional radiotherapy and chemotherapy are all promoting the decline of immune function, which may make the two more imbalanced;

5. traditional therapy damages the central immune organs, Thymus has been inhibited in cancer, and chemotherapy inhibits the bone marrow, like "adding frost into snow." The entire central immune organ is damaged and not effectively protected;

6. Traditional therapy is a damage therapy, which has a certain impact on the patient's disease resistance, but is not effectively protected;

7. Traditional therapy ignores the anti-cancer ability of the human body and neglects the anti-cancer system's anti-cancer system (NK cell population, K cell population, LAK cell population, macrophage cell population, TK cell population).

The effects of anti-cancer cell factors IFN, IL-2, TNF, and LT in the host were ignored. And it was neglecting the role of tumor suppressor genes and tumor suppressor genes in the host (there are oncogenes and tumor suppressor genes, cancer metastasis genes and tumor suppressor genes) and neglecting the role of neurohumoral system and endocrine hormones in the host, neglecting the role of anti-cancer institutions and their influencing factors in the human body, as well as its role in regulating, balancing, and stabilizing the host's own anti-cancer, neglecting the intrinsic factors of the body's own anti-cancer has not been activated, mobilized, but can only be pursued to kill cancer cells;

8. the goal of traditional therapy is relatively simple, just kill cancer cells. Not all of them meet the actual conditions of the biological characteristics of cancers that are currently recognized such as cancer cell invasion behavior; metastasis and multiple steps; the cause of recurrence, latent months, recurrence in several years. At present, it has been recognized that anti-tumor drugs are not necessarily resistant to metastasis, and anti-metastatic drugs are not necessarily anti-tumor.

How to do? What should it be done? There are problems with the above. Further research should be conducted in depth, basic experimental research and clinical research should be carried out, and reforms should be deepened, and thinking should be updated and knowledge should be updated. Update observations, advance in reform, and be brave in innovation.

Innovation must challenge traditional concepts, overcome its shortcomings, correct its deficiencies, and make it more perfect.

Innovation must challenge the status quo and transcend the status quo. Innovation should also take a different approach and find new ways to overcome cancer.

FOREWORD (5)

- These series of monographs are not written with a pen, but are made with work.

- The contents of these monographs all come from clinical practice experience and lessons, review, reflect, and practice real knowledge.

- The contents of these monographs are all based on the results of experimental research in their own laboratories.

- The contents of these monographs are real records from experiment to clinical, and then from clinical to experimental research thinking and scientific practice. The summary of experimental research and clinical verification data has risen to the theoretical essence, and new discoveries, new understandings, and new theories are proposed. These clinical practical innovation theories can be used to guide clinical treatment. All should be transferred to clinical applications through translational medicine to guide clinical treatment work and benefit patients.

- The contents of these monographs:

All of them are more than half a century of treatment practice experience and 20 years of experimental research data summary, collation, collection of books, scientific research results, scientific and technological innovation series, are their own materials, some of which are international initiatives, original innovation. Some are internationally advanced, independent innovation, and have independent intellectual property rights.

- The contents of these series of monographs:

fully compliant with transformation or translational or conversion medicine content.

Our 28-year research route is from clinical → experimental → clinical → re-experiment → re-clinical, back to clinical to solve clinical practical problems, our research model is fully in line with this new medical research model.

Conversion or Transformation or Translational medicine

Translational medicine has developed rapidly in the world in recent years. This new medical research model advocates patient-centered, discovers and raises questions from clinical work, conducts in-depth basic research, and then quickly shifts basic research results to clinical applications to improve overall medical care and ultimately benefit patients.

Academician Chen Yu has analyzed the connotation of translational medicine:

First of all, translational medicine is a science that explores the mechanisms of disease occurrence, development, and health protection promotion through laboratory-to-clinical and clinical-to-laboratory two-way channels to explore new prevention strategies.

Secondly, it is necessary to transform scientific research results into interventions, techniques, and programs that can be used for clinical or public health, so that they can be popularized.

The World Health Organization proposes that medicine in the 21st century should not continue to focus on diseases, and human health should be the main research direction. Academician Chen Yu pointed out:

In order to transform the health care model, it is necessary to shift from the treatment of the late stage of the major illness to the prevention, and move the barrier forward and sink the center of gravity. Strengthening preventive medical research is a major issue in China's transformation of the global medical model.

The focus of translational or transformation medicine research in China, the modernization and internationalization of traditional Chinese medicine and traditional Chinese medicine is one of the key contents of translational medicine research in China.

THE LIBRARY OF CANCER PREVENTION AND ANTI-CANCER MEDICAL RESEARCH

First

Professor Xu Ze (XZ-C)'s Research collected works on Cancer Prevention and Cancer Treatment Research

XZ-C proposes: How to overcome cancer? How to prevent cancer? How to treat cancer?

XZ-C cancer treatment new concept

<u>The Names and Contents</u> of Collection Books for Cancer Research

(Monograph)

First volume

Conquer cancer and launch the total attack----cancer prevention and cancer control and cancer treatment at the same time and at the same level and at the attention

Second volume

Walked out of the new way of cancer treatment with immune regulation and control of the combination of Chinese and Western medicine for and treating cancer" (Part 1) and (Part 2)

Third volume

The research of XZ-C immunomodulation anticancer traditional Chinese medicine – the experimental research and clinical validation

Fourth volume

Build up the Multidisciplinary of conquering cancer and the Science Base of Cancer-Related Research ---- the Science City"

Fifth volume

Innovation of Clinical Application theory of Cancer Prevention and Treatment Research in the 21st Century"

Volume VI

Create the research institute of cancer prevention and carry out cancer prevention system engineering

Dawning C plan

Dawning A•B•D Program

Pollution Prevention and pollution treatment and cancer prevention and anti-cancer

Shuguang Research Program

Shuguang scientific research spirit

Medical is benevolence, to set up is first

Volume seventh

Condense wisdom and conquer cancer - for the benefit of mankind" (volume I and II)

Volume eighth

The Road to Overcome Cancer

Volume IX

On Innovation of Cancer Treatment

Volume tenth

New understanding and new model of cancer treatment

Volume Eleventh

New Concepts and New Methods for Cancer Metastasis Treatment

Volume twelve

New Progress in Cancer Treatment

Volume Thirteenth

New Concepts and New Methods for Cancer Treatment

[Note: Each volume is a published monograph on cancer medical research]

Note:

1. *XZ-C is Xu Ze-China, because science is borderless, but scientists are national and intellectual property.*

2. *Cancer is a disaster for all mankind. It must evoke the struggle of the people all over the world. Therefore, 10 of these series are exclusively in English, distributed worldwide, and published on Amazon.com.*

3. *Corresponding author: Professor Xu Ze, China • Hubei • Wuhan Wuchang • No. 66 Village, Wuhan*

Second

Professor Xu Ze (XZ-C) summed up and collected, condensed wisdom, and put forward the "1- 8 of the new road to conquer cancer" to facilitate clinical application.

How to overcome cancer? How to prevent cancer? How to treat cancer? How to overcome cancer and to launch the general attack of cancer?

In the past 30 years, our scientific research achievements and technology innovation series are in the direction of conquering cancer research. In this series of "Monographs", the following arguments are first proposed internationally, all of which are original papers, internationally pioneered, and have reached the forefront of the world.

XZ-C's scientific thinking, scientific research design, academic thought, and scientific dedication of conquering cancer and launching attack were summarized the following monographs.

Professor Xu Ze (XZ-C) put forward the "new concept of cancer treatment" and published the 1-8 monographs "walked out of the new road to overcome cancer"

1, "Walked out of the new road to overcome cancer" – 1 (1)

Conquer cancer and launch the total attack of cancer – cancer prevention, cancer control, cancer treatment at the same lever and at the same time and at the same attention"

2, "Walked out of the new road to overcome cancer" - 2 (two) (volume 1) - 3 (three) (volume 2)

Walked out of the new way of immune control, Chinese and Western medicine combined with cancer treatment"

(Volume 1) and (Volume 2)

3, "Walked out of the new road to overcome cancer" - 4 (four)

"XZ-C immunomodulation anticancer Chinese medicine research"

—— Experimental research and clinical verification

4, "Walked out of a new road to overcome cancer" - 5 (five)

"Creating a Science City for Scientific Research Bases for Cancer Multidisciplinary and Cancer Research"

5, "Walked out of the new road to overcome cancer" - 6 (six)

"The 21st Century Cancer Prevention Research Clinical Application Theory Innovation"

6, "Walked out of a new road to overcome cancer" - 7 (seven) (volume 1) - 8 (eight) (volume 2)

XZ-C proposed "Creating an Environmental Protection and Cancer Prevention Research Institute" and carrying out cancer prevention system engineering (volume 1) and (volume 2)

—— Scientific anti-pollution, pollution control and scientific cancer prevention and anti-cancer

—— Twilight or Dawn cancer prevention research plan and Shuguang scientific research spirit

—— Medical is benevolence, Setting up moral is first

Third

Professor Xu Ze (XZ-C) published the monographs on cancer research:

3 monographs, Chinese version, domestic issue.

15 monographs, English version, global distribution.

Professor Xu Ze continued to research after he retired, and Science has continued to achieve the following series of scientific research results.

In 1996, I was 63 years old and I was retired. After I retired, I have been living in a small building for 20 years. I have been working alone and fighting alone. I have continued a series of experimental studies and clinical verification observations. I have achieved the following series of scientific research results. The following monographs have been published.

3 monographs, Chinese version, domestic issue

15 monographs, English version, published by Washington AuthorHouse, global distribution, AuthorHouse network distribution.

These 18 monographs are the result of four difficult stages of research, four hardships, one foot and one step of a scientific research, four different stages of scientific research, and four different levels of mountain peaks.

1). Xu Ze (the first monograph published in the 67-year-old flower year) "New understanding and new model of cancer treatment"

Hubei Science and Technology Press, January 2001

2). Xu Ze (the second monograph published in the 73-year-old ancient rare year) "New concept and new method of cancer metastasis treatment"

Published by Beijing People's Military Medical Press, January 2006

In April 2007, the People's Republic of China Publishing Office issued the "Three One Hundred" original book certificate.

3). Xu Ze, etc (the third monograph in the 78-year-old ancient rare year) "New Concepts and New Methods of Cancer Treatment" in Chinese version.

Published by Beijing People's Military Medical Press, October 2011

Later, the American medical doctor Dr. Bin Wu and others translated into English, and the English version was published in Washington, DC on March 26, 2013.

4). Xu Ze, etc, the third monograph in English was published "New Concept and New Way Of Treatment of Cancer", published in Washington, March 2013, full English version, international distribution

5). Xu Ze, etc, the fifth monograph was published at the age of 82, "On Innovation of Treatment of Cancer", published in Washington, December 2015, full English version, global distribution

6). Xu Ze, etc, the sixth monograph was published at the age of 83, "New Concept and New Way of Treatment of Cancer Metastais"

It is published in August 2016, Washington published a full English version, global distribution

7). Xu Ze, etc, the seventh book was published at the age of 83, "The Road To Overcome Cancer"

Published in Washington, DC in December 2016, full English version, global distribution

8). Xu Ze, etc published the eighth monograph at the age of 86, "Condense Wisdom and Conquer Cancer for the Benefit of Mankind"

Volume 1 : How to overcome cancer? How to prevent cancer? In December 2017 it was published in Washington, June 2018, in English, globally distributed

Volume 2: How to overcome cancer? How to treat cancer?

In February 2018 it was published in Washington, June 2018, in English, globally distributed

9). Xu Ze, etc, the ninth monograph was published in the age of 87) **"The New progress in Cancer Treatment"**

Published in Washington, June 2018, in English, globally distributed

10). Xu Ze, etc, published the eleventh monograph in the age of 87, **"Conquer Cancer and Launch The Total attack to Cancer" - prevention cancer, anti-cancer, cancer treatment at the same time and at the same level and at the same attention"**

Published in Washington, November 2018, full English version, global distribution

11). Xu Ze, etc, the eleventh monograph was published in the year of 87 years old, **"Walked out of the New Road to Conquer Cancer" "Walking out of the new way of cancer treatment with immune regulation and control of combination of Chinese and Western medicine"**, which is published in Washington, February 2019 (Volume 1 and volume 2), full English, global distribution.

12). Xu Ze, etc in the 87th year published the twelfth monograph" **The Reseach on Anticancer Traditional Chinese medication With Immune Regulation and Control ---- Experimental Research and Clinical Validation**

Published in Washington, January 2019, full English version, global distribution

13). Xu Ze, etc in the 87th year published the thirteenth monograph **"Innoration on Clinical Application Theory of Cancer Prevention and Treatment Research in the 21st Century"**

Published in Washington, March 2019, full English version, global distribution

14). Xu Ze, etc in the 87-year-old year of the fourteenth publication **"Build up the Multidiseiplinary and the Scientific City of Scientific Research Base with Related to Cancer Research For Conquering Cancer -- Promoting the new pregresses in Oncology in 21st century**

Published in Washington, April 2019, full English version, global distribution

15). Xu Ze, etc in the year of the 87-year-old, who had the publication of the fifteenth monograph **"Create the Research institute of the Environ Protection and Cancer Prevention and Carry out Cancer Prevention System Engineering"**

—— Opening the New Era of 21st Century cancer prevention Research and Cancer Prevention System Engineering (Volume 1)

Published in Washington, June 2019, full English version, global distribution

INTRODUCTION (1)

How to overcome cancer, how to prevent cancer

How can I treat cancer?

XZ-C found problems and raised problems from follow-up results (Hint: how to prevent postoperative recurrence and metastasis is the key to improve long-term outcomes after surgery)

↓

Pathfinding (to overcome cancer, where is the road? How do you find it?)

↓

Pathfinding and footprinting (anti-cancer, anti-cancer metastasis research and scientific research results, scientific and technological innovation series)

↓

Published cancer monographs (3 Chinese editions are exclusively distributed nationwide, 15 full English editions are published worldwide)

↓

Participate in the International Conference on Oncology (attend the AACR Academic Conference, Washington)

↓

Visiting the Stirling Cancer Institute in Houston, USA (2009)

↓

Basic and clinical research on anti-cancer and anti-cancer metastasis in the past 30 years

↓

More than 12,000 clinical application experience in 20 years

$\downarrow$

Walked out of the level of an immune regulatory molecule, Chinese and Western medicine combined with a new road to cure cancer

$\downarrow$

—— Walking out of a new road to overcome cancer, "Chinese-style anti-cancer", Chinese and Western medicine combined with immune regulation and treatment of cancer

- Published the English monograph "The Road to Overcome Cancer"

December 6, 2016, published in Washington, DC, global distribution, Amazon website distribution.

$\downarrow$

- Published the English monograph "Condense Wisdom and Conquer Cancer"

Published in December 2017 (volume 1), published in February 2018 (the next volume), published in Washington, USA, full English version, global distribution, Amazon website.

- Published the English monograph "Conquer Cancer and launch The Total Attack to Cancer"------ cancer prevention, cancer control, cancer treatment at the same time and at the same level and at the same attention)

In November 2018, the United States published in Washington, DC

INTRODUCTION (2)

The challenge of the times

The development of medicine in the 21st century should be the century of conquering cancer.

Nowadays, cancer is not only a household name or each family aware and each household knows, but also a problem that is often encountered in life. When it comes to cancer, it is always inevitable, and there is even a sense of cancer. In the long years, mankind has struggled with the disease and achieved a another victory. The plague, typhoid, cholera, smallpox, and plague that threatened human life in the past have caused humans to die in batches. Before the 19th century, when the smallpox was in a hurry, the smallpox won the alias of "God of Death."

In the Song Dynasty of China, vaccination was carried out with vaccinia, and later spread to Europe. Since then, the smallpox has been conquered. Tuberculosis was considered "incurable disease" decades ago. Streptomycin was invented in 1944, and Isoniazid was invented in 1945. Tuberculosis is not terrible.

In short, the diseases that once caused people to die in batches were eliminated and controlled one by one. Today's cancer has risen to become the main disease endangering human health. Coupled with the rapid development of modern industry, the three wastes are increasing, and cancer poses more and more serious challenges to human life. Therefore, it should be proposed to overcome cancer and launch a general attack.

Pollution prevention and pollution control and pollution treatment can achieve the effect of first-class cancer prevention and anti-cancer. Scientific pollution prevention, pollution control, scientific cancer prevention, anti-cancer resolutely fight well and win three major pollution battles.

XZ-C proposed an initiative to establish the "Innovative Environmental Protection and Cancer Prevention Research Institute" and carry out cancer prevention system engineering.

—— Open a new era of cancer prevention research and cancer prevention system engineering in the 21ˢᵗ century.

A SMALL SUMMARY

XZ-C proposes :

To create an environmental protection and cancer prevention research institute and carry out cancer prevention systems engineering and opening 21st Century Cancer Research

How to overcome cancer? How to overcome conquer cancer and launch the general attack of cancer?

How can I prevent cancer? How do I develop cancer prevention research?

How to prevent pollution and pollution?

How to scientifically prevent cancer and control cancer?

To overcome the cancer research work, the purpose is to make people's health

Keep away from cancer, and also a great pioneering work or great initiative for future generations to seek health and welfare.

—— To establish an overall framework for the fight against cancer, to create a science city that overcomes the research base of cancer multidisciplinary and cancer-related research, which is the only way to overcome cancer

—— Proposed the overall design, plan, plan, blueprint and implementation rules of Science City

------ Equivalent to designing an overall framework for Chinese characteristics to overcome cancer

------- The following is the implementation of XZ-C's outline of how to overcome cancer:

The main project to implement the outline of how to overcome cancer is:

The structural work:

To conquer cancer and to launch the general attack of cancer, to focus on prevention, control, and treatment together and at the same attention

To create a scientific research base for multidisciplinary and cancer-related research – The Science City

Two-wing project:

A wing - how to overcome cancer? How to prevent cancer?

----- It is to reduce the incidence of cancer

B wing - how to overcome cancer? How to treat cancer?

---- It is to improve cancer cure rate

The Aims:

A: *To reduce the incidence of cancer*

B: *To improve cancer cure rate, prolong patient survival, and improve patient quality of life*

If it is to implement and realize the overall design of cancer, planning blueprints, it is possible to overcome cancer.

How to implement, how to achieve this general guideline to overcome cancer, programs, plans, blueprints? It should be set up to "the cancer attack team of conquering cancer and launching the general attack."

It is invite famous experts, professors, academic leaders or leading scientists to support scientists, entrepreneurs, leaders, and volunteers who have overcome the general attack on cancer, and invite them to work together to make an unprecedented event in human history, "to overcome the general attack of cancer," and "to create A science city that conquers cancer, for the benefit of mankind.

The Preparation of setting up:

"The first science city in the country to overcome cancer research base"

"The world's first science city to conquer cancer research base"

Chapter 1

The Source Background and Experience
of the Scientific Research Topics

(1) The source background and the course of the completion of the project (the tortuous path)

My three new monographs are actually the key scientific and technological projects I have undertaken during the" Eighth Five" Plan period-------------------the Project name was:

"The Experimental and Clinical studies of further exploring prevention cancer and anti-cancer Chinese herbal medicine for the prevention and treatment of anti-metastasis on liver cancer, gastric cancer and precancerous lesions with the combination of Chinese and western herbal medicine." The special topic name of Thematic contract of "Eighth Five" National Technology and Science Research plan was :

"Clinical and Experimental Research on Treatment of Gastric Cancer and Precancerous Lesions by Chinese and Western Medicine" was headed or was in charged by the National Science and Technology Commission.

In April 1991, the author submitted an application to the State Science and Technology Commission for key scientific and technological projects during the "Eighth Five Plan" period. The project name is "further explore the experimental and clinical research on the prevention and treatment of anti-cancer and anti-cancer Chinese herbal medicine for the prevention and treatment of precancerous lesions of gastric cancer, liver cancer and gastric cancer." In June, Director of Hubei Provincial Science and Technology Commission Tian organized the three project leaders of the province to apply for the National Science and Technology Commission (1 person from Tongji Medical College, 1 from Hubei Medical College, 1 from Hubei College of Traditional Chinese Medicine) to go to Beijing to report to the Chinese Medicine Administration of the Ministry of Health.

Two months later, Director Tian of the Provincial Science and Technology Commission and three project leaders went to Beijing to report further to the Ministry of Health on design and acceptance of the project. **Two months later, when the project task was issued and the "Eighth Five National Science and Technology Research Project Contract" was being signed formally, Professor Xu Ze suddenly developed acute myocardial infarction, anterior wall and high wall myocardial infarction. After rescue and treatment, he was hospitalized for half a year, and he was relieved after a half-year break after leaving the hospital. The National Science and Technology Commission will also be stranded and suspended.**

In 1993, Professor Xu Ze's physical condition gradually recovered and also thought about the idea of continuing to study the content of the subject. It was because the author has followed up a lots of the postoperative patients with the radical resection and the results showed that postoperative recurrence and metastasis of cancer were the key factors affecting the long-term outcome after radical resection. The clinical basis and effective methods for preventing postoperative recurrence and metastasis must be studied. It was determined to do some research work that should be done within this capacity. However, there were thoughts but no research funding, so I began to find ways to raise funds for research. In 1993, my wife retired, she applied for a clinic, and her meager income was the starting point for research funding or her meager income started as a research fund. Kunming mice were purchased from the Animal Center of the Medical College for animal experiments, animal cages and related equipment and instruments were prepared, and animal experiments were started. The meager income of the clinic is used to support Professor Xu Ze's animal experiments and scientific research, and to save money in careful calculation or carefully save on applications. Six rooms on the second floor were used for animal experiments. In 1996, Professor Xu Ze was 63 years old and applied for retirement. After that, with the support of this meager income, a series of experimental research and clinical verification work were carried out. After 16 years of hard work and hard work, we finally completed the research project of the State Science and Technology Commission. We collected experimental and clinical research materials, data and summaries, and published three monographs:

1). "New understanding and new model of cancer treatment", Xu Ze, published by Hubei Science and Technology Press, January 2001, Xinhua Bookstore issued;

2). "New Concepts and New Methods for Cancer Metastasis Treatment", Xu Ze, published by the People's Military Medical Press, January 2006, issued by the National Xinhua Bookstore. In April 2007, the General Administration of Press of the People's Republic of China issued the "Three One Hundred" original book certificate.

3). "New Concepts and New Methods of Cancer Treatment" by Xu Ze and Xu Jie, published by Beijing People's Military Medical Press in October 2011. Later, the American medical staff Dr. Bin Wu and others translated into English. The English version was published in Washington, DC on March 26, 2013, and is distributed internationally.

(2) Some experiences

In the past, the author carried out scientific research work in medical colleges, with the guidance of superiors and the help of colleagues, and the laboratory conditions were excellent, undertook the National Natural Science Foundation of China, the National Science and Technology Commission project, provincial science and technology commission project. Two scientific research achievements have been made, one is the domestic advanced level and the other is the international advanced level. He won the second prize of Hubei Province Science and Technology Achievements and won the first prize of Hubei Provincial Health Science and Technology Achievements.

But now it is different. Under such special circumstances, in a clinic or outpatient center, first there is no condition, second there is no equipment, how can we carry out and complete the national task? The author has the following brief experience.

1. Self-reliance and self-raising or self-reliant and self-financing. For the patient service to treat the patient and to work in outpatient and the outpatient income is used as research funding.

2. Keep outpatient medical records and follow up throughout the process.

3. Establish special scientific research collaborations, collaborate and cooperate according to scientific research plans.

4. Establish detailed medical records (including epidemiological data of patients), and analyze in depth the success of each treatment, the failure lessons and the particularity of the condition.

5. Scientific research cooperation strategy of sharing equipment, sharing equipment and sharing results, and not adding large-scale instruments and equipment, and collaborating with the medical college affiliated school, the high-precision equipment inspections are carried out in the medical college affiliated hospital.

6. Selecting scientific frontier topics, failing to apply and to declare the subject (because it has been nearly ancient and rare), and to report the results to the Ministry, the province, and the city.

7. In the private clinic office the old professors can also carry out and complete research projects by fully utilizing the advanced equipment conditions of colleges and universities and combining decades of clinical experience through research and cooperation with universities and colleges, sharing of instruments and equipment, and the strategy of sharing results,

After 20 years of hard work under the heat and cold, I carried out a series of experimental research and clinical verification work, and finally basically completed the "Eighth Five Plan" research project of the National Science and Technology Commission that I applied for. I have compiled experimental and clinical research materials, data, conclusions, and summaries, and have written more than 100 research papers. Since there is no research funding, it is not possible to publish the magazine according to the paper, but it is published according to the new book. Two monographs were published successively. The third book of "New concepts and new methods of cancer treatment" is now published. These three monographs are our difficult moving and the difficult climbing, three different stages with one step and one footprint; is the results from the different levels, three different peaks, which are a series of coherent scientific research steps and scientific research processes.

The above briefly describes the background and ins and outs of my three monographs:

From the discovery of the results of a clinical follow-up to the findings of experimental tumor research; from the review of clinical medical practice cases to the analysis, evaluation and reflection of postoperative adjuvant chemotherapy cases, the drawbacks of traditional chemotherapy were discovered.

Looked for anti-cancer and anti-metastatic new drugs from natural medicines (Chinese medicines):

From performing in vitro and in vivo experiments on cancer-bearing models to the discovery and production of XZ-C series of immunomodulatory Chinese medicines, to go to clinical validation. Now more than 12,000 cases have been clinically validated for more than 16 years.

From the experimental basic research and clinical verification observation moving up to the theoretical understanding, a series of innovative theories are proposed, some are original innovations, and a series of reform measures for traditional therapies are proposed, and the strategies and strategic prospects for conquering cancer are proposed, such as some of the above scientific research contents and scientific research results are the research papers of the original innovative intellectual property that were first reported internationally. All of them are filled in my three monographs and published in the form of books.

Note:

Attachment:

3. Introduction to the Institute of Experimental Surgery, Hubei College of Traditional Chinese Medicine (see page of this book)

4. Science and technology research topics

Chapter 2

Briefly describe the scientific research process of anti-cancer research

1. **Briefly describe the scientific research process of anti-cancer research**

In 1985, I conducted a petition with more than 3,000 patients who were underwent the radical resection of various chest/thoracic surgery and general surgery. The results showed that most patients relapsed and metastasized about 2-3 years after surgery, and some even metastasized within a few months after surgery. I realized that the operation was successful, and the long-term efficacy was unsatisfactory. Postoperative recurrence and metastasis were the key factors affecting the long-term efficacy of the operation.

Therefore, a question is also raised:

Studying prevention and treatment of postoperative recurrence and metastasis is the key to improving postoperative survival.

Therefore, clinical basic research must be carried out, and without breakthroughs in basic research, clinical efficacy is difficult to improve. So we established the Institute of Experimental Surgery and spent 15 years conducting a series of experimental research and clinical validation work from the following three aspects:

1). **Exploring the pathogenesis of cancer, the mechanism of invasion and the mechanism of recurrence and metastasis, and exploring and performing the experimental research on looking for the effective measures to control invasion, recurrence and metastasis.**

My colleagues and I have been conducting experimental tumor research for four years in our laboratory. The selection of research projects is to ask questions from the clinical, to attempt to explain some clinical problems through experimental research, or to solve some clinical problems, all of which are clinical basic research.

2). The experimental research of looking for the new drug of anti-cancer, anti-metastatic, anti-recurrence from natural medicine Chinese herbal medicine.

The existing anticancer drugs not only kill cancer cells but also kill normal cells, and have serious side effects. *__Our laboratory uses a tumor suppressor test in cancer-bearing mice to find new drugs that inhibit cancer cells without affecting normal cells from natural Chinese herbal medicines.__*

Our lab spent the entire three years, for 200 kinds of Chinese herbal medicines commonly used in traditional anti-cancer prescriptions and anti-cancer prescriptions reported in various places, the anti-tumor or tumor inhibition screening experiments in the cancer-bearing animals were carried out one by one. The result:

__It was screened out 48 traditional Chinese medicines that have a good tumor inhibition rate. At the same time, it has a good effect of increasing immune function, and finds the traditional Chinese medicine TG which can inhibit the new micro-vessels.__

3). Clinical verification work:

Through the above four years to explore the basic experimental research on the mechanism of recurrence and metastasis, after three or three years of experimental research on natural medicines and Chinese herbal medicines, it was found a batch of XZ-C1-10 anti-cancer immune regulation and control chinese medicine, through the clinical validation of more than 12,000 patients with advanced or postoperative metastatic cancer in 20 years. The application of XZ-C immunomodulation of traditional Chinese medicine has achieved good results, improved quality of life, improved symptoms, and significantly prolonged survival.

Recently, I have reviewed, analyzed, reflected, and experienced the results and findings of my clinical research on clinical practice for more than 60 years, from experiment to clinical, from clinical to experimental, the experimental research and clinical verification data were summarized and collected and organized and published into three monographs:

1)). "New understanding and new model of cancer treatment", published by Hubei Science and Technology Press, Xu Ze, January 2001.

2)). "New Concepts and New Methods for Cancer Metastasis Treatment", Beijing People's Military Medical Press, Xu Ze, January 2006. In April 2007, the General Administration of the People's Republic of China issued the "Three One Hundred" original book certificate.

3)). "New Concepts and New Methods of Cancer Treatment", published by Beijing People's Military Medical Press, Xu Ze, October 2011. Later, the American medical doctor Dr. BinWu translated into English. The English version was published in Washington, DC on March 26, 2013, and is distributed internationally.

2. Ideological understanding and scientific research thinking of our scientific research journey

The thinking and scientific thinking of our scientific research journey in cancer research for 28 years can be divided into four stages:

1) The first stage 1985-1999

- Identify problems from follow-up results → ask questions → study questions;

- From reviewing, analyzing, reflecting, and discovering the problems of current cancer traditional therapies, further research and improvement are needed;

- Recognize that there are problems, change your mindset, and change your mindset;

- Summarize the materials, collate, collect and publish the first monograph "New Understanding and New Model of Cancer Treatment" published by Hubei Science and Technology Press in January 2001.

2) The second stage After 2001 -

- *Positioning the goals of the study and the "target" of cancer treatment on anti-metastatic, pointing out that the key to cancer treatment is anti-metastatic;*

- Conducted a series of anti-cancer metastasis, recurrence experimental research and clinical basis and clinical validation research, and rose to theoretical innovation, and proposed new ideas and methods for anti-metastasis;

- Summarize the materials, collate, collect and publish the second monograph "New Concepts and New Methods for Cancer Metastasis Treatment" published by People's Military Medical Press in January 2006, issued by Xinhua Bookstore.

- In April 2007, he was awarded the "Three One Hundred" Original Book Award by the General Administration of Press and Publication of the People's Republic of China.

3) The third stage After 2006 -

- **Study the goals and priorities of the research on the prevention and treatment of the whole process of cancer occurrence and development;**

- Closely combined with clinical practice, propose reforms and innovations, scientific research and development in response to the problems and shortcomings of current clinical traditional therapies;

- Recognize that the strategy of cancer prevention and treatment must move forward, the way out for anti-cancer treatment is "three early", and the way out for anti-cancer is prevention;

- I have been engaged in oncology surgery for 60 years, more and more patients, the incidence of cancer is rising, and the mortality rate remains high. I deeply understand that cancer should not only pay attention to treatment, but also pay attention to prevention, so as to block it at the source. I conducted a series of related research, did the summary materials and collation and collection and publication of the third monograph "New Concepts and New Methods for Cancer Treatment", published by the People's Military Medical Press in October 2011, and published by Xinhua Bookstore. Later, the American medical professional Dr. Bin Wu translated into English. The English version was published in Washington, DC on March 26, 2013.

4) The fourth stage After 2011 -

- Now is the fourth stage of our research work, which is being developed and carried out; the research work has been to be performed through step by step, positioning the research goal or "target" to reduce the incidence of cancer and to improve the cure rate and to prolong the survival period.

- We have been working on cancer research for 28 years:

The experimental research and clinical research work in the first three stages are mainly to research the new drugs in the treatment aspects and the new methods and new technologies of diagnosis and the new concepts and new methods of treatment.

- But today, in the second decade of the 21st century the cancer is still awkward. The more patients are treated, the higher the incidence rate and the higher the mortality rate.

I am deeply aware that cancer should not only pay attention to treatment, but also pay attention to prevention, in order to stop at the source.

- The current tumor hospital or oncology hospital model is fully focused on treatment, focusing on middle-stage and late-stage patients, the efficacy is poor, it is to exhaust human resource and financial resources, and it failed to reduce the incidence rate. The more the patient is treated, the more the patient comes. The status quo is:

The road that has passed in a century is to attention to or to rectify the treatment with ignoring prevention, or only to treat cancer without prevention at all. For many years we have only been working on cancer treatment. However, work on cancer prevention has been done very little and almost nothing has been done. As a result, the incidence of cancer continues to rise.

Through review, reflection, cliché about cancer prevention and anti-cancer work, what research or work have we done on cancer prevention for a century? What has it been achieved?

The teaching content in the medical school textbook does not pay attention to cancer prevention knowledge;

The setting-up hospital model has not paid attention to the setting up of cancer prevention science;

The scientific research projects in medical schools or hospitals have not paid attention to cancer prevention scientific research projects;

The Journal of Oncology Medicine does not pay attention to cancer prevention work papers.

In short, cancer prevention has not been taken seriously, and prevention has not been taken seriously. The prevention of the old-fashioned talks is mainly based on failure to pay attention.

How to do? How to reduce the incidence of cancer? How to improve the cure rate of cancer? How to reduce cancer mortality? How to prolong the survival period? How to improve the quality of life?

It should launch the general attack of conquering cancer and put the prevention and treatment at the same level and at the same attention and at the same time.

The goal of conquering cancer should be:

To reduce morbidity, improve cure rate, reduce mortality, prolong survival, improve quality of life, and reduce complications.

- At present, the global hospitals and hospitals in China are all devoted to treatment, attention to treatment and light prevention, or only treatment without prevention.

XZ-C believes that this mode of hospitalization or cancer treatment is unlikely to overcome cancer and it is impossible to reduce the incidence.

Global hospitals and hospitals in China must carry out an overall strategic reform of cancer treatment, shifting focusing on treatment into focusing on prevention and treatment at the same level and attention.

- Therefore, we propose to a general plan and design to overcome cancer and launch the total attack. XZ-C (Xu Ze-China) proposed to launch a general attack, which is to carry out the three-stage work of cancer prevention, cancer control and cancer treatment at the same time and the same level.

It is to propose the "Necessity and Feasibility Report for Overcoming cancer and launching the General Attack of Cancer."

It is to propose "XZ-C Scientific Research Plan for Overcoming cancer and launching the General Attack of Cancer"

3. Why do I study cancer and propose to launch a general attack and to prepare to build a "science city to overcome cancer"?

It is because:

1). In 1985, I conducted a petition to more than 3,000 patients who had undergone chest and abdominal cancer surgery. I found that most patients relapsed or metastasized within 2-3 years after surgery. Therefore, it is necessary to study methods to prevent postoperative recurrence and metastasis in order to improve the long-term efficacy after surgery.

2). I suddenly had an acute myocardial infarction in 1991. After the treatment was improved and recovered, it was not advisable to go to the operating table again. It was quiet and I went to the small building to concentrate on scientific research.

3). Through experimental research, it was found that thymus atrophy and immune function are low, which is one of the causes and pathogenesis of cancer, and it needs to be further expanded and studied in depth.

4). Through experimental research and clinical validation, after more than 12,000 clinical trials in 28 years, I found this new "Chinese-style anti-cancer" road of the modernization of Chinese medicine with the combination of Chinese and western medicine at the molecular level, which entered into and walked out the new path of the immunomodulation with the combination of the western medicine and the traditional Chinese medicine at the molecular level to prevent thymic atrophy, promote thymic hyperplasia, protect bone marrow hematopoietic function, and improve immune surveillance for conquering cancer, then to stay perversion and to research persistently.

Therefore, it is to propose to overcome cancer and launch the general attack on cancer, prepare to build a "science city" to overcome cancer. **The Attempt is to achieve:**

Reduce the incidence of cancer; improve the cure rate of cancer; prolong the survival of cancer patients; achieve "three early" (early detection, early diagnosis, early treatment), can be cured in the early stage; to achieve prevention, control, and treatment at the same time and at the same level and at the same attention; both prevention and treatment at the same time and level can only overcome cancer and reduce the incidence of cancer.

All basic research must be for the clinical, to improve the patient's efficacy and benefit patients. The criteria for assessing the efficacy of cancer patients should be: The survival period is prolonged, the quality of life is good, and the complications are few.

I came to Wuhan in 1951 and entered the Central South Tongji Medical College. I graduated from Tongji Medical College in 1956 and was assigned to the Affiliated Hospital of Hubei College of Traditional Chinese Medicine. I was the director of surgery and the director of the Institute of Experimental Surgery of Hubei College of Traditional Chinese Medicine.

In 1991, due to sudden acute myocardial infarction, after emergency treatment, I recovered after half a year of hospitalization. It was because he can no longer go to the stage for surgery, I become calm and hide in the small building to conduct basic and clinical research on cancer. Due to the good equipment conditions of my experimental surgical laboratory, a large number of experimental studies on the etiology, pathology, pathogenesis, and cancer metastasis mechanism of cancer were carried out, and the experimental screening of anti-cancer Chinese herbal medicine in the cancer-bearing animal model was conducted.

I was 63 years old in 1996 and applied for retirement. After retiring, I continued my scientific research, and Science will not stop. I have been living in a small building for 20 years, fighting alone (no one cares after retirement, no one knows in the unit and organization, no one asks, no one supports), single-handedly, self-reliant, from the year of the flower to the age of the ancient ; in the year of more than eighty years, I am still persevering and keep perseverance so that a series of experimental studies and clinical validation observations continued. Finally, we have achieved a series of scientific research achievements and technological innovation series.

The experimental and clinical data, information, conclusions, and summaries were collected, and more than 100 scientific research papers were written and published in the new book.

I have published 18 series of monographs that focus on cancer research. Three of them are in Chinese and 15 are in English.

The English version is published in Washington and distributed worldwide.

The book proposes a series of new concepts and new methods to overcome cancer, puts forward the theory of cancer treatment innovation, proposes the road to overcome cancer, and forms the theoretical system of immune regulation and control and treatment, which is the theoretical basis and experimental basis for cancer immunotherapy. It is undergoing clinical application observation and verification, and embarking on the new path to overcome cancer. Why is the English version? It is because cancer is a disaster for all mankind, the people of the world must work together for it. I took my 60 years of medical practice, 30 years of scientific research and clinical verification work of the experimental research of conquering cancer research and the scientific thinking and scientific understanding and skills and lessons and wisdom to contribute to the people, for the benefit of mankind.

I am 87 years old this year. I am the chief designer of the XZ-C research project, "Conquering cancer and launching the General Attack on Cancer and Building Science City for Scientific Research Bases to Conquer Cancer."

I will use my academic, knowledge, wisdom and strength to fully participate in the preparation of the "the Science City of conquering Cancer" practice, to build a "the hospitals for the global demonstration of prevention and treatment", to prevent and control and treat cancer at the same level, to build a good laboratory and multidisciplinary Cancer Research Group.

It is to change the mode of running a school from paying attention to treatment and ignoring defense into prevention, control, and treatment at the same level and at the same attention and at the same time.

It is to change the treatment mode from paying attention to the treatment for the middle and late stage or severe illness of treatment into focusing on "three early" (early detection, early diagnosis, early treatment) precancerous lesions, early carcinoma in situ. This will benefit mankind and will open up a new era of anti-cancer research, making China's prevention and treatment of cancer and medical care into the forefront of the world.

4. **After 30 years of basic and clinical research on cancer with the direction of research as "to overcome cancer", we deeply understand that in order to achieve the purpose of cancer prevention and control:**

1), it must launch the general attack.

That is to say, the three stages of cancer prevention, cancer control and cancer treatment at the same time; the three carriages go hand in hand so as to reduce the incidence of cancer, improve cancer cure rate, reduce cancer mortality, and prolong the survival of cancer patients.

If it only is to treat without prevention, or only pays attention to treatment with light prevention, it can never overcome cancer because it can't reduce the incidence, and the patients become more and more because it does not reduce the incidence, the more patients are treated and the more it will have the patients.

How to launch a general attack and implement cancer prevention + cancer control + cancer treatment?

It is necessary to establish a hospital with prevention and treatment of cancer with development and prevention and treatment during the whole process of cancer development and occurrence. It is to change the current hospital mode that can only attention to the treatment without prevention. It is to change the current treatment model which only aims at the middle-stage or late-state cancer.

2). It is necessary for the government to lead and for the experts and scholars to work hard, and for the masses to participate, and thousands of households can participate in it. At present, China is building an innovative country. It is the government-led, mass participation, national mobilization, and the work of thousands of households. This is great timing. If it can carry out medical scientific research to overcome cancer, prevent cancer and control cancer, it will certainly improve the awareness of cancer prevention among the whole people, and achieve the effect of preventing cancer and cancer control. It will receive the effects of significantly reducing the incidence of cancer in China, our province and our city.

3). Why is it to launch a general attack?

It is because the status quo is:

a. The current mode of running a hospital is to pay attention to or to rectify the treatment with light prevention and/ or only have the treatment without prevention ; the more the patient is treated and the more the patients show up.

b. The current treatment mode is mainly in the middle and late stages of cancer, and the effect is very poor.

c. The current radiotherapy and chemotherapy cannot cure, and can only be alleviated. Cancer is still progress during 4 weeks of mitigation period, and the curative effect is very poor. There are still problems and drawbacks.

It is necessary to emphasize early diagnosis, early treatment, and early rehabilitation:

a. It is to change the mode of running a hospital for prevention, control, and treatment at the same attention

b. It is to change the treatment mode into "three early", precancerous lesions.

c. The way out for anti-cancer is prevention, research, and cancer prevention research.

5. **I have been conducting basic research and clinical validation for cancer research for 30 years, both of which are carried out in laboratories and hospitals.** Why is it to think of applying for government support now?

It is because 90% of cancers are related to the environment, the occurrence of cancer is closely related to people's clothing, food, housing, travel and living habits. Therefore, I deeply think that cancer prevention and cancer control work is not only done by medical personnel and experts and scholars which can be done. It must rely on the government's major policy. The current environmental pollution is serious and the ecosystem is degraded, which may be closely related to the rising incidence of cancer.

The treatment of cancer depends on medical personnel and researchers to study new drugs and new treatment techniques.

However, about cancer prevention and control, how to reduce the incidence of cancer, cancer prevention work must rely on the government's major policy, rely on government leadership and mastership and rely on the experts, scholars, and mass participation so as that it can be carried out.

The current status quo is:

1). The more patients are treated, the higher the incidence is, and 90% is related to the environment. We deeply understand that cancer should not only pay attention to treatment, but also pay more attention to prevention, in order to stop it at the source, and it must prevent and treat at the same attention.

2). The current diagnostic method, B-ultrasound, CT, MRI, is currently the most advanced diagnostic means, but once diagnosed, mostly in the middle stage and late-stage, the effect is very poor. Research must be done to find new methods, new reagents, and new technologies for early diagnosis. Early cancer can be cured if it can be diagnosed in early stages and precancerous lesions. Therefore, the way out for cancer treatment is "three early". (early detection, early diagnosis, early treatment).

What should I do next?

Now it is to propose to overcome cancer and launch a general attack. I hope to get support from leaders at all levels. I know that in order to achieve the purpose of cancer prevention, control, and treatment, the government leaders, government masters, experts, and scholars must work hard, and the masses participate and thousands of households participate in.

About 11922 people in China are diagnosed with cancer every day, and 8 people are diagnosed with cancer every minute. Therefore, to study the scientific research work of launching the general attack on cancer, it should not walk slowly, it should run forward and save the wounded.

According to the "2015 China Cancer Statistics" report published by the National Cancer Center, in 2015, the number of new cancer cases in China was about 4.292 million yuan, that is, it should avoid empty talking and should do the hard work, and should always start to walk. No matter how far the road to conquer cancer is, it should always start.

6. **I have been studying in 2013→2014→2015, formulating basic ideas and designs on how to overcome cancer, formulating the theoretical basis and experimental basis for how to overcome cancer, developing the plan and blueprint and the route and the guidelines and the methods for how to overcome cancer. It came up with:**

1). "XZ-C Scientific Research Plan for Overcoming cancer and launching the General Attack of Cancer"

2). "Report on the Necessity of Preparing for the Hospital of Prevention and Treatment of Cancer in the Whole Process"

3). "The report of the necessity and feasibility of at the same time as building a well-off society – it is suggesting "taking a ride to scientific research" - conducting medical scientific research of cancer prevention and treatment and performing the work for cancer prevention and cancer control"

4). "Planning and the overall design of building the Science City for overcoming the cancer and launching the general attack."

These four scientific research projects were first proposed internationally which are opening up thenew areas of anti-cancer research. Professor Xu Ze proposed to the general attack of conquering cancer, which is unprecedented work. As of July 2015, it was formulated as the "Dawning C-type plan". That is, the dawn is morning light, Chaoyang, C type = China, that is, the plan of overcoming cancer with "Chinese model". The "four items" report is generally for "to overcome cancer and to launch a general attack" and for "establish a science city of conquering cancer."

How to implement this plan of conquering cancer in detail?

I have elaborated the overall design, master plan, specific program research team talents, etc. planning and blueprint.

It came up with Total Design • Blueprint of "Science City for Overcoming cancer and launching the General Attack of Cancer"

It was to come up with the overall design and preparation work of Science City

It is to established a trial area for the cancer working group (station)

It is to set up :

1). The Academic Committee of Conquering Cancer

2). The preparation group of the science city (the medical, teaching, research, development science city for conquering cancer and launching the general attack of cancer)

7. **This work is underway. We have been walking on cancer research of conquering cancer in the 3-4 years, and it is to only slowly moving forward step by step.**

On January 12, 2016, US President Barack Obama proposed the National Cancer Plan in his State of the Union address:

Conquer cancer

The name of the program: "Cancer moon shot"

Goal: Conquer cancer

Nature: National plan to overcome cancer

The person in charge of the plan: Vice President Biden

We have been on the road of conquering cancer for 3-4 years, but only individuals are living in small buildings and fighting alone, step by step, just slowly moving forward.

Now US President Barack Obama announced the National Cancer Plan in his State of the Union address:

Conquer cancer.

It is implemented by the vice president. Vice President Biden is actively implementing it. He goes to the cancer centers in the United States every month to preach: "Cancer moon shot".

On June 29, 2016, the National Cancer Lunar Plan was broadcast to the United States at the White House. Calling on all American scientists to gather wisdom and overcome cancer.

This international scientific research situation is a gratifying situation, and the situation is compelling and inspiring. In this case, the government must be called upon to ask the government to lead and lead the work to support this unprecedented work for the benefit of mankind.

This is a big event. This is an unprecedented event that benefits mankind.

Therefore, XZ-C proposes to move forward together and head to the scientific hall of cancer.

Chapter 3

Briefly describe the academic thinking and scientific research thinking of my scientific research process

This is gradually recognized in my scientific research journey in the past 28 years of the research of conquering cancer engaged in. It is our journey of scientific research to complete the application of the "Eighth Five". It is a series of coherent scientific research steps, scientific research stages, scientific research levels, continuous integration, step by step, and different understandings at different stages.

Scientific research is like climbing, and when you reach a mountain peak, you can see a layer of scenery. A mountain is taller than a mountain, and a mountain is better scenery than a mountain scenery.

Following the scientific development concept, the ideological understanding and scientific thinking of my scientific research journey can be divided into three stages:

(1) The first stage (1985-1999)

New discoveries and new insights :

It was to find out or discover the existing problems – asking questions – innovative thinking, changing ideas.

In 1985, I conducted a petition to more than 3,000 patients who had undergone chest and abdominal cancer surgery. I found that most patients relapsed or metastasized 2-3 years after surgery. Postoperative recurrence and metastasis are the key factors affecting the long-term efficacy of surgery. Clinical basic research to prevent cancer recurrence and metastasis must be carried out. Without breakthroughs in basic research, clinical efficacy is difficult to improve. Since experimental surgery is a key to open the medical exclusion zone, we established a tumor animal laboratory, set up an experimental surgical laboratory, and conducted a series of experimental tumor research:

Performed cancer cell transplantation; Established a cancer animal model; Explored the mechanisms and laws of cancer invasion, metastasis, and recurrence; looked for effective measures to regulate and to control the cancer invasion, recurrence and metastasis.

The new discovery

From experimental tumor research it was found:

1. *Removal of the thymus can produce a cancer-bearing animal model. The conclusion of the study:*

the occurrence and development of cancer has a positive relationship with the thymus of the host.

2. *When we studied the relationship between cancer metastasis and immunity in our laboratory, the experimental results suggest that metastasis is related to immunity.*

3. *Experimental studies have found that as the cancer progresses, the host's thymus is progressively atrophied.*

For further research, the Institute of Experimental Surgery of Hubei College of Traditional Chinese Medicine was established in March 1991 on the basis of the Experimental Surgery Laboratory. Professor Xu Ze is the director, and the academician Qiu fazu was the advisor. The goal and mission of his research is to become "conquer cancer" as the main direction.

In 1994, we established a special outpatient center for oncology clinics. Through the review of clinical medical practice cases and the analysis, evaluation and reflection of postoperative adjuvant chemotherapy, it was found or revealed the existing problems:

1). Some patients with postoperative adjuvant chemotherapy failed to prevent recurrence;

2). Some patients did not prevent metastasis after adjuvant chemotherapy;

3). Some patients have chemotherapy that promotes immune failure.

From the analysis and reflection of clinical practice case, why does the patient's postoperative chemotherapy fail to prevent recurrence and metastasis?

From the analysis of cancer cells in the cancer cell cycle, analysis and reflection from the inhibition of immunity by chemotherapeutic drugs, analysis and reflection from the drug resistance of chemotherapeutic drugs, it was found that there are problems:

1). There are still some important misunderstandings in current chemotherapy;

2). There are still several major contradictions in current chemotherapy, which need further research and improvement.

From the follow-up results, it was found that postoperative recurrence and metastasis is the key to affect the long-term efficacy of surgery. Therefore, we also raised an important question for us:

Clinicians must pay attention to and study the prevention and treatment of postoperative recurrence and metastasis in order to improve the long-term efficacy of postoperative.

From 1985 to 1999, we conducted a series of experimental and clinical research, and reviewed, analyzed and reflected, summed up the positive and negative experiences and lessons of success and failure, and then compiled and published the first monograph "New understanding and new model of cancer treatment", published in January 2001 by Hubei Science and Technology Publishing House, Xinhua Bookstore.

(2) The second stage (after 2001)

The research goals and the "targets" of cancer treatment was positioned on anti-metastatic, it is pointing out that the key to cancer treatment is anti-metastasis.

After 2001, our research work was that **it is in-depth analysis of what the key to the postoperative recurrence and metastasis is**?

Looking back from the 1970s, in view of the recurrence and metastasis rate after cancer surgery, in order to prevent postoperative recurrence and metastasis, a series of adjuvant chemotherapy after surgery was used, and even chemotherapy was started before surgery. But the results are not satisfactory. Recurrence and metastasis still occur soon after surgery. Or there is metastasis while chemotherapy, the more the chemotherapy and the more metastasis. Some cases contribute to immune failure due to intensive chemotherapy. These are all worthy of our clinicians should seriously and objectively think and analyze how cancer treatment work should prevent recurrence and anti-metastasis in order to obtain good long-term therapeutic effects.

Today, the most important problem in cancer treatment is how to resist metastasis. Metastasis is already the bottleneck of cancer treatment.

If the problem of cancer metastasis after radical surgery in patients cannot be solved, cancer treatment can no longer leap forward.

Therefore, the key to current cancer research is anti-metastasis. The core problem of cancer treatment is to resolve metastasis and recurrence.

One of the keys to cancer treatment is anti-cancer metastasis. Metastasis is only a phenomenon. How does it to clearly understand the process, steps and mechanisms of cancer cell metastasis? We should try to understand why cancer cells metastasize? How is it transferred? What are the steps, routes, process shapes and how is the fate of the transfer? What is the molecular mechanism of cancer cell metastasis? Where is the weak link in the process of cancer cell transfer? Which or which link or part is stroke or blocked can achieve the purpose of anti-metastasis?

We spent more than three years experimenting with animal models of cancer metastasis, observing and tracking the regularity of cancer cells on the way to metastasis, looking for ways to interfere with and prevent cancer cells from metastasizing.

Through the review, analysis and evaluation of a large number of cases in clinical practice, we propose:

1. The key to current cancer research is anti-metastasis;

2. Cancer appears in three forms in the human body, and the third form is cancer cells on the way to metastasis;

3. The goal of cancer treatment should be directed to these three forms;

4. "Two-point, one-line theory" cancer treatment in the whole process of cancer development, not only should pay attention to two points, but should also pay attention to cutting off the front line;

5. The specific measures to prevent metastasis should be to carry out the surrounding, chasing, blocking and intercepting of cancer cells during the transfer. It is put forward that in the third field of anti-cancer *metastasis treatment, the "main battlefield" of cancer cells on the way to quenching metastasis is in the blood circulation, and it is important to improve immune regulation and immune monitoring.*

By 2005, we compiled a large amount of data from the above experimental research and clinical verification, summarized, collected and published the second monograph "New Concepts and New Methods for Cancer Metastasis Treatment" published by People's Military Medical Press in January 2006, issued by Xinhua Bookstore. In April 2007, the company won the "Three One Hundred" Original Book Awards issued by the General Administration of Press of the People's Republic of China.

(3) The third stage (after 2006)

The research focuses on the prevention and treatment of the whole process of cancer occurrence and development. It closely combined with clinical practice, it aims at the problems and drawbacks of current clinical traditional therapy, and proposes reform and innovation, research and development. It is recognizing that the strategy of cancer prevention and treatment must move forward, the way out for cancer treatment is "three early", and the way out for cancer is prevention.

The second monograph is moving forward and further based on the first monograph of scientific research, which is positioning **that the "target point" of cancer treatment is anti-metastasis.**

It is pointed out that the key to cancer treatment is anti-metastasis. But metastasis is only the last stage of the whole process of cancer development, *it is only a local problem* in the whole process of cancer, and it cannot reduce the incidence of cancer and **may reduce the mortality rate**.

After 2006, we realized that the goal of cancer treatment is all necessary for the treatment of severely ill patients in the middle and late stages, but the curative effect is very poor. The more new patients are treated, the more the patients we have. Once diagnosed, it is in the middle and late stage, and the effect is not good. In order to overcome cancer, it must be "three early" and must be prevented in order to reduce the incidence of cancer and cancer mortality.

The way out for cancer treatment is "three early", and the study of "three early" must be strengthened.

The occurrence and development of cancer experience the stage of susceptibility - precancerous lesions - the invasive stage. At present, the treatment of cancer in oncology or tumor centers in various cancer hospitals or major hospitals in China, mainly in the middle and late stages, and the treatment effect is poor. If the middle and advanced patients can be operated on, they will be treated surgically. If surgery is not possible, they can only be evaluated. Therefore, the way out for cancer treatment should be "three early", early detection, early diagnosis, early treatment. Early patients generally have better therapeutic effects and improve the therapeutic effect, which inevitably reduces the cancer mortality rate. Therefore, we must pay attention to the study of early diagnosis methods and treatment methods, but also must pay attention to the treatment of precancerous lesions to reduce the middle and late stage patients in the invasion stage.

If we can treat well in precancerous lesions or early stage cancer, the number of patients who progress to invasion and metastasis will decrease, which will also reduce the incidence of cancer. Therefore, we believe that the current local cancer hospitals or oncology departments, mainly in the treatment of middle and late patients, even if the treatment results are good, can only reduce the mortality rate, however it is neglecting the precancerous lesions in the susceptible stage and/or neglecting the early patients, it is unlikely to reduce the incidence of cancer or it is impossible to reduce cancer incidence rate, therefore, we believe that we must pay attention to the occurrence of cancer, the prevention and treatment of the whole process of development, is a strategic overall concept, we must update our thinking and change our mindset.

I have been engaged in oncology surgery for 59 years, and more and more patients, the incidence of cancer is also rising, which makes me deeply understand that cancer should not only pay attention to treatment, but also pay attention to prevention, in order to stop at the source. Therefore, I deeply understand that the cancer treatment is in the "three early days". It is necessary to strengthen the research of "three early" (early detection, early diagnosis, early treatment*). The way to fight cancer is prevention, and research on preventive measures must be strengthened.*

As mentioned above, the focus of cancer prevention and treatment strategy is shifted forward. Its meaning has two aspects, one is to change lifestyle, to improve environmental pollution and other preventive measures, and the other is to treat precancerous lesions and stop its development to the invasive or mid-late period.

(4) The fourth stage (after 2011)

Putting the focus of cancer prevention and treatment strategies forward and carrying out anti-cancer research to reduce the incidence of cancer, Professor Xu Ze proposed:

the initiative to create an environmental protection and cancer prevention research institute and carry out cancer prevention system engineering and open a new era of cancer prevention research and cancer prevention system engineering in the 21st century.

1. **Why did I propose to create an environmental protection and cancer prevention research institute and carry out an cancer prevention system project?**

At present, the cancer hospital or oncology department is all to pay heavy attention to treatment with ignoring prevention or only to treat without prevention.

I entered the Central South Tongji Medical College in 1951. It has been 68 years since then, and I have experienced and witnessed the whole process of cancer prevention and control work in China for a century. Looking back at the 20th century, although hospitals in China and around the world are also preventing cancer and anti-cancer work, in fact, the focus is on the treatment of primary cancers that have formed cancerous lesions and the treatment of anti-metastasis, all of which are invasive, middle stage and late stage, and the treatment effect is poor.

So far in the second decade of the 21st century, hospitals all over the world, the oncology departments of the provincial cancer hospitals and the affiliated hospitals of various universities in China, the oncology departments of the top three hospitals are all treatment hospitals, the cancer hospitals are all clinical treatment work, the hospital model is treatment hospitals, and the academic journals of oncology are also clinically diagnosed or clinically based, although there are several journals for cancer prevention and treatment. But there are very few articles on cancer prevention work.

In short, the oncology departments of the cancer hospitals and affiliated hospitals of the 20th century are all attention to treatment with light prevention or only have treatment without prevention.

Looking back, reflecting, old-fashioned cancer prevention and anti-cancer work, what research or work did we do in cancer prevention for a century? What has it been achieved?

The status quo is:

The road that has passed in a century is to pay attention to treatment with light prevention, or only to treatment without prevention. Cancer prevention and anti-cancer are human business and careers and causes, but over the years we have only been working and researching on anti-cancer and cancer treatment. However, work on cancer prevention has been done very little and almost nothing has been done.

There is no emphasis on cancer prevention knowledge in the teaching content of medical school textbooks.

The hospital or the hospital model did not pay attention to the setting up of cancer prevention science.

There is no emphasis on cancer prevention research projects in medical research projects in medical schools or hospitals. The Journal of Oncology Medicine does not pay attention to cancer prevention work papers. In short, cancer prevention has not been taken seriously, and prevention has not been taken seriously.

Old-fashioned cancer prevention and anti-cancer work and that old-fashioned prevention is the main focus did not pay attention to and were implemented.

2. **How to launch a general attack to overcome cancer? How can cancer prevention research work be carried out?**

XZ-C (Xu Ze-China - China Xu Ze) proposed the general attack, which is that the work for the three stages of cancer prevention and cancer control and cancer treatment should fully developed and synchronized, that is, it is to carry out and to start up cancer prevention research work. And it is the most important and it is the top priority.

As everyone knows:

How to reduce cancer mortality? How to improve the cure rate? How to prolong the survival period?

The way out for cancer treatment is "three early" (early detection, early diagnosis, early treatment), the effect of early cancer treatment is good and works well and it can be fully cured. <u>In particular, cancer lesions are well treated and can be cured.</u>

3. The way out to control cancer is prevention, and research on preventive measures must be strengthened.

Cancer has become the world's largest public health problem, and compared with other chronic diseases, cancer prevention and control will face even greater challenges.

In the past 30 years, the cancer mortality rate in China has shown a clear upward trend, and it has become the first cause of death for urban and rural residents. On average, one out of every four deaths has died of cancer.

Cancer is not only a serious threat to human health, but also an important factor in the rise in medical costs. China's annual direct cost for cancer treatment is nearly 100 billion yuan. The patient and the society as a whole bear a huge economic burden. Many patients have spent tens of thousands or even hundreds of thousands of dollars, and have not achieved corresponding effects. As a result, both human and financial are empty, cancer mortality is still the first, what should I do? It is worthy of our clinician analysis, reflection, and research. How is the research road to go? It is sure to recognize the problems that exist in current treatments.

Although countries have invested heavily in the treatment of cancer patients, the 5-year survival rate of some common cancers has not improved significantly in the past 20 years.

How to do?

The way out of controlling control cancer is prevention. Prevention and intervention are the top priority in the public health field. In recent years, it has been recognized that more than 90% of cancers are caused by environmental factors. Protecting and restoring a good environment is an important part of preventing cancer. One third of cancers are preventable.

The relationship between environment and cancer is extremely close. Environmental pollution can cause various carcinogens to enter the human body or various carcinogenic factors affect the human body. *How to prove the relationship between environmental pollution and cancer has been confirmed by many examples in history.*

Air pollution in environmental pollution can increase the incidence of lung cancer. In industrialized countries, harmful gases such as power generation, steelmaking, automobiles, aircraft, fuel, energy, and large amounts of smoke are emitted into the atmosphere, polluting the air, leading to an increase in the incidence and mortality of lung cancer.

Water pollution in environmental pollution and cancer:

water pollution is mainly caused by industrial and agricultural production and urban sewage. Water pollution can induce or promote cancer.

Chemical carcinogenesis in environmental pollution is also closely related to the incidence of cancer. 80-90% of human cancers are related to environmental factors, among which are mainly chemical factors.

Studying the sources of environmentally-friendly carcinogens and studying how to eliminate such pollution is a very important issue in the prevention of cancer. Prevention of cancer must prevent pollution and control pollution.

I think that energy saving and emission reduction, pollution prevention and pollution control are the first-level prevention of cancer and it is to block the occurrence of cancer at the source. And think this is a good time to help "overcome cancer". I am convinced that building a well-off society will surely achieve the effects of preventing cancer and cancer, and achieving good results, so that the people can be healthy and stay away from cancer.

In order to overcome cancer and conduct cancer prevention and cancer control research, it is necessary to carry out basic and clinical research on anti-cancer metastasis and recurrence, and carry out joint research on multidisciplinary cooperation. It is necessary to establish Wuhan Anticancer Research Association.

With the strong support of the academician Qiu Fazu, Xu Ze, Li Huizhen and other professors applied for preparation. After approval by the higher authorities of Wuhan, the Wuhan Anticancer Research Association was established on June 21, 2009, then it was to establish a professional committee for cancer metastasis treatment and recurrence treatment.

Chapter 4

The formation course of new concepts and new methods of cancer treatment

First

From the follow-up to the establishment of experimental surgical research room

Since 1985, the author has conducted a petition to more than 3,000 patients with chest and abdominal cancer after surgery which was performed by my own. It was found that most patients relapsed or metastasized in 2 to 3 years, and some even relapsed, metastasized and died after several months and one year after surgery.

These patients are often not returned to the original surgical surgery center after surgery for review, instead, go to the oncology department or the tumor hospital for chemotherapy and chemotherapy.

- Through large-scale follow-up, the author found an important problem, that is, postoperative recurrence and metastasis are the key factors affecting the long-term efficacy of surgery.

- Therefore, we also recognize that research on the prevention and treatment of postoperative recurrence and metastasis of cancer is the key to improving the long-term efficacy of surgery, which is the key to improve the postoperative survival of patients.

- Therefore, clinicians must conduct clinical basic research to prevent cancer recurrence and metastasis. Without breakthroughs in basic research, clinical efficacy is difficult to improve.

Based on the follow-up results, the next research goals were determined:

1). In order to prevent postoperative recurrence and metastasis so as to improve long-term postoperative efficacy, clinical basic research must be carried out;

2). In order to study prevention of recurrence and metastasis, the experimental tumor models must be established for experimental research.

Therefore, we established an experimental surgical laboratory to conduct experimental tumor research, perform cancer cell transplantation, establish a tumor animal model, and carry out a series of experimental tumor research.

- Explore cancer recurrence, metastasis mechanisms and patterns, and explore the relationship between tumors and immune and immune organs, as well as immune organs and tumors.

- Explore ways to suppress progressive atrophy of immune organs and rebuild immunity when tumor progression.

- Look for effective measures to regulate and to control cancer invasion, recurrence, and metastasis.

- The experimental screening of 200 anti-cancer Chinese herbal medicines commonly used in the literature for the tumor inhibition rate in the cancer-bearing solid tumors animal was performed.

- Search for anti-cancer, anti-metastatic, anti-recurrence new drugs from natural medicines, and use modern science and technology to conduct in-depth research and discovery of cancer prevention and anti-cancer Chinese herbal medicines.

--------- Screening of the anti-cancer Chinese herbal medicines in the traditional understanding of the anti-cancer rate in a strict, scientific and repeated cancer-bearing animal model.

It was to eliminate the effect of no stability, and 48 kinds of XZ-c immunomodulatory anti-tumor Chinese medicines with good curative effect were screened out.

- Based on the success of animal experiments, it has been applied to clinical practice. After 12 years of clinical trials of a large number of clinical cases, the curative effect is remarkable.

Second

The new discoveries

1. Found from the results of follow-up

(1) Postoperative recurrence and metastasis are the key factors affecting the long-term efficacy of surgery. Therefore, we also raised an important issue, that is, clinicians must pay attention to and study the prevention and treatment measures for postoperative recurrence and metastasis, so as to improve long-term postoperative outcomes.

(2) Clinical basic research on recurrence and metastasis must be carried out. Without breakthroughs in basic research, clinical efficacy is difficult to improve.

2. Found from experimental tumor research

(1) Excision of the thymus can produce a model of cancer-bearing animals, and injection of immunosuppressive drugs can also contribute to the establishment of a cancer-bearing animal model.

The conclusions of the study clearly demonstrate that the occurrence and development of cancer has a clear relationship with the immune function of the host's immune organs, thymus and immune organs.

(2) Whether is it immune function decrease first and then easy to get cancer or It is cancer occurrence first and then it causes the low immune function?

Our experimental results are that the immune system is first low and then easy to have cancer. If the immune function is not reduced first, it is not easy to be vaccinated successfully.

The results suggest that improving and maintaining good immune function and protecting the thymus of the immune organs is one of the important measures to prevent cancer.

(3) When studying the relationship between metastasis and immunity of cancer, an animal model of liver metastasis was established, which was divided into two groups, group A and group B. Group A used immunosuppressive drugs, and group B did not. The result was that the number of intrahepatic metastases in group A was significantly higher than that in group B.

The experimental results suggest that metastasis is associated with immunity, low immune function or the use of immunosuppressive drugs can promote tumor metastasis.

(4) When investigating the effects of tumors on immune organs,

it was found that as the cancer progressed, the thymus showed progressive atrophy. Immediately after inoculation of cancer cells, the thymus of the host showed acute progressive atrophy, cell proliferation was blocked, and the volume was significantly reduced.

The experimental results suggest that the tumor will inhibit the thymus and cause the immune organs to shrink.

(5) It was also found through experiments that some of the experimental mice did not have a successful vaccination or the tumor grew very small, and the thymus did not shrink significantly.

In order to understand the relationship between tumor and thymus atrophy, when transplanted solid cancer in a group of experimental mice grew into the size of the thumb, it was removed. After 1 month of dissection, the thymus did not undergo progressive atrophy.

Therefore, it is speculated that a solid tumor may produce a factor that is not yet known to inhibit the thymus, which is temporarily called "cancer suppressor factor", which needs further study.

(6) The above experimental results prove that the progression of the tumor will cause the thymus to progressively shrink.

Can be there some ways to prevent the host's thymus from shrinking?

Therefore, we began to use immune organ cell transplantation to restore the experimental function of immune organs.

In the study of suppressing/inhibiting the thymus atrophy of the immune organs during the progress of tumors and looking for ways to restore the function of the thymus and rebuild the immune system, the experimental study of transplantation of fetal liver, fetal spleen and fetal thymus cells to restore immune function was performed by using mice.

The results showed that S, T, L three-level or three types cells were transplanted together, and the complete tumor regression rate was 40% in the near future or the short-term, and the long-term tumor complete regression rate was 46.67%. The tumor completely disappeared and survived for a long time.

(7) When investigating the effect of tumor on the spleen of the immune organs of the body, it was found that the spleen had an inhibitory effect on tumor growth in the early stage of the tumor, and in the late stage of the tumor, the spleen also showed progressive atrophy.

The experimental results suggest that the effect of spleen on tumor growth is bidirectional, with some inhibition in the early stage and no inhibition in the late stage. Spleen cell transplantation can enhance the inhibition of tumors.

(8) The results of follow-up suggest that controlling metastasis is the key to cancer treatment. There are many steps and links in the current known cancer cell metastasis. To stop one of the links can prevent their metastasis. In 1986, the author's laboratory carried out microcirculation research work. Microcirculation microscopy was used to observe microvascular formation and flow rate and flow rate of tumor nodules in transplanted mice.

(9) We design looking for anti-tumor angiogenesis drugs from natural medicines. The Olympus microcirculation microscopy system was used to observe the neovascularization process and count the flow rate and flow rate of the arterioles and venules. And the TG of Huang Lateng ethyl acetate extract was found from Chinese herbal medicine to carry out experiments to inhibit blood vessel formation.

It was found that on the first day of vaccination there was no neovascularization; on the second day microscopic neovascularization was observed, and TG reduced the density of neovascularization into and out of the tumor.

(10) From the large number of tumor-bearing animal models in the laboratory, it was also found that the experimental tumors inoculated subcutaneously in some

tumor-bearing mice grew larger, the central tissue structure of the transplanted solid tumor is more different from the surrounding cancer cells. The center of the nodule is mostly sterile necrosis or liquefaction, and the surrounding area is still active cancer cells. Therefore, in the clinical treatment work, measures for treating sterile necrosis can be employed.

According to the results of laboratory experiments, it was found that resection of the thymus can produce a cancer-bearing animal model. *The thymus progressive atrophy was found in cancer, and it was found that immunity is related to the occurrence and development of cancer, and low immunity is related to the metastasis of cancer.*

It was found that excision of the thymus can produce a model of cancer-bearing animals, and it is found that the thymus is progressively atrophied during cancer, and it is found that immunity is related to the occurrence and development of cancer, and low immunity is related to the metastasis of cancer.

The purpose of the next study and treatment determined is to:

1). to prevent thymus atrophy, increase thymus weight, increase immunity, that is, the principle of treatment of protection of Thymus and protection of bone marrow of hematopoiesis or producing the blood.

2). Based on the above experimental findings, data and information, the experimental basis and theoretical basis of new concepts and methods for anticancer and anti-metastasis treatment were established, namely, preventing progressive atrophy of the thymus, protecting the thymus, increasing the weight of the thymus, increasing immunity, and protecting the bone marrow and promoting the production of bone marrow stem cells and immunogenic cells and improving immune surveillance.

3). It was to settle down the experimental basis and theoretical basis of establishing principles, directions, and guidelines for the treatment Established based on new concepts and methods. That is, biological immunotherapy or XZ-C immunomodulation therapy.

How can it be to stop the thymus from shrinking and protecting the thymus?

After three years of basic laboratory research, the thymus progressive atrophy was discovered during cancer; mouse with excision of the thymus can be inoculated with cancer cells to produce a cancer-bearing animal model. Immunization decrease is associated with the occurrence, development and metastasis of tumors. According to the experimental data and information, it is determined that the treatment goal is to try to protect the thymus, increase the weight of the thymus, prevent thymus atrophy, increase immunity, protect Thymus and increase immune function, and protect the marrow from producing blood. ***The theoretical basis for the new concept of anti-cancer and anti-metastatic treatment, the theoretical system of new methods and clinical practice have been established.***

What method can be used to prevent thymus atrophy and protect the thymus?

Through experiments, the author found that when the fetal Thymus, fetal liver and fetal spleen stem cell in the same kind of fetal rat were transplanted, the tumor disappearance rate reached 46.7% and achieved good results. However, the results of this experiment are difficult to be used in clinical practice because human homologous fetal cells cannot be obtained.

So it was to begin to look for drugs that prevent thymus atrophy and protect the thymus from natural medicines.

Third

The experimental research on finding new anticancer and anti-metastatic drugs in natural medicines

The experimental methods of finding new drugs for anti-cancer and anti-metastasis from natural medicines were the followings:

1. In vitro screening experiment

The cancer cells were cultured in vitro to observe the direct damage of the drug to the cancer cells, and the inhibition rate of cell proliferation caused by cytotoxicity was measured.

2. Tumor inhibition rate in tumor-bearing animals

Each batch of experiments consisted of 240 Kunming mice, divided into 8 groups, 30 in each group. Groups 1 to 6 were experimental groups, each group was screened for 1 traditional Chinese medicine, the seventh group was blank control group, and the eighth group was treated with fluorouracil or cyclophosphamide as a control group. The whole group of mice was treated with EA~C or S180 or H22 cancer cells 1×107/ml. After 24 hours of inoculation, each rat was orally fed with crude biological powder according to the body weight of 1000mg/kg, 1/d feeding for 4 weeks. It was to observe survival, adverse reactions, calculate prolonged survival, and calculate tumor inhibition rate.

Among the 200 kinds of crude drugs screened by experiments, 48 of them have certain or even good tumor inhibition rate, and the inhibition rate of cancer cells is 70%-90% or more, and the other 152 kinds of traditional Chinese medicines have no inhibition rate for cancer.

After optimized combination, the tumor inhibition rate experiment in the tumor-bearing animal model was carried out to form XZ-C1~XZ-C10 immunoregulatory particles. XZ-C1 can significantly inhibit cancer cells, but does not affect normal cells.

XZ-C4 can protect the Thymus and increase immune function and improve immune function. XZ-C8 can protect the marrow to produce blood, improve the quality of life, increase appetite, enhance physical fitness and prolong survival term.

Fourth

Clinical validation work

1. After 7 years of scientific experiments in the laboratory, it was to screen from natural medicines and to constitute XZ-C immunomodulatory of anti-cancer, anti-metastasis Chinese medicine with the protection of Thymus and increase of immune function, the protection of bone marrow to produce blood, promoting the blood circulation and dissolving the blood stasis, and the clinical validation work is carried out on the basis of the success of the animal experiment or on the basis of the success of animal experiments, clinical validation work was carried out.

2. Since 1985, one side of the tumor-bearing mouse tumor-bearing animal experiment, clinical efficacy in the outpatient clinic.

3. Since 1985, on the one hand, the tumor-bearing mice were tested in the tumor-bearing mice, and on the other hand, the efficacy was verified in the outpatient clinic. However, there are few patients, and there is no medical record in the outpatient clinic (the medical records are all issued to patients), and it is impossible to accumulate scientific research materials. It must take the road of scientific research and cooperation.

4. Set up an anti-cancer research collaboration group, take the road of scientific research and cooperation, and jointly set up the research road, and set up the Dawn or Shuguang Oncology Clinic.

5. Resume outpatient medical records, fill in complete and detailed outpatient medical records, obtain complete information of clinical verification, facilitate analysis and statistics, and be conducive to outpatient clinical research to improve medical quality.

6. The outpatient cases were kept, and they were followed up regularly. The experience and lessons of the diagnosis and treatment of this case were analyzed briefly to observe the long-term effects.

7. The oncology clinic outpatient medical records are designed in a tabular format, which contains all relevant medical information and relevant epidemiological data to facilitate statistical analysis of possible pathogenic factors.

8. After more than one year of follow-up, outpatient medical records, the medical records are summarized, and the large table analysis is carried out. The contents of the large table include the contents of the outpatient medical record form, which are concise and detailed, and detailed.

The Twilight Oncology Clinic has been verified for 14 years, and the large table has accumulated more than 10,000 outpatient clinical data for outpatient clinical research.

9. The cases and Outpatient medical records which follow up more than 1 year are all written into medical records summary and add on the big table analysis, each item in the large form contains the contents of the outpatient medical record form. That is to be concise and detailed, and that has both the detailed and throughout. Dawning or Twilight Oncology Clinic has been verified for 14 years. The large table has accumulated nearly 10,000 outpatient clinical data for outpatient clinical research.

10. From experimental research to clinical research, from clinical to experimental, the collaborative group has experimental research bases and clinical application verification bases. The former is in the medical school laboratory, and the latter is in the Twilight Oncology Clinic. From experiment to clinical, that is, based on the success of experimental research, it is applied to the clinic, and new problems are found in the clinical application process. Further basic research is carried out, and new experimental results are applied to clinical verification.

For example, outpatients with liver cancer with portal vein tumor thrombus, renal cancer patients with inferior vena cava tumor thrombus. Some are CT reports, and some are pathological sections of surgically removed specimens. **In fact, the cancer plug is the cancer cell group on the way to transfer, is the third manifestation of cancer in the human body. After we found** a cancer thrombus problem, we began the experimental study of cancer thrombus formation. It was to look for new ways to fight against cancerous plugs and dissolve cancerous plugs. As a result, we found four kinds of traditional Chinese medicines that help to dissolve cancerous plugs and found out their active ingredients.

Such experiments → clinical → re-experiment → re-clinical, continuous cyclical rise, after 12 years of clinical practice experience, awareness continues to rise, it was to sum up practice; after conducting analysis and reflection and evaluation, it has risen to the theory and proposes new understanding, new thinking, and new treatment ideas.

11. In the past 12 years, through a large number of outpatient consultations after analysis, evaluation, reflection, a series of clinical problems was found, further research and improvement is needed.

12. From the review, analysis and reflection of a large number of outpatient medical records, it is recognized that postoperative adjuvant chemotherapy in many patients fails to prevent recurrence and even promotes immune failure. This indicates that chemotherapy needs further research and improvement.

13. From the review, analysis and reflection of a large number of outpatient medical records, it is recognized that many patients have recurrence and metastasis soon after surgery. The design of "radical surgery" needs further research and improvement. *How to do the intraoperative tumor-free technology to prevent and treat the shedding and planting of cancer cells in the thoracic cavity or*

abdominal cavity or surgical field cancer cells is an important measure to prevent postoperative recurrence and metastasis.

14. Through the collaborative group to focus on a large number of cases of treatment practice, evaluation, analysis, reflection, and experience the following points:

(1) Current postoperative adjuvant chemotherapy:

Many patients fail to prevent cancer recurrence and metastasis.

(2) The focus of anti-cancer should be anti-metastasis and recurrence, which is the key to improve the long-term efficacy of postoperative patients.

(3) The "threshold" of anti-cancer should be "three early".

(4) Anti-cancer recurrence must start from the surgery:

From the data of outpatients, some radical hospitals underwent radical surgery without rules and regulation, therefore, the recurrence is early and the abdominal cavity is widely metastasized or there were recurrence early and extensive intra-abdominal metastasis. The education and learning of standardized and regulated cancer surgery should be strengthened.

(5) Some patients with postoperative cancer have weak constitution and it is 4 cycles of chemotherapy or 6 cycles of chemotherapy, which promotes the decline of immune function and even exhaustion. Why do you want 4 cycles or 6 cycles, and what is the theoretical basis or experimental data?

The theoretical basis of laboratory experimental research with 4 courses of chemotherapy or 6 courses of treatment has not been found in domestic and foreign literatures.

15. Through review, analyze, reflect, evaluate from 14 years of access to a large number of outpatients, the diagnosis of current cancer mainly relies on pathological sections. However, pathological sections must be obtained after surgery, intraoperative or endoscopic biopsy or puncture, which is in the middle and late stages. **Therefore, we should try to study new methods of early diagnosis and new tumor markers.**

16. Looking back or Judging from the positive performance of CT, MRI, and color Doppler examinations in a large number of outpatients, once CT, MRI, color

Doppler, etc. see the place, most of the patients are mostly in the advanced stage, and some have lost the opportunity for surgery. Therefore, we should try to study and find new new technologies, new markers and new diagnostic methods that can be discovered early.

17. Clinical efficacy observation:

On the basis of experimental research, since 1994 the medications have been applied to clinically various types of cancer, which mostly patients are with stage III or IV. That is, advanced cancer that cannot be removed by exploration; recent or long-term metastasis or recurrence after various cancer operations; liver metastasis, lung metastasis, brain metastasis, bone metastasis or cancerous pleural effusion and cancerous ascites in various advanced or late-stage cancers; various cancer palliative resection, exploration can only do gastric thoracic anastomosis or colostomy can not be removed; patients who are not suitable for surgery, radiotherapy or chemotherapy.

XZ-C immunomodulation anticancer Chinese medicine has been clinically applied for 14 years, and systematic observation has achieved obvious curative effect. No adverse reactions were observed after long-term use. Clinical observations have proven that XZ-C immunomodulatory Chinese medicine can comprehensively improve the quality of life of patients with advanced cancer, improve the body's immunity, control cancer cell proliferation, consolidate and enhance the long-term efficacy after surgery or chemotherapy or radiotherapy.

18. **Oral administration and external application of XZ-C drug have a good effect on softening and reducing body surface metastasis.** Combined with intervention or intubation pump treatment, it can protect the liver, kidney, bone marrow hematopoietic system and immune organs, and improve immunity.

In the Dawning or Twilight Oncology Clinic, 4,698 patients with stage III, IV or metastatic recurrent cancer were treated for long-term follow-up or follow-up.

19. **The evaluation of the quality of life of patients with advanced cancer with taking XZ-C immunomodulatory Chinese medicine :**

The patients were all middle-advanced patients. After taking the drug, the improvement of symptoms was 93.2%, the mental improvement was 95.2%, the appetite was improved by 93%, and the physical strength was increased by 57.3%. The overall quality of life of patients with advanced cancer was improved.

The 42nd Annual Meeting of the American Society of Clinical Oncology (ASCO) proposed that comprehensive assessment of the quality of life of loyalists is one of the main treatment goals. A total of 223 articles in the 2006 ASCO conference papers were related to the quality of life of patients, accounting for 5.8 of the total number of papers. %, quality of life has become an important factor that people must consider when choosing a treatment strategy.

For understanding the purpose of anti-tumor treatment, as people continue to improve the quality of life of cancer loyalists as one of the main purposes of treatment, a large number of studies have begun to take the impact of treatment on quality of life as the main evaluation indicators.

A total of 223 articles in the ASCO conference papers in 2006 were related to the quality of life of patients, accounting for 5.8% of the total number of papers. Quality of life has become an important factor that must be considered when people choose treatment strategies. The understanding of the purpose of anti-tumor treatment has made people increasingly improve the quality of life of cancer patients as one of the main purposes of treatment. A large number of studies have begun to take the impact of treatment on quality of life as the main evaluation index.

20. XZ-C anti-cancer analgesic effect:

Pain is a more obvious and painful symptom in patients with advanced cancer. General analgesics have little effect on cancer pain, and narcotic analgesics are addictive and analgesic. XZ-C anti-cancer analgesic cream has strong analgesic effect and lasts for a long time. After 298 cases of clinical verification, the effective rate was 78.0%, and the total effective rate was 95.3%. Repeated use did not show obvious adverse reactions, no addiction, and the analgesic effect was stable. It is an effective treatment for cancer patients to relieve pain and improve their quality of life.

21. Efficacy evaluation:

Paying attention to the short-term efficacy and imaging indicators, and paying more attention to the long-term efficacy of survival, quality of life and immune indicators. The goal is to have a long life and good quality of life. During the course of medication, it is necessary to pay attention to changes in self-conscious symptoms and improvement of self-conscious symptoms for more than one month, otherwise it is invalid. It is effective to pay attention to the spirit, good appetite, and quality of life

(Carson's score) for more than one month, otherwise it will be invalid. The evaluation criteria for solid tumor mass were classified into 4 grades according to the size of the tumor, that is, the grade 1 mass disappeared, the grade II mass was reduced by 1/2, the grade III mass became soft, and the grade IV mass did not change or increase.

Chapter 5

The scientific research routes and research methods for the new concepts and methods of related cancer treatment

Science is the end of the world. Our scientific research work has always followed the scientific development concept, based on known science, future-oriented medicine, and looking forward. After 16 years of hard work, we will practice the scientific concept of development, face the frontiers of science, and strive for innovation and progress. To overcome cancer, we must advance under the guidance of scientific development concept; we must go from the clinical, through experimental research, to the clinical, to solve the actual problems of patients; we must seek truth from facts, use facts, use data to speak; it must constantly self-transcend, self-advance In scientific research, we should emancipate our minds, break away from traditional old ideas, stand on independent innovation, and original innovation; our route of scientific research in decades is to discover problems → ask questions → study problems → solve problems or explain problems, the road was walked out like this, it is step by step, and it is difficult to climb or travel, under the guidance of the concept of scientific development, we hope to embark on an innovative road of anti-cancer and anti-metastasis with Chinese characteristics and independent intellectual property rights.

Our model of oncology research is patient-centered, it is to find and ask questions from clinical work, and to conduct in-depth basic research in animal experiments, then turn the basic research results into clinical applications so as to improve the overall level of medical care, patients will ultimately benefit.

Why would it get on the theoretical innovation?

It is because all clinical treatment, medication, and diagnosis must have a reasonable theoretical basis and theory guides the clinic.

Through the review and reflection of the practice of clinical tumor surgery for half a century, the author deeply realized that the current "oncology" is the most backward subject in various medical disciplines. Why?

It is because the etiology, pathogenesis, pathophysiology of oncology are not well understood, the oncology discipline is still a virgin land for scientific research, and it needs a lot of basic scientific research, clinical verification research and the combination of basic and clinical research.

Since 1985, the author has followed up more than 3,000 postoperative patients with thoracic and abdominal cancer whom I did surgery on by my own.

It was found that most patients relapsed or metastasized in 2 to 3 years, and some even relapsed and metastasized and died within 1 year after surgery. Through large-scale follow-up, an important problem has also been found, that is, postoperative recurrence and metastasis are the key factors affecting the long-term efficacy of surgery. Therefore, the author recognizes that research on prevention and treatment of postoperative metastasis and recurrence of cancer is the key to improving the long-term efficacy of surgery. Then the experimental surgery laboratory was established, and a series of studies on experimental tumors were carried out:

It took 4 years to study the mechanism and law of cancer metastasis and find an effective method for anti-cancer metastasis;

It took another three years to screen the anti-tumor rate of 200 kinds of traditional anti-cancer Chinese herbal medicines through strict scientific cancer-bearing animal models. It turns out that 48 kinds of XZ-C immunomodulatory anti-cancer and anti-metastatic traditional Chinese medicines with good anti-cancer rate were screened out. Based on this experimental study, it has been applied to nearly 10,000 patients with advanced cancer in the past 18 years, and achieved good results.

On the basis of clinical verification, combined with half a century of clinical experience and skills and reflection, it rised up to the theory and put forward a number of new understandings and new concepts and new theories. These experimental research and clinical verification data, information, collection were summed into these monographs.

The new discoveries, new theories, and new concepts proposed in the book are mostly independent intellectual property rights of independent innovation and original innovation. These new insights, new theoretical insights, and new concepts have the important academic significance and important academic value. It will have an important impact on the development of oncology medical science, which may benefit patients with millions of cancer metastasis and come out with a new path to overcome cancer.

How is it to find measures to prevent cancer cell metastasis, and how is it to explore it?

In the research of anti-cancer, traditional Chinese medicine is China's advantage, and it is to develop the role of this advantage in anti-metastasis research, to give full play to China's advantages and to catch up with the international advanced level. The XZ-C immunomodulation anti-cancer anti-metastatic Chinese medicine introduced in this book has been tested and screened in vivo for 3 years in a tumor-bearing animal model. It has been clinically validated and applied for 16 years, not only for the benefit of millions of cancer metastasis patients, but also get billions of economic benefits for the country.

This book is independent innovation or original innovation, is at the level of molecular tumors, is from clinical to experimental, is from experimental to clinical, taking the combination with the molecular level of Chinese medicine and Western medicine, it has embarked on the new road with Chinese characteristics against cancer and anti-metastasis.

First

The research route

The clinical research work of our Dawn or Twilight Oncology Clinic is conducted in accordance with the following scientific research routes:

1. The outlines:

It was to find the problem

Through high-volume patient follow-up, the key factors found to affect the long-term efficacy of surgery are postoperative recurrence and metastasis.

$$\downarrow$$

It was to pose the problem

It is proposed that recurrence and metastasis must be studied to improve the long-term efficacy;

It is to propose that the goal or "target" of the research should be how to resist metastasis.

↓

It was to research the problem

It established a research institute to conduct a series of projects and experiments and explored transfer mechanisms and found anti-recurrence and metastasis techniques and new drugs.

It screened out 48 kinds of traditional Chinese medicines with certain anti-cancer and anti-metastatic effects from 200 kinds of traditional Chinese medicines.

↓

It was to solve the problem

Carried out clinical verification and clinical research, explored the law of cancer metastasis and found a new model of anti-metastasis treatment, and rised to the theory of independent innovation and new anti-metastasis treatment mode and new scheme.

2. This study is all from clinical → experimental → clinical → re-experiment → re-clinical, back to the clinical to solve the problem.

3. The theory and practice are closely combined. This topic which is selected was all from the clinical, to find the key point of clinical problems and the point of clinical breakthroughs, after experimental research and clinical verification, and then applied to the clinic to solve clinical practical problems

4. This study was to take the road of combining Chinese and Western medicine → macroscopic combination → molecular level combination and use modern cancer cell molecular transfer mechanisms and the newest eight-step, three-stage theory, search for and screen anti-metastatic drugs with protecting the immune organs and activating cytokines and immune factors from 200 ancient Chinese medicines. It modernized ancient Chinese medicine with international standards and combined modern medicine with ancient Chinese herbal medicine at the molecular level and BRM level.

5. It is evidence-based medicine, seeking truth from facts, scientific, speaking with facts, argumentation, and evaluable experimental research and clinical validation data.

6. The efficacy evaluation criteria, long-term efficacy:

It is the long living life and the clinical observation for 3 to 5 years, or even 8 to 10 years, then it can be used to initially evaluate the long-term efficacy.

Second

The research methods

The Anti-Cancer Recurrence and Metastasis Research Laboratory and the Shuguang Oncology Clinic opened and adhered to the following scientific research methods for clinical research:

1. Self-reliance and self-financing.

See the patients in the outpatient center and the income of the patient fee was as a research funding.

2. It established an outpatient medical record cabinet, keep medical records, and follow up throughout. After many years of long-term follow-up, the phone can always answer questions at any time, guide dietary precautions, and guide how to recover, such as follow-up form, intervention + Chinese medicine follow-up form.

3. It establish a scientific research collaboration group, established scientific research collaborations for specific projects, and collaborated and cooperated according to scientific research plans, such as scientific research tables.

4. It established detailed medical records, including patient epidemiological data, and analyze in depth the success and failure lessons of each treatment and the specificity of the condition, such as analysis data.

5. Stage summary analysis was performed in all cases from 6 months to 1 year. Cases that have been reviewed for more than 3 years are excerpted from medical

records, written medical records, and analyzed treatment experiences and lessons, such as abstract medical records.

6. Established a large form of disease with item-by-item statistical analysis item such as the big form posted on the wall included the epidemiological data on various cancers, the data of cancer metastasis rules and the treatment experience and lessons of each case.

7. The scientific research cooperation strategy of instrument sharing, equipment sharing, and results sharing were used.

It doesn't need to add large-scale instruments and equipment, but cooperate with the medical college affiliated school. The high-precision equipment inspection and the molecular level examination are carried out in the medical college.

4. Do not ask for money from the top (not to the Ministry, the province, the city to declare the subject and research funding). And it reported to the provinces and cities on high-level advanced scientific research results of independent innovation and original innovation and independent intellectual property rights and scientific review or scientific assessment of academic achievements.

Third

The academic value and academic status

Science is the end of the world. Our scientific research work has always followed the scientific development concept, based on known medicine, facing the future of medicine, and looking forward. After 12 years of hard work, we have implemented the scientific concept of development, facing the forefront of science, striving for innovation and progress.

1.

1. Modern molecular tumor metastasis mechanism	Ancient Chinese herbal medicine screening

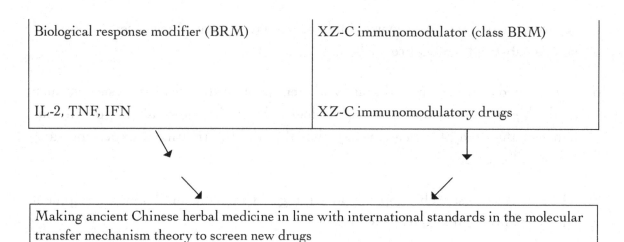

2.

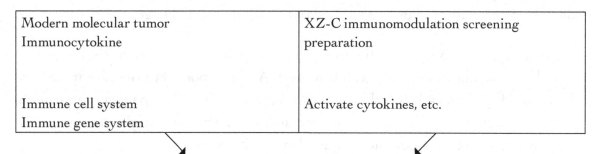

XZ-C is a combination of Chinese and Western medicine at the molecular level

3. **The new concept of cancer treatment:**

Primary tumor ▶ metastatic cancer on the way to metastasis ▶ Metastase lesion

A   B   C

Handle with these three(A, B, C) ▶ make theory completion, possiblyconquer cancer

The traditional concept:

Primary focus ⟶ Metastase lesion

Isolated both ⟶ The theory is incomplete and it cannot conquer cancer

4.

Initially found out the development of oncology, research and development, research direction; review, reflection, summary, saw a slight dawn.

The successful experience and failure lessens

↓

Find out the existing problem

↓

Facing the present and recognizing that the understanding of cancer in the 20th century, the diagnosis of cancer, and the treatment of cancer are all at the cellular level.

↓

It found out the direction of the way forward, and proposed the understanding of cancer in the 21st century, the conclusion of cancer, and the treatment of cancer. All of them should be at the molecular level.

↓

From the beginning of cell malignancy change to the diagnosis of CT, MRI, B-ultrasound and other imaging, there is a large distance between blank space and time. At present, there is no effective detection method. The next step should be to find an effective detection method for this time segment to achieve early diagnosis.

↓

The "target" in the 21st century is precancerous lesions and micrometastases. It is the world of molecular, genetic diagnosis, molecular immunity, molecular biology, traditional Chinese medicine, and gene therapy.

↓

Take an innovative road of anti-cancer transfer with Chinese characteristics and independent intellectual property rights

Fourth

Shuguang scientific research spirit

Hard work

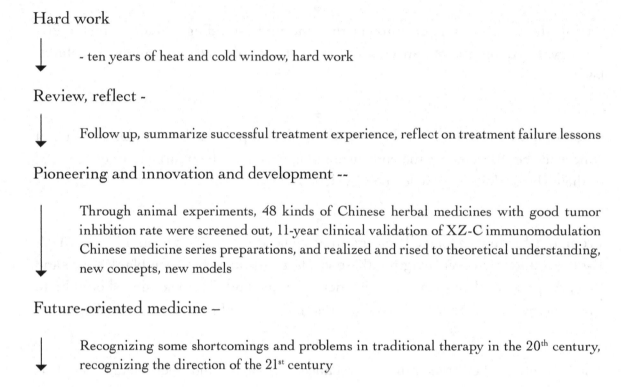

- ten years of heat and cold window, hard work

Review, reflect -

Follow up, summarize successful treatment experience, reflect on treatment failure lessons

Pioneering and innovation and development --

Through animal experiments, 48 kinds of Chinese herbal medicines with good tumor inhibition rate were screened out, 11-year clinical validation of XZ-C immunomodulation Chinese medicine series preparations, and realized and rised to theoretical understanding, new concepts, new models

Future-oriented medicine –

Recognizing some shortcomings and problems in traditional therapy in the 20th century, recognizing the direction of the 21st century

Looking forward

Chapter 6

Task, Mission, Opportunities and Challenges of Anticancer Research

First

Conducting research on anti-cancer metastasis is an urgent need

(1) It must know the current problems

1). The basic problem is that the traditional three major treatments have been applied for nearly a hundred years, and the mortality rate of cancer patients is still the first.

What should we do? It is to analysis, reflection and research.

2). The problem of postoperative recurrence is still very serious.

Patients and their families are afraid of recurrence after surgery, and some patients are worried about the whole day after surgery. Oh, it's not a day. How the surgeon should prevent recurrence and prevent postoperative metastasis is worthy of our study.

3). Metastasis is the core problem of cancer and the key to survival. Everyone is afraid of cancer metastasis. How should it be to effectively prevent cancer metastasis, control cancer cell metastasis? Basic and clinical research should be conducted.

(2). Be sure to recognize the problems in current treatment

1). Chemotherapy needs further research and improvement. Does postoperative adjuvant chemotherapy prevent recurrence? whether is it to prevent metastasis? And how can it help prevent postoperative recurrence and metastasis? These are all worthy of our thinking and research, so we take our own data and experience and do further research and improvement.

2). Radiotherapy needs further research and improvement, and radiotherapy is for local treatment and metastasis is systemic problems. How to play its role in anti-metastatic treatment and how to further research and improve are worth thinking about.

3). The design of "radical surgery" needs further research and improvement to reduce postoperative recurrence and metastasis. Since it is a "radical cure", why has it not achieved the goal of radical cure? Since lymphatic dissection has been done, why is there a metastasis? These require further study. How to pay attention to intraoperative tumor-free technology, how to reduce and prevent intraoperative cancer cell detachment, how to reduce intraoperative promotion of cancer cell metastasis, and how to reduce dissemination from the tumor vein are all issues that clinicians should pay attention to in practice. The operation should be light, stable and accurate, and basic experimental research should be carried out, and experimental observation and study on the tumor-bearing animal model should be carried out. The first thing in surgery is to prevent metastasis.

Second

Conducting anti-cancer metastasis research is the need for the development of oncology

1. "Oncology" is the most backward discipline in the current medical sciences. It is because the etiology, pathogenesis, pathophysiology of oncology are not well understood. The oncology discipline is still a scientific virgin land for scientific research, and it needs a lot of basic scientific research.

2. Although countries have invested heavily in the treatment of cancer patients and although it has been using traditional three major treatments for nearly a hundred years, however, the mortality rate of cancer is still the first cause of death for urban and rural residents in China. The reasons are mainly the following:

(1) The cause of cancer is not fully understood:

People still lack sufficient understanding of pathogenesis and cancer cell metastasis mechanisms.

(2) There is still insufficient understanding of the complex biological behavior of cancer.

(3) The treatment plan is still quite blind.

(4) The diagnostic method is backward. Once found, it is in the middle and late stages, and the treatment effect is poor.

(5) Many large hospitals have not established laboratories, and cannot carry out basic research on cancer, anti-cancer metastasis, and recurrence. It is necessary to carry out basic research on cancer-bearing animal models. It is necessary to establish various cancer metastasis animal models in nude mice to study the laws and mechanisms of cancer cell metastasis (the author's laboratory uses pure Kunming mice to make cancer-bearing animal models, about 10,000 Times), it is because without a breakthrough in basic research, clinical efficacy is difficult to improve.

Third

Under the guidance of the scientific development concept, take the innovative road of scientific research of anti-cancer metastasis with Chinese characteristics

Academic research on cancer metastasis focuses on the study of unknown knowledge. Researchers should look ahead and face the science of the future. Science is the end of the world.

Scientific research must transcend previous old knowledge with a developmental perspective. Constantly updated, constantly surpassing, constantly developing, and constantly advancing.

As clinical medical workers, especially professors and chief physicians, we have dual tasks on our shoulders. One is to treat patients; the other is to develop medicine. Publishing a paper is to develop medicine, and adding bricks to the medical science hall.

1). The core issue of the research is based on "research", to develop medicine, use the vision of development, use the spirit of innovation, look forward, and face the future of medicine, study the prevention and treatment of cancer metastasis. Oncology in the 20th century is at the cellular level, and 21st century oncology should be at the molecular level. The research and development of oncology must constantly surpass the knowledge of predecessors. One generation is more than one generation, and blue is better than blue. The medical experts of the older generation are willing to be ladders and welcome to pass over on academics, technology and achievement.

2). Research should be based on patients, based on research on new outcomes and new methods that benefit patients, improve medical quality, reduce patient suffering, and prolong patient survival. Medical quality refers to the medical effect. The medical effect of cancer patients is that they live for a long time, the quality of life is good, and the patients suffer little.

Fourth

What to do and how to do it?

1.   Doing what?

It is to carry out basic research in biology of molecular biology and genetic engineering, to conduct clinical basic research and conduct clinical follow-up retrospective analysis; to conduct evidence-based medicine. There are evaluable experimental studies and clinically validated data to evaluate the long-term efficacy of the evaluation study. It is to explore cancer metastasis, recurrence mechanisms and effective measures to find regulation. Animal experimental surgery is extremely important in the development of medicine. It is the key to opening the medical exclusion zone and can promote the development of medical undertakings. Many new drugs and new technologies are applied to the clinic based on the success of animal experiments.

2.   How is it to do it?

Our research route is:

1). Discover the problem → ask a question → study the problem → solve the problem or explain the problem.

2). Theory and practice are closely integrated. The topic which is selected of this study comes from the clinical, to find the key point or focus of clinical problems and the points of clinical breakthroughs, after experimental research and clinical verification, and then applied to the clinic to solve clinical practical problems.

3). Take the road of combining Chinese medicine and Western medicine ------ Macroscopic combination-----through Experimental research-------Molecular level binding.

4). The combination of tumor basic and clinical research will surely play a leading role in the fight against cancer.

5). We should be in the field of our existing advantages, give play to China's advantages and catch up with the international advanced level. In the field of cancer research, traditional Chinese medicine and the combination of Chinese and Western are the advantages of China and give play to this advantage.

The role of cancer research should be a strategic vision of international significance.

3.   Anti-cancer research requires a group of research elites. It is to undertake scientific research on research topics and micro-metastasis, and they have been working in the clinical first field for many years with rich clinical experience, these scientific elites will be the locomotives for the development of oncology.

The new research work on anti-cancer metastasis should be based on scientific research, development, transformation of results, and the path of production, learning and research. It is to take the banner of the scientific development concept, standing on the forefront of oncology, and advancing toward the general direction of research and development, we will surely achieve fruitful results in overcoming cancer.

4. All of them are scientific research elites, and some are even leading talents in science and technology. It must take the lead in research results. We must take the road of innovation in anti-cancer transfer with Chinese characteristics and make achievements in the fight against cancer metastasis research.

Let us advance together on the scientific research road, and keep on the road of science. It is facing the future of science, looking forward, developing and innovating.

Chapter 7

Research on cancer treatment reform and development

First

How is it to summarize, organize and express clinical research materials?

The use of the table format to describe scientific research materials or scientific research papers can be both concise and detailed, making them easy to read and understand. The use of the table format to describe scientific research materials or scientific research papers can be both concise and detailed, making them easy to read and understand. Through decades of painstaking and meticulous clinical research work, the large amount of scientific research materials and experimental data obtained are summarized, collated and collected, and expressed in a tabular narrative. They are concise and clear, and the readers can understand the core content in ten minutes.

China is a country with a population of 1.4 billion people and is therefore a major resource for cancer cases. There are a large number of cancer cases in China for clinical observation and analysis. In the daily clinical work, clinicians carefully observe the condition, carefully analyze and analyze, and actively explore research. After long-term practice of medical experience, there will be some discoveries, developments, and continuous advancement. Medical research is to improve clinical diagnosis and treatment, improve medical quality and medical level, so clinical research work is also an important part of clinical work.

1. Save the outpatient medical records, accumulate the outpatient consultation, treatment, rehabilitation and follow-up materials, fill in the complete and detailed tabular outpatient medical records, to obtain the complete data of clinical

verification, easy to analyze and statistics. If the outpatient medical records are not saved, the analysis, statistics, and follow-up of the outpatient diagnosis in the outpatient clinic will not be possible. The outpatient medical records were retained to observe long-term efficacy. Restoring and retaining outpatient medical records will help clinic clinical research and improve medical quality.

2. Establish a list of cancer treatments for outpatients. The results are complete and detailed. All patients who have been re-examined for more than 3 months have completed the large form. After years, they will continue to register and fill in the large form in order to sort, collect, organize and count a large amount of data.

3. How to summarize, summarize, organize, analyze, demonstrate and express clinical research materials and laboratory research materials?

This book summarizes, collects, organizes, and classifies a large number of scientific research materials and experimental data based on more than 50 years of clinical medical practice and combined with 30 years of laboratory cancer research. They are all clinical and experimental materials, all of which are made by work. Actually, it is a collection of scientific research results or a series of scientific research results.

The author proposed new findings, new ideas, new treatment concepts and new treatment methods through experimental research and clinical practice experience, combining with the clinical verification of a large number of clinical cases in the past half century, the review, analysis, evaluation and self-reflection of clinical practice cases of traditional therapy, summarizing the positive and negative experiences and lessons of their clinical practice.

How is it to collect, sort, classify and summarize so many clinical and experimental scientific research materials, so many scientific research papers, theoretical innovations and recent developments? The author uses a tabular format to describe scientific research materials or scientific research papers, making them easy to read, easy to understand, and easy to guide.

Second,

One of the researches on new concepts and new methods of cancer treatment

The Study on New Concept and Way of Treatment of Carcinoma (1)

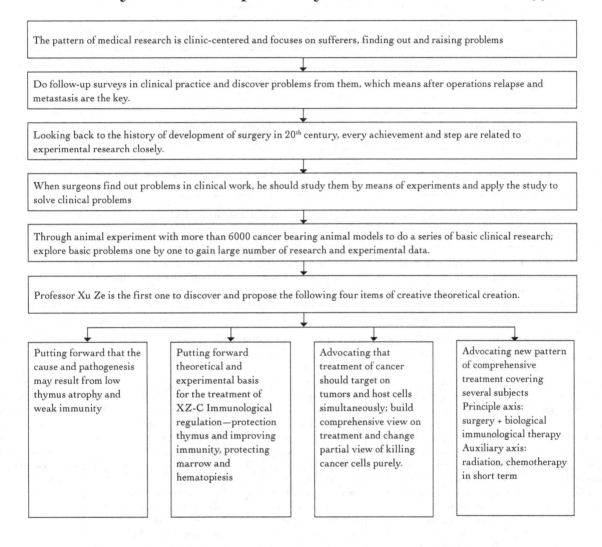

The pattern of medical research is clinic-centered and focuses on sufferers, finding out and raising problems

Do follow-up surveys in clinical practice and discover problems from them, which means after operations relapse and metastasis are the key.

Looking back to the history of development of surgery in 20th century, every achievement and step are related to experimental research closely.

When surgeons find out problems in clinical work, he should study them by means of experiments and apply the study to solve clinical problems

Through animal experiment with more than 6000 cancer bearing animal models to do a series of basic clinical research; explore basic problems one by one to gain large number of research and experimental data.

Professor Xu Ze is the first one to discover and propose the following four items of creative theoretical creation.

Putting forward that the cause and pathogenesis may result from low thymus atrophy and weak immunity

Putting forward theoretical and experimental basis for the treatment of XZ-C Immunological regulation—protection thymus and improving immunity, protecting marrow and hematopiesis

Advocating that treatment of cancer should target on tumors and host cells simultaneously; build comprehensive view on treatment and change partial view of killing cancer cells purely.

Advocating new pattern of comprehensive treatment covering several subjects
Principle axis: surgery + biological immunological therapy
Auxiliary axis: radiation, chemotherapy in short term

Third

Two of the research of new concepts and methods of cancer treatment

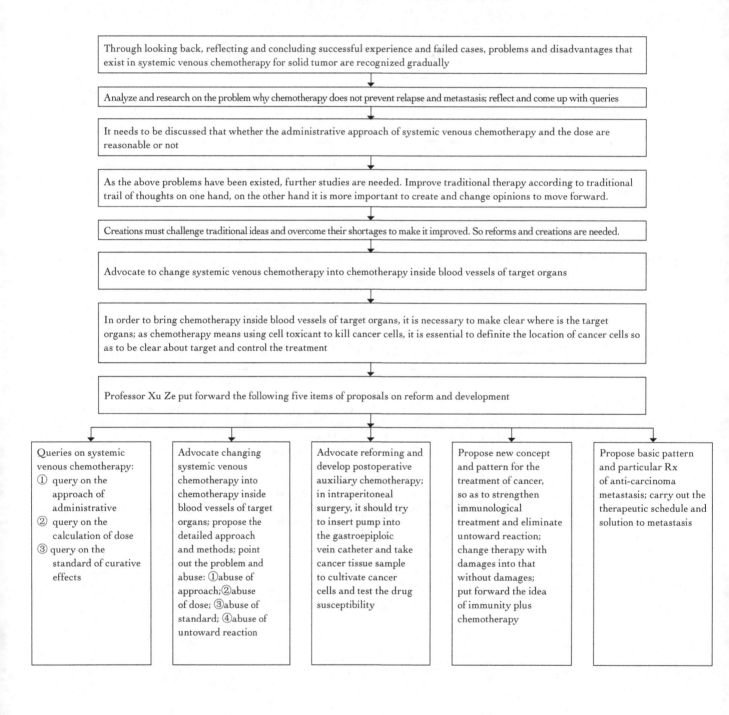

Through looking back, reflecting and concluding successful experience and failed cases, problems and disadvantages that exist in systemic venous chemotherapy for solid tumor are recognized gradually

Analyze and research on the problem why chemotherapy does not prevent relapse and metastasis; reflect and come up with queries

It needs to be discussed that whether the administrative approach of systemic venous chemotherapy and the dose are reasonable or not

As the above problems have been existed, further studies are needed. Improve traditional therapy according to traditional trail of thoughts on one hand, on the other hand it is more important to create and change opinions to move forward.

Creations must challenge traditional ideas and overcome their shortages to make it improved. So reforms and creations are needed.

Advocate to change systemic venous chemotherapy into chemotherapy inside blood vessels of target organs

In order to bring chemotherapy inside blood vessels of target organs, it is necessary to make clear where is the target organs; as chemotherapy means using cell toxicant to kill cancer cells, it is essential to definite the location of cancer cells so as to be clear about target and control the treatment

Professor Xu Ze put forward the following five items of proposals on reform and development

| Queries on systemic venous chemotherapy: ① query on the approach of administrative ② query on the calculation of dose ③ query on the standard of curative effects | Advocate changing systemic venous chemotherapy into chemotherapy inside blood vessels of target organs; propose the detailed approach and methods; point out the problem and abuse: ①abuse of approach;②abuse of dose; ③abuse of standard; ④abuse of untoward reaction | Advocate reforming and develop postoperative auxiliary chemotherapy; in intraperitoneal surgery, it should try to insert pump into the gastroepiploic vein catheter and take cancer tissue sample to cultivate cancer cells and test the drug susceptibility | Propose new concept and pattern for the treatment of cancer, so as to strengthen immunological treatment and eliminate untoward reaction; change therapy with damages into that without damages; put forward the idea of immunity plus chemotherapy | Propose basic pattern and particular Rx of anti-carcinoma metastasis; carry out the therapeutic schedule and solution to metastasis |

Fourth

Three of the research on new concepts and new methods of cancer treatment

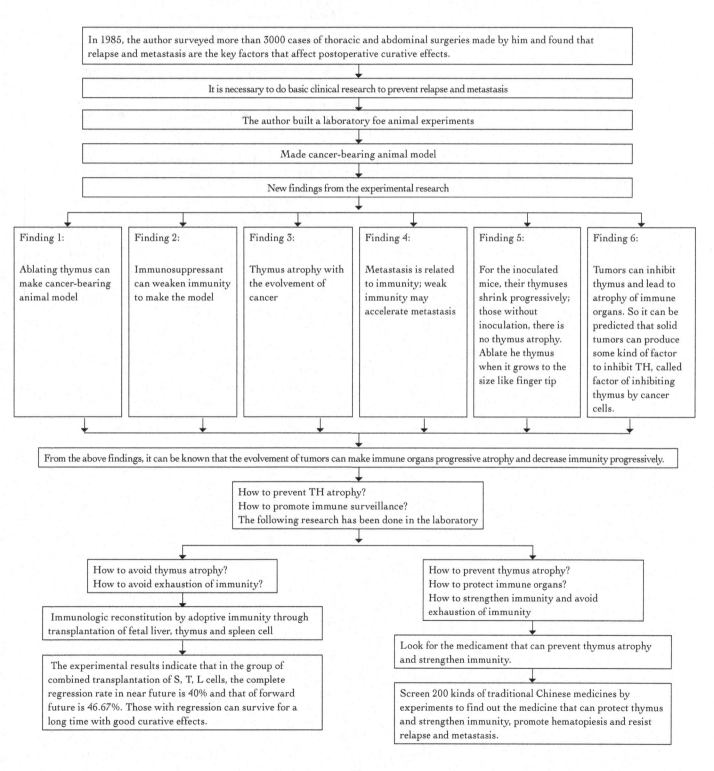

In 1985, the author surveyed more than 3000 cases of thoracic and abdominal surgeries made by him and found that relapse and metastasis are the key factors that affect postoperative curative effects.

It is necessary to do basic clinical research to prevent relapse and metastasis

The author built a laboratory foe animal experiments

Made cancer-bearing animal model

New findings from the experimental research

Finding 1:

Ablating thymus can make cancer-bearing animal model

Finding 2:

Immunosuppressant can weaken immunity to make the model

Finding 3:

Thymus atrophy with the evolvement of cancer

Finding 4:

Metastasis is related to immunity; weak immunity may accelerate metastasis

Finding 5:

For the inoculated mice, their thymuses shrink progressively; those without inoculation, there is no thymus atrophy. Ablate he thymus when it grows to the size like finger tip

Finding 6:

Tumors can inhibit thymus and lead to atrophy of immune organs. So it can be predicted that solid tumors can produce some kind of factor to inhibit TH, called factor of inhibiting thymus by cancer cells.

From the above findings, it can be known that the evolvement of tumors can make immune organs progressive atrophy and decrease immunity progressively.

How to prevent TH atrophy?
How to promote immune surveillance?
The following research has been done in the laboratory

How to avoid thymus atrophy?
How to avoid exhaustion of immunity?

Immunologic reconstitution by adoptive immunity through transplantation of fetal liver, thymus and spleen cell

The experimental results indicate that in the group of combined transplantation of S, T, L cells, the complete regression rate in near future is 40% and that of forward future is 46.67%. Those with regression can survive for a long time with good curative effects.

How to prevent thymus atrophy?
How to protect immune organs?
How to strengthen immunity and avoid exhaustion of immunity

Look for the medicament that can prevent thymus atrophy and strengthen immunity.

Screen 200 kinds of traditional Chinese medicines by experiments to find out the medicine that can protect thymus and strengthen immunity, promote hematopiesis and resist relapse and metastasis.

↓

| Experimental articles can not be published |

↓

| Screen and look for natural medicament from traditional Chinese herbs through animal experiment. |

↓

The experiments for screening in the laboratory: ①screening experiment by the rate of inhibiting tumors in vitro; ②screening experiment by the rate of inhibiting tumors in vivo of cancer-bearing animal model

From a series of experimental research on tumors with cancer-bearing animals over 7 years, there is a deeply-felt that it is necessary to persist in research on resisting cancerometastasis with Chinese characteristics, namely the combination of experimental research and clinical verification. It is essential to do experimental research on tumors, or it is difficult to improve clinical curative effects.

● Experimental oncology is the basis of research on preventing cancer, which promote the research in China to step further and deeper

● Experimental surgery plays an important role in developing medical science, which is a key to open the forbidden zone of medical science

● Methods of preventing many diseases result from animal experimental research. After acquiring stable achievements, they can be applied in clinic to promote the development of medicine.

Fifth

Four of the research on new concepts and new methods of cancer treatment

(1)

Theoretical innovation content of Clinical Applied Oncology

(introduction)

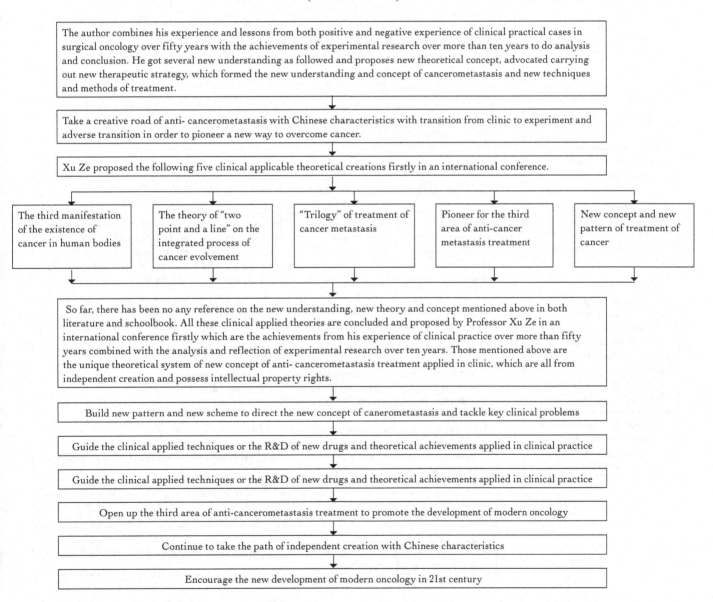

The author combines his experience and lessons from both positive and negative experience of clinical practical cases in surgical oncology over fifty years with the achievements of experimental research over more than ten years to do analysis and conclusion. He got several new understanding as followed and proposes new theoretical concept, advocated carrying out new therapeutic strategy, which formed the new understanding and concept of cancerometastasis and new techniques and methods of treatment.

Take a creative road of anti- cancerometastasis with Chinese characteristics with transition from clinic to experiment and adverse transition in order to pioneer a new way to overcome cancer.

Xu Ze proposed the following five clinical applicable theoretical creations firstly in an international conference.

| The third manifestation of the existence of cancer in human bodies | The theory of "two point and a line" on the integrated process of cancer evolvement | "Trilogy" of treatment of cancer metastasis | Pioneer for the third area of anti-cancer metastasis treatment | New concept and new pattern of treatment of cancer |

So far, there has been no any reference on the new understanding, new theory and concept mentioned above in both literature and schoolbook. All these clinical applied theories are concluded and proposed by Professor Xu Ze in an international conference firstly which are the achievements from his experience of clinical practice over more than fifty years combined with the analysis and reflection of experimental research over ten years. Those mentioned above are the unique theoretical system of new concept of anti- cancerometastasis treatment applied in clinic, which are all from independent creation and possess intellectual property rights.

Build new pattern and new scheme to direct the new concept of canerometastasis and tackle key clinical problems

Guide the clinical applied techniques or the R&D of new drugs and theoretical achievements applied in clinical practice

Guide the clinical applied techniques or the R&D of new drugs and theoretical achievements applied in clinical practice

Open up the third area of anti-cancerometastasis treatment to promote the development of modern oncology

Continue to take the path of independent creation with Chinese characteristics

Encourage the new development of modern oncology in 21st century

(2)

Theoretical innovation content of Clinical Applied Oncology
(The specific expansion or development)

1. Xu Ze (XU ZE) first proposed a doctrine or a new theoretical understanding in the international arena, that is to say, there are three manifestations of cancer in the human body, and the third form of its presence in the human body is the cancer cell group on the way to metastasis.

It is necessary to update thoughts and change concepts to overcome cancer that therapeutics of cancer should have comprehensive therapeutic concept

---

(1)　Two manifestations in traditional therapeutics of cancer:

1st manifestation—primary lesion
2nd manifestatio—metastatic lesion

---

(2) Three manifestations of cancer existing in human bodies in Xu Ze's theory:
1st manifestation—primary lesion
2nd manifestation—metastatic lesion
3rd manifestation—cancer cells, crowd of cancer cells on the way of metastasis and micro cancer embolus

---

Traditional therapeutics is targeted on these two manifestations:

One is to the 1st manifestation — primary lesion
The other is to the 2nd manifestatio—metastatic lesion

The new concept holds that the aims or the "targets" of treatment should point to these three manifestations:
1. to the 1st manifestation—primary lesion
2. to the 2nd manifestatio—metastatic lesion
3. to cancer cells, crowd of cancer cells on the way of metastasis and micro cancer embolus

---

The new concept holds that cancer cells exist in human bodies in three manifestations, which is more complete and comprehensive. It illustrates the dynamic connection, causal relation and subordination among the three manifestations, so it is a complete therapeutics of cancer that explains the whole process of cancer evolvement and gives answer to the question how to control the whole process of canerometastasis in all its aspects. This new theory sheds a great deal of light on the solution to cancer.

The traditional therapeutics has been used for more than 100 years, which separates the above two targets and ignore the dynamic connection, causal relation and subordination between them . If there is no prevention of cancer cells that are on the way of metastasis, cancerometastasis can not be controlled. Thus, traditional therapeutics holds that there are only two manifestations, which is partial and defective.

Once the new theory or the new understanding was proved effective and recognized by public, it will cause a series of reforms and renovations of oncotherapy (especially for the cancer cells that are on the way of metastasis) as chain reaction.

---

① it will cause the reform and renovation of the concept of oncotherapy.
② it will bring into the significant reforms and renovations of diagnostic methods
③ it will lead to important reforms and renovation of research and development of anti-cancer and anti-metastasis drugs.
④ it will result in reforms updates of the pattern and methods of oncotherapy.
⑤ it will cause the reform and renovation that guide the research on metastasis and relapse from oncology of cellular pathomorphology on cellular level to molecular organism and genetic expression on molecular level.

Because this problem has been neither recognized by people, nor attached with adequate attention without any reference in literature and schoolbooks.

Why it is necessary to come up with that the third manifestation is the crowd of cancer cells on the way of metastasis?

2. Xu Ze (XU ZE) first proposed another new theory or new theoretical understanding at the international conference. That is, the "two points and one line" theory of the whole process of cancer development. In the treatment of cancer, the past and present have only recognized and valued the "two points" and neglected the "first line." In fact, the treatment of cancer should not only pay attention to the "two points", but also pay more attention to the "first line." ***Cutting off the "first line" is the key to anti-cancer metastasis.***

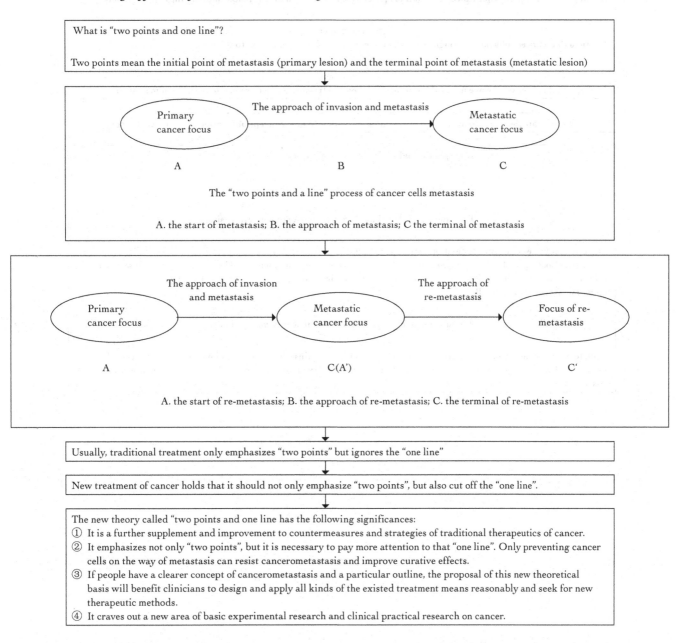

What is "two points and one line"?

Two points mean the initial point of metastasis (primary lesion) and the terminal point of metastasis (metastatic lesion)

The "two points and a line" process of cancer cells metastasis

A. the start of metastasis; B. the approach of metastasis; C the terminal of metastasis

A. the start of re-metastasis; B. the approach of re-metastasis; C. the terminal of re-metastasis

Usually, traditional treatment only emphasizes "two points" but ignores the "one line"

New treatment of cancer holds that it should not only emphasize "two points", but also cut off the "one line".

The new theory called "two points and one line has the following significances:
① It is a further supplement and improvement to countermeasures and strategies of traditional therapeutics of cancer.
② It emphasizes not only "two points", but it is necessary to pay more attention to that "one line". Only preventing cancer cells on the way of metastasis can resist cancerometastasis and improve curative effects.
③ If people have a clearer concept of cancerometastasis and a particular outline, the proposal of this new theoretical basis will benefit clinicians to design and apply all kinds of the existed treatment means reasonably and seek for new therapeutic methods.
④ It craves out a new area of basic experimental research and clinical practical research on cancer.

3. Xu Ze (XU ZE) first proposed the "Trilogy" of anti-cancer metastasis treatment worldly

Try to strike or destroy each steps of metastasis

Conclude the "eight steps" of cancerometastasis and divide them into three stages

1st stage: the stage from the point that cancer cells fall off parent tumors to the moment before moving into blood vessels **2nd stage:** the stage that cancer cells pass through the wall and move into blood circulation to work **3rd stage:** the stage that cancer cells wave out of the wall and land on the tissue of target organs, namely form metastasis

Three strategies of resisting cancerometastasis according to new concept of treatment of cancer (trilogy)

Therapeutic goal of the 1st stage of anti-cancerometastasis: prevent cancer cells move into blood vessels **Therapeutic goal of the 2nd stage of anti-cancerometastasis:** activate immune cells in blood circulation to protect thymus function; improve immunity and immune surveillance so that cancer cells floating in blood circulation can be captured, phagocytosed and then killed by immune cells. The second stage is the major battlefield of annihilating the cancer cells in blood circulation, as well as the major strategy to intervene in and inhibit metastasis of cancer cells **Therapeutic goal of the 3nd stage of anti-cancerometastasis:** regulate tissue immunity of local microenvironment, which makes against the growth and implantation of cancer cells; inhibit blood vessels to produce factors, which is the strategy of intervention that focuses on inhibiting the formation of new vessels

4. Xu Ze is the first to put forward the third area of anti-cancerometastasis treatment internationally.

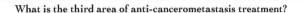

What is the third area of anti-cancerometastasis treatment?

All treatments aimed at primary cancer are called the first area of the treatment of cancer

All treatments aimed at metastatic cancer are called the second area of the treatment of cancer

All treatments aimed at the third manifestation of cancer existing in human bodies, namely the treatment of cancer cells on the way of metastasis, are called the third area of the treatment of cancer for human beings.

(1) The essentiality of proposing the third area of anti-carcinoma treatment:

as cancer cells that are in the process of metastasis are the third manifestation in human bodies, it is necessary to prevent and kill them. So it is essential to open up the third area.

(2) The possibility of intercepting the cancer cells on the way of metastasis:

the key of incepting metastasized cancer cells during the process lies in breaking down the inhibition of immune system by tumors and activating effective immune response especially that based on T cells.

(3) A large amount of immune surveillance cells in circulatory system:

As immune cells is the effective to kill cancer cells added with wallop and shearing force of blood stream, it is difficult for individual or signle cancer cells to survive. In order to avoid being killed by immune cells, cancer cells will adhere to PLT and stick to the wall of blood vessels, then pass through micrangium or microvessels.

(4) The particular scheme of Xu Ze's treatment of cancerometastasis:

To develop the third area of treatment of cancer; intervene in and intercept cancer cells on the way of metastasis and annihilate them to control cancerometastasis; to open up the third area; to promote the development of modern therapeutics of tumors

5. **Xu Ze 's new concept and new model for the treatment of cancer, namely, strengthening immunotherapy and improving the adverse reactions of chemotherapy.**

(1) Adverse reactions of traditional chemotherapy

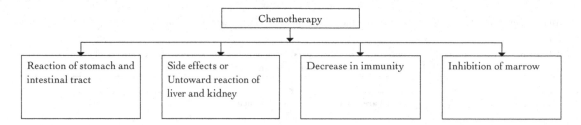

(2) The defense methods in the treatment of cancer with new concept, that is, <u>which is to take effective actions to protect host cells.</u>

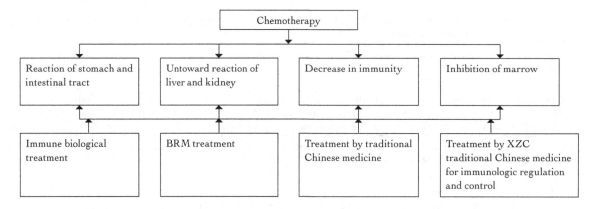

(3) Changing intermittent treatment into continuous treatment

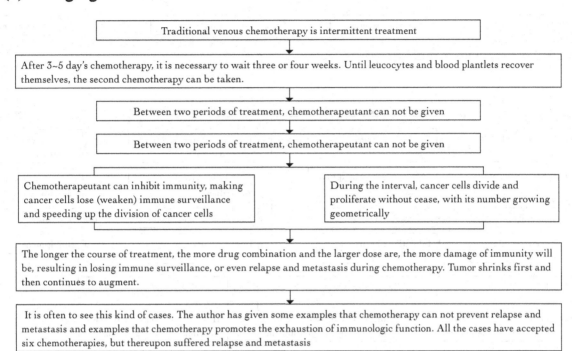

| Traditional venous chemotherapy is intermittent treatment |

After 3~5 day's chemotherapy, it is necessary to wait three or four weeks. Until leucocytes and blood plantlets recover themselves, the second chemotherapy can be taken.

Between two periods of treatment, chemotherapeutant can not be given

Between two periods of treatment, chemotherapeutant can not be given

| Chemotherapeutant can inhibit immunity, making cancer cells lose (weaken) immune surveillance and speeding up the division of cancer cells | During the interval, cancer cells divide and proliferate without cease, with its number growing geometrically |

The longer the course of treatment, the more drug combination and the larger dose are, the more damage of immunity will be, resulting in losing immune surveillance, or even relapse and metastasis during chemotherapy. Tumor shrinks first and then continues to augment.

It is often to see this kind of cases. The author has given some examples that chemotherapy can not prevent relapse and metastasis and examples that chemotherapy promotes the exhaustion of immunologic function. All the cases have accepted six chemotherapies, but thereupon suffered relapse and metastasis

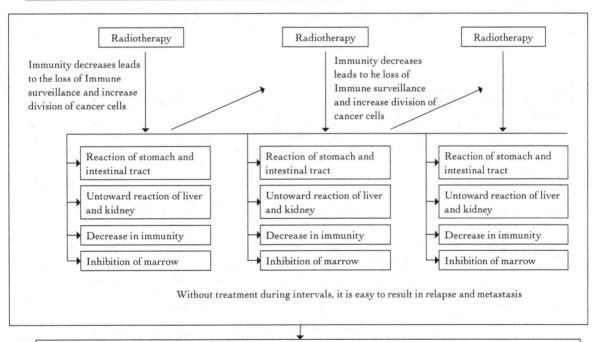

How to do? The author holds that the pattern of treatment between two periods should be changed into the following, namely chemotherapy plus continuous immunotherapy

New concept and pattern of the treatment of cancer belong to successive treatment using treatment by XZ-C1+XZ-C4 traditional Chinese medicine for immunologic regulation and control or BRM treatment during intervals

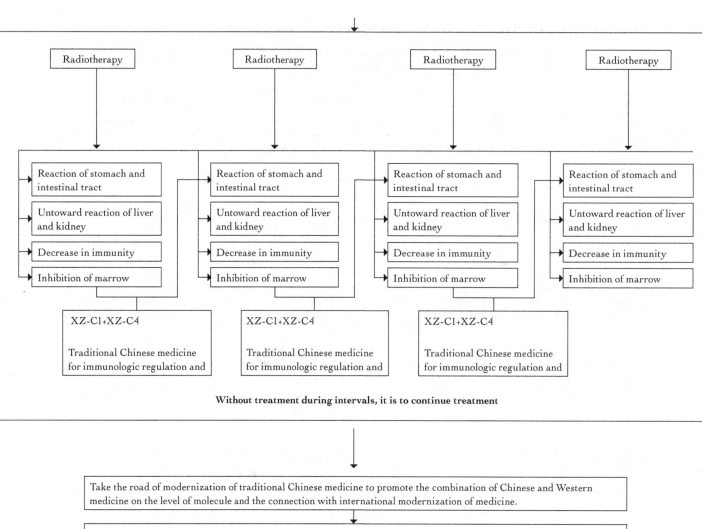

Without treatment during intervals, it is to continue treatment

Take the road of modernization of traditional Chinese medicine to promote the combination of Chinese and Western medicine on the level of molecule and the connection with international modernization of medicine.

Invasion and metastasis of cancer are decided by two factors, which are the biological characteristics of tumor cells and the effect of host cells to confinement factors. Comparing these two factors, if they are balanced, then the cancer is controlled; if not, the cancer evolves.

Traditional radiotherapy and chemotherapy can weaken immunologic function and render them more unbalanced

New pattern of the treatment of cancer means trying to improve immunity and raise immunity to attain balance, so as to benefit the prevention of cancer and strengthen immune surveillance.

Therefore, the author advocates immunochemotherapy, namely the combination of chemotherapy and treatment for immunologic regulation and control, in which these two treatments complement each other. They should be practical partners

Take the creative path of resisting cancerometastasis with Chinese characteristics

Take the road of modernization of traditional Chinese medicine to promote the combination of Chinese and Western medicine on the level of molecule and the connection with international modernization of medicine.

Sixth

Five of the Research on New Concept and Way of Treatment of Carcinoma

The detail or particular experimental projects or programs of Professor Xu Ze's unique or exclusive research on and development of XZ-C traditional Chinese medicine for immunologic regulation and control of anti-cancer and anti-metastasis are the following:

Goal:

It is to find out and pick up the traditional Chinese herbs for anti-cancer and anti-metastasis.

Purpose:

It is to pick out the "intelligent anticancer drugs" that can be taken orally during a long period with high selectivity but without drug resistance and untoward reactions

Approach:

It is from experimental research to clinical research, applying the successful animal experiments to clinical practice.

Methods:

The author has done the screening test on 200 kinds of traditional Chinese herbs that were thought to have anti-cancer effects by traditional Chinese medicine with the expectation to find out new anti-cancer and anti-metastasis drugs.

The author has done the following experimental research on the rate of tumor inhibition of traditional Chinese herbs

1. Cultivate cancer cells in vitro to do screen test on the rate of traditional Chinese herbs' inhibition of tumors	Make the model with cancer-bearing animals inoculated with EAC or S-180 or H22 cancer cells to do screen test on the rate of traditional Chinese herbs' inhibiting tumors in vivo

(1) screen test on inhibiting tumors in vitro: Cultivate cancer cells in vitro and observe the direct damage of cancer cells by drugs	(1) Screen test on inhibition of tumor in vivo: Make animal model, namely inoculate mice with EAC or S-180 or H22 caner cells

(2) Screen test inside a test tube: Cultivate cancer cells inside test tubes and add crude drugs (500μg/ml); observe the inhibition of cancer cells	(2) Grouping: Divide 240 mice into 8 groups in each experiment with 30 mice in a group; the 7th group is for blank control and the 8th group is used as control group with fluorouracil or cyclophosphane

(2) Screen test inside a test tube: Cultivate cancer cells inside test tubes and add crude drugs (500μg/ml); observe the inhibition of cancer cells	After 24 hours from inoculation, feed the mice with specific dose of rough medical powder in a long period and observe the lifetime and untoward reactions; calculate the percentage of those whose lifetimes are prolonged and the rate of inhibiting tumors

Take screen tests on the 200 kinds of traditional Chinese herbs that are thought to have anti-cancer effects by traditional Chinese medicine one by one	(3) Experimental results: 48 kinds of traditional Chinese herbs do have certain rate of inhibiting tumors and 26 of them have better effects of inhibiting tumors

Take screen tests on the 200 kinds of traditional Chinese herbs that are thought to have anti-cancer effects by traditional Chinese medicine one by one	(3) Experimental results: 48 kinds of traditional Chinese herbs do have certain rate of inhibiting tumors and 26 of them have better effects of inhibiting tumors

Cultivate and test cancer cells with fibrous cell for comparison under the same condition	Optimize and regroup those 48 kinds of traditional Chinese herbs with high rate of inhibiting tumors

(3) Experimental results: 48 kinds of traditional Chinese herbs with high rate of tumor –inhibition, other 152 kinds (that are thought to have good anti-cancer effects traditionally) have no effects on inhibiting tumors	Repeat the above experiment and the experiment on immunity

Take a further step to make cancer-bearing animal model to do screen test on the rate of inhibiting tumors in vivo	Develop Xu Ze China1~ Xu Ze China10 pharmaceutics of traditional anti-cancer Chinese medicine for immunologic regulation and control with Chinese characteristics (XZ-C1~XZ-C10)

The particular experimental program on the immunologic function of XZ-C traditional Chinese anti-carcinoma herbs for immunologic regulation and control on the level of molecule:

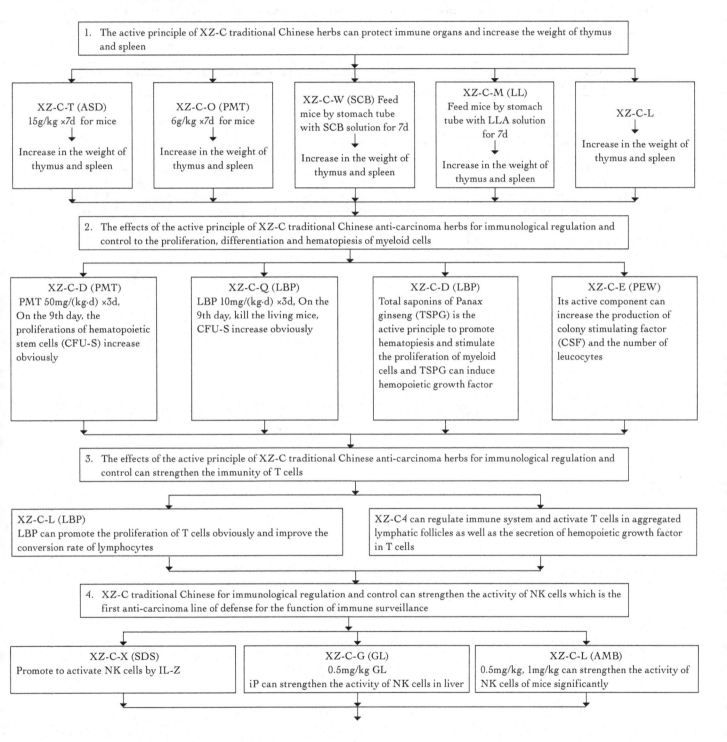

1. The active principle of XZ-C traditional Chinese herbs can protect immune organs and increase the weight of thymus and spleen

| XZ-C-T (ASD) 15g/kg ×7d for mice ↓ Increase in the weight of thymus and spleen | XZ-C-O (PMT) 6g/kg ×7d for mice ↓ Increase in the weight of thymus and spleen | XZ-C-W (SCB) Feed mice by stomach tube with SCB solution for 7d ↓ Increase in the weight of thymus and spleen | XZ-C-M (LL) Feed mice by stomach tube with LLA solution for 7d ↓ Increase in the weight of thymus and spleen | XZ-C-L ↓ Increase in the weight of thymus and spleen |

2. The effects of the active principle of XZ-C traditional Chinese anti-carcinoma herbs for immunological regulation and control to the proliferation, differentiation and hematopiesis of myeloid cells

| XZ-C-D (PMT) PMT 50mg/(kg·d) ×3d, On the 9th day, the proliferations of hematopoietic stem cells (CFU-S) increase obviously | XZ-C-Q (LBP) LBP 10mg/(kg·d) ×3d, On the 9th day, kill the living mice, CFU-S increase obviously | XZ-C-D (LBP) Total saponins of Panax ginseng (TSPG) is the active principle to promote hematopiesis and stimulate the proliferation of myeloid cells and TSPG can induce hemopoietic growth factor | XZ-C-E (PEW) Its active component can increase the production of colony stimulating factor (CSF) and the number of leucocytes |

3. The effects of the active principle of XZ-C traditional Chinese anti-carcinoma herbs for immunological regulation and control can strengthen the immunity of T cells

| XZ-C-L (LBP) LBP can promote the proliferation of T cells obviously and improve the conversion rate of lymphocytes | XZ-C4 can regulate immune system and activate T cells in aggregated lymphatic follicles as well as the secretion of hemopoietic growth factor in T cells |

4. XZ-C traditional Chinese for immunological regulation and control can strengthen the activity of NK cells which is the first anti-carcinoma line of defense for the function of immune surveillance

| XZ-C-X (SDS) Promote to activate NK cells by IL-Z | XZ-C-G (GL) 0.5mg/kg GL iP can strengthen the activity of NK cells in liver | XZ-C-L (AMB) 0.5mg/kg, 1mg/kg can strengthen the activity of NK cells of mice significantly |

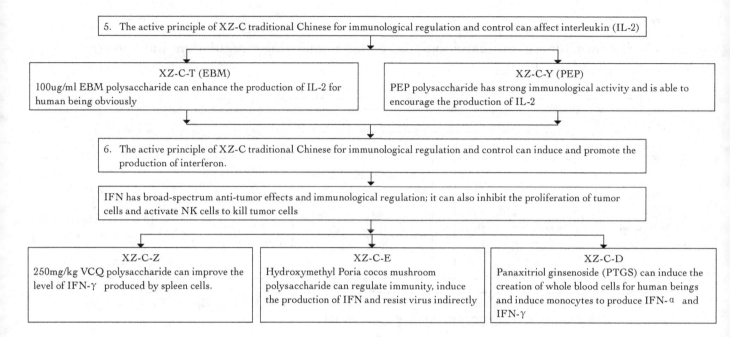

5. The active principle of XZ-C traditional Chinese for immunological regulation and control can affect interleukin (IL-2)

XZ-C-T (EBM)	XZ-C-Y (PEP)
100ug/ml EBM polysaccharide can enhance the production of IL-2 for human being obviously	PEP polysaccharide has strong immunological activity and is able to encourage the production of IL-2

6. The active principle of XZ-C traditional Chinese for immunological regulation and control can induce and promote the production of interferon.

IFN has broad-spectrum anti-tumor effects and immunological regulation; it can also inhibit the proliferation of tumor cells and activate NK cells to kill tumor cells

XZ-C-Z	XZ-C-E	XZ-C-D
250mg/kg VCQ polysaccharide can improve the level of IFN-γ produced by spleen cells.	Hydroxymethyl Poria cocos mushroom polysaccharide can regulate immunity, induce the production of IFN and resist virus indirectly	Panaxitriol ginsenoside (PTGS) can induce the creation of whole blood cells for human beings and induce monocytes to produce IFN-α and IFN-γ

Treatment of tumors by biological response modifier (BRM) and analogous BRM traditional Chinese medicine

BRM opens up the new area of biological treatment of tumors. Currently, it has been regarded as the fourth modality of treatment of tumors which is widely appreciated in medical field.

What is BRM?
Oldham founded biological response modifier, namely theory of BRM in 1982 and proposed the fourth modality of cancer treatment, namely biological treatment later on this basis.

According to BRM theory:
Normally, tumors and the defense of organism are in dynamic equilibrium. The occurrence and even metastasis of tumors result from this dynamic equilibrium. If the disordered state can be adjusted to the normal, it is possible to control the growth of tumors and make them fade away.

According to the research on the mechanism of XZ-C traditional Chinese anti-carcinoma medicine for immunological regulation and control exclusively studied and developed by the author, cancer invasion and metastasis are decided by the comparison of two factors, which is:

Biological characteristics of cancer cells ⎫ balance leads to control

Effects of host cells by the constraints ⎭ unbalance leads to the evolvement of cancer

Taking the road of modernization of traditional Chinese medicine is good for the combination with traditional Chinese and Western medicine on the level of molecule and the connection with the modernization of international medicine.

The mechanism of XZ-C traditional Chinese anti-carcinoma medicine for immunological regulation and control is similar to that of BRM

The effects of biological response modifier include the following:

(1) To strengthen the defense mechanism of host cells or to weaken the immunodepression of cancer-bearing host cells so as to achieve immune response
(2) To add natural or biological active substance with genetic recombination to strengthen the defense mechanism of host cells
(3) To modify tumor cells and induce the strong response of host cells
(4) To promote the proliferation and mature of tumor cells and normalize them
(5) To alleviate untoward reaction of radiotherapy and chemotherapy and strengthen the resistance of host cells

The main pharmacological action of XZ-C traditional Chinese anti-carcinoma medicine is to resist cancer and strengthen immunity, whose mechanism is similar to that of BRM

(1) To activate the system of immune cells and strengthen the defense mechanism of host cells to achieve the immune response to cancer cells
(2) To activate the system of immune cytokine of the organismal anti-cancer mechanism to improve immune surveillance
(3) To protect thymus and strengthen immunity and to protect hematopiesis of marrow
(4) To alleviate the untoward reactions of radiotherapy and chemotherapy
(5) To augment thymus and gain the weight to prevent its progressive atrophy and to improve immunity and immune surveillance

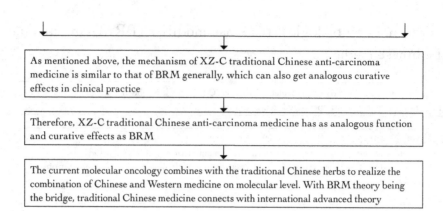

As mentioned above, the mechanism of XZ-C traditional Chinese anti-carcinoma medicine is similar to that of BRM generally, which can also get analogous curative effects in clinical practice

Therefore, XZ-C traditional Chinese anti-carcinoma medicine has as analogous function and curative effects as BRM

The current molecular oncology combines with the traditional Chinese herbs to realize the combination of Chinese and Western medicine on molecular level. With BRM theory being the bridge, traditional Chinese medicine connects with international advanced theory

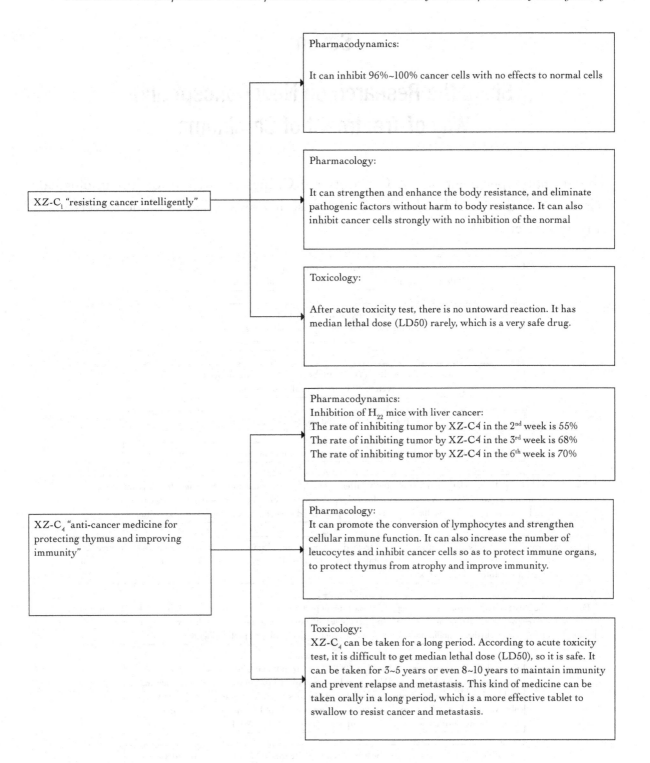

XZ-C$_1$ "resisting cancer intelligently"

Pharmacodynamics:

It can inhibit 96%~100% cancer cells with no effects to normal cells

Pharmacology:

It can strengthen and enhance the body resistance, and eliminate pathogenic factors without harm to body resistance. It can also inhibit cancer cells strongly with no inhibition of the normal

Toxicology:

After acute toxicity test, there is no untoward reaction. It has median lethal dose (LD50) rarely, which is a very safe drug.

XZ-C$_4$ "anti-cancer medicine for protecting thymus and improving immunity"

Pharmacodynamics:
Inhibition of H$_{22}$ mice with liver cancer:
The rate of inhibiting tumor by XZ-C4 in the 2nd week is 55%
The rate of inhibiting tumor by XZ-C4 in the 3rd week is 68%
The rate of inhibiting tumor by XZ-C4 in the 6th week is 70%

Pharmacology:
It can promote the conversion of lymphocytes and strengthen cellular immune function. It can also increase the number of leucocytes and inhibit cancer cells so as to protect immune organs, to protect thymus from atrophy and improve immunity.

Toxicology:
XZ-C$_4$ can be taken for a long period. According to acute toxicity test, it is difficult to get median lethal dose (LD50), so it is safe. It can be taken for 3~5 years or even 8~10 years to maintain immunity and prevent relapse and metastasis. This kind of medicine can be taken orally in a long period, which is a more effective tablet to swallow to resist cancer and metastasis.

Seven

Six of the Research on New Concept and Way of Treatment of Carcinoma

The animal experiment of XZ-C traditional Chinese medicine for immunological regulation and control has been successful, so it was applied to clinic to verify its curative effects.

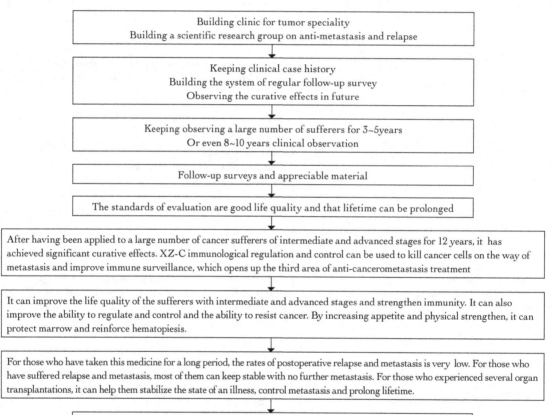

Building clinic for tumor speciality
Building a scientific research group on anti-metastasis and relapse

Keeping clinical case history
Building the system of regular follow-up survey
Observing the curative effects in future

Keeping observing a large number of sufferers for 3~5years
Or even 8~10 years clinical observation

Follow-up surveys and appreciable material

The standards of evaluation are good life quality and that lifetime can be prolonged

After having been applied to a large number of cancer sufferers of intermediate and advanced stages for 12 years, it has achieved significant curative effects. XZ-C immunological regulation and control can be used to kill cancer cells on the way of metastasis and improve immune surveillance, which opens up the third area of anti-cancerometastasis treatment

It can improve the life quality of the sufferers with intermediate and advanced stages and strengthen immunity. It can also improve the ability to regulate and control and the ability to resist cancer. By increasing appetite and physical strengthen, it can protect marrow and reinforce hematopiesis.

For those who have taken this medicine for a long period, the rates of postoperative relapse and metastasis is very low. For those who have suffered relapse and metastasis, most of them can keep stable with no further metastasis. For those who experienced several organ transplantations, it can help them stabilize the state of an illness, control metastasis and prolong lifetime.

Clinical information: from 1994 to Nov. 2002, XZ-C traditional Chinese medicine has been used in 4698 cases of III stage, IV stage, relapse and metastasis, in which 3051 cases are male and 1647 cases are female with the oldest being 86 years old and the youngest being 11 years old. All these have been above III stage according to TNM of International Union against Cancer by histopathology diagnosis or type-B ultrasonic, CT or MRI.

Curative effects: symptoms can be alleviated that life quality has been improved and lifetime has been prolonged. Among those 4277 cases who have taken XZ-C traditional Chinese medicine for more than three months, those with advanced cancer have had improvement of symptoms in different degree. The effective rate has researched 93.2% with general information in table 34-1, the improvement of life quality is seen in table 34-2, and the changes in tumors have been showed in table 34-3 and analgesia in table 34-4

Table 1 The general information about 4277 cases of relapse and metastasis

		Liver cancer	Lung cancer	Gastric cancer	Cardia Cancer	Rectal and anal cancer	Colon cancer	Breast cancer	Cancer of pancreas
Cases		1021	752	668	624	328	442	368	74
Male: Female		4:1	4.4:1	2.25:1	3.1:1	1:1	2.1:1	All female	3.2:1
Focus	primary	694(68.8%)	699(93.9%)	-	-	-	-	-	-
	metastatic	327(31.2%)	53(6.1%)	-	-	-	-	-	-
General parts of metastasis		from lung (2%) from gorge (27.2%)	lymph nodes metastasis in clavicle (11.6%)	from liver (23.8%) from lung (3%)	from clavicle (13.1%)	rate of relapse (14.8%)	from liver (16.0%)	lymph nodes metastasis in clavicle (17.5%)	from liver (11.7%)
		from cardia (19.5%) from recta (31.2%)	from brain (3.1%) from marrow (4.6%)	from peritoneum(29.1%) from clavicle (6.1%)	from liver (8.3%)	from liver (7.0%)	from peritoneum (6.0%)	lymph nodes metastasis in armpit (15.0%) from bone (5.0%)	behind peritoneum (39.1%)
Age (year)	popular (%)	30-39 (76.2)	50-69 (71.6)	40-49 (73.4)	40-69 (80.4)	40-49 (75.2)	30-69 (88.0)	40-59 (65.9)	40-59 (70.0)
	youngest	11	20	17	30	27	27	29	34
	oldest	86	80	77	77	78	76	80	68

↓

Table 2 The life qualities of the sufferers with advanced cancer among the 4277 cases with comprehensive improvement in observation of curative effects

	Spirit	Appetite	Physical strengthen	Improvement of general situation	Gain in weight	Improvement of sleep	Improvement of mobility and alleviation of movement restriction	Living by oneself and ambulating normally	Recovery of the ability to do light muscular work
Cases with improvement	4071	3986	2450	479	2938	1005	1038	3220	479
Percentage (%)	95.2	93.2	57.3	11.2	68.7	23.5	24.3	75.3	11.2

↓

Table 3 The changes in metastatic nodes after the external application of XZ-C medicine among 56 cases

	The enlargement of lymph nodes in cervical clavicle			
	Disappear	Shrink by 1/2	Become to be soft	No changes
Cases	12	22	14	8
Percentage (%)	21.4	39.2	25.0	14.2
Total effective rate	85.7			

↓

Table 4 the situation of analgesia after oral administration and external application of XZ-C medicine among 298 cases

Clinical performance	Analgesia			
	Alleviated lightly	Alleviated obviously	Disappear	No effects
Cases	12	22	14	8
Percentage (%)	21.4	39.2	25.0	14.2
Total effective rate	85.7			

On the aspect of improving life quality (according to KPS)

The average score is 50 before administration; it increases to 80, even 90 or 100 after 3 months

Analysis of lifetime: it is difficult to compare clinical sufferers as their stadiums and degrees are different. In this group, all sufferers are above third stage with different organ transplantations and dysfunctions. According to former statistics in this sort, the medium lifetime is about six months. In this group, the longest case is 14-years with the average lifetime of other cases being more than 1 year.

The sufferer in one case who experienced relapse and re-ablation after surgery of liver cancer has been taking XZ-C medicine for 14 years; that in another one case of liver cancer has been taking XZ-C medicine for ten and a half years; the sufferers in three cases that the lung cancer can not be cut off have been taking this medicine for three and a half years; two cases of cancer of gastric remnant taking XZ-C medicine for 8 years; three cases of rectal cancer with postoperative relapse have been taking XZ-C for 3 years; one case of mastocarcinoma with metastasis from liver and rib has been taking it for 8 years and another one case of renal carcinoma with postoperative relapse has been taking it for 9 and a half years. These sufferers have rechecked in clinic, got the medicine and taken them so as to keep the state of illness stable with lifetime being prolonged obviously.

Analysis of prolonging lifetime:

(1) without surgeries, radiotherapies and chemotherapies, cases that have been taking XZ-C traditional Chinese medicine for immunological regulation and control solely for 5 years are: ①Di, central type carcinoma of lung in left top lung accompanied by metastasis in left lung, has been taking XZ-C1+XZ-C4+XZ-C7 for 5 years; ② Huang, with esophageal carcinoma has been taking this medicine for 5 years; ③ Huang with cancer in the middle place of oesophagus has been taking this medicine for 5 years; ④ Huang, with primary massive type cancer has been taking this medicine for 5 years; ⑤ Qi, primary liver cancer, has been taking this medicine for 5 years.

(2) Typical cases whose cancer can not be cut off by exploratory surgeries and can not use radiotherapies and chemotherapies to treat, have been taking XZ-C traditional Chinese medicine for immunological regulation and control for 4 years: ① Cheng, with tumors after abdominal distention which can not be cut off by exploratory surgery, has been taking this medicine for 4 years; ② Fang, with cancer of pancreas which can not be cut off by exploratory surgery, has been taking XZ-C medicine for 7 years; ③ Li, with primary massive type liver cancer that can not be cut off by exploratory surgery in Tongji Hospital, has been taking XZ-C medicine for 4 years; ④ Ke, with primary liver cancer that can not be cut off by exploratory surgery in the PLA general hospital, has been taking XZ-C medicine for 5 years.

Chapter 8

What research work have we carried out? what scientific research results and scientific and technological innovation series have been achieved?

Briefly describe anti-cancer research and scientific research results, scientific thinking, academic thinking, and scientific contribution or dedication

In the past 30 years, our research results and scientific and technological innovation series, which focus on the direction of cancer research as conquering cancer, are the first in the world. All of them are original papers, internationally pioneering and internationally leading, and have reached the forefront of the world.

Its main contents are as follows:

The following is that Professor Xu Ze (XZ-C) has first proposed in the world:

These 30 items were first proposed internationally.

(1) Professor Xu Ze (XZ-C) first proposed at the international level:

It was first proposed internationally:

"Thymus atrophy, immune dysfunction is one of the causes and pathogenesis of cancer"

(2) It was first proposed at the international level:

"*Protection of Thymus and Increase of Immune Function* ' Theoretical Basis and Experimental Basis of XZ-C Immunoregulation Treatment"

(3) The first international initiative:

"Cancer treatment should change the concept and establish a comprehensive treatment concept"

(4) The first international initiative:

"A new model for the combination of multidisciplinary treatment of cancer"

(5) First proposed at the international level:

"Analysis, evaluation and questioning of systemic intravenous

(6) First proposed at the international level:

It is to initiative for the treatment of abdominal solid tumors with systemic intravenous chemotherapy as **target organ intravascular chemotherapy** ; it is to initiative to reform for traditional chemotherapy

(7) First proposed at the international level:

"There are three main forms of cancer in the human body"

(8) First proposed at the international level:

"Two Points and One Line" in the Whole Process of Cancer Development

(9) First proposed at the international level:

"Three Steps of Anticancer Metastasis Treatment"

(10) First proposed at the international level:

"Developing the third field of cancer metastasis treatment"

How is it to overcome cancer? XZ-C proposes to overcome conquer and launch the general attack of cancer, this is unprecedented work as the following:

(11) First proposed at the international level:

"XZ-C Scientific Research Plan for overcoming cancer and launching the General Attack of Cancer"

(12) First proposed at the international level:

"Necessity and Feasibility of overcoming cancer and launching the General Attack of Cancer"

(13) First proposed at the international level:

"Preparing to build the hospital with cancer prevention and treatment during the whole process of cancer occurrence and development"

(14) First proposed at the international level:

"To build the designation for the general attack of conquering cancer and to build the basic design of the Science City"

(15) First proposed at the international level:

"Overcoming cancer and launching the general attack of cancer – prevention and control and treatment at the same attention and at the same level and at the same time"

—— Changed the mode of hospitalization of heavy treatment and light defense

(16) First proposed at the international level:

"Preparing to build a scientific science city to overcome cancer"

----- -   established an overall framework for conquering cancer

(17) First proposed at the international level:

"Walked out of a new path to overcome cancer" to prevent postoperative recurrence and metastasis

(18) Independently developed XZ-C immunomodulation anticancer traditional Chinese medicine series products

(19) First proposed at the international level:

How is it to overcome cancer? XZ-C proposed "Dawning C-type plan No.1-6"

(20) First proposed at the international level:

How is it to overcome cancer?

XZ-C proposed: Cancer is a disaster for all mankind. It is necessary for the people of the world to work together and China and US joint to do the research

"Cancer moon shot" (US) and "Dawning C-type plan" (China)

- Moving forward together, heading for the science hall to overcome cancer

Why is it said to move forward together? What is it the common? It is to analyze that China and the United States each have their own advantages and it is to take complementary advantages.

(21) Over the past 100 years internationally, the history of that conquering cancer has been proposed:

-- ------- Two US presidents have successively proposed a national plan to "conquering cancer"

------— A Chinese physician XZ-C proposed a general design, plan, specific plan, blueprint for conquering cancer, and published 15 monographs (English version, global release)

(22) How is it to overcome cancer?

XZ-C proposes two wheels, A wheel, B wheel

(23) How to overcome cancer?

XZ-C proposes need A wheel, A runway

B wheel, B runway

(24) First proposed at the international level:

How to overcome cancer?

XZ-C proposes to need three targets for A, B and C.

(25) XZ-C proposes that several treatments rules and laws and principles of traditional Chinese medicine can be applied to the treatment of tumors.

(26) It was proposed for the first time in the world:

XZ-C proposes:

To overcome cancer, it is necessary to create an environmental protection and cancer prevention research institute and carry out prevention cancer system engineering, which is the first time in the world.

To conduct cancer prevention research, to find cancer-causing factors, to detect the source of carcinogens or carcinogenic factors, and to try to prevent damage to these human body by carcinogenic factors.

The Cancer Research Institute should conduct cancer prevention research:

a. The relationship between air pollution and cancer;

b. Water pollution and cancer;

c. Soil pollution and cancer;

d. Chemical, physical, biological factors and cancer;

e. Diet, lifestyle, clothing, food, housing, travel, house decoration, etc. with cancer,

It is to study these sources of pollution and try to stop at the source.

(27) XZ-C proposes that research ethics should be advocated, medicine is benevolence, and ethics is the first.

Research ethics:

Products should have ethical standards

Standard:

The bottom line should not be harmful to human health

Basic ethics:

All products and people are harmless and do not harm people's health, especially for children, and do not allow carcinogens.

(28) Post-study review

--- - How is it to implement, how is it to achieve this general design, plan, plan, blueprint for cancer?

(29) How is it to carry out "to overcome cancer and to launch the general attack of cancer" in Hubei and Wuhan?

(30) First proposed at the international level:

XZ-C proposes Dawning cancer prevention program A, B and D which is to carry out pollution prevention and pollution control, cancer prevention and anti-cancer.

As stated above, our research work is at the forefront of the world, and it is already a first-class discipline. Under the guidance of Xi Jinping's new era of socialism with Chinese characteristics, we should make great strides forward, new era, new journey, new weather, new actions, and brave the struggle of the new era.

In short, if the above items can be implemented and realized, they should be able to overcome cancer.

(1) The goal of conquering cancer:

It is to reduce the incidence of cancer, improve the cure rate of cancer, reduce the cancer mortality, significantly prolong the survival of patients and improve the quality of life.

(2) It is to achieve and to reach the followings:

1/3 can be prevented, 1/3 can be cured, and 1/3 can prolong life through treatment.

I hope some universities can create this first-class discipline which consider "overcoming cancer" as the research direction.

It is to suggest:

The scientific research in Huazhong University of Science and Technology, Wuhan University, Hubei University of Traditional Chinese Medicine and other alma mater [Note] should be pushed to the forefront of the world, and it is to build up the first batch of first-class disciplines which the direction of the research is to conquer cancer in China and the world. Guided by the socialist thought with Chinese characteristics in Xi Jinping's new era, it is to strive to take the road of innovation in China's distinctive anti-cancer metastasis, to adhere to the road of independent innovation with Chinese characteristics, to adhere to take the path of the combination of Chinese and Western medicine with the "Chinese-style anti-cancer" independent innovation. I hope that in Hubei and Wuhan, the first batch of first-class disciplines which the research direction is to overcome cancer research will be established in the whole country and in the world. It is to make new achievement to the conquer cancer, the contribution is in the modern age or in the present and it will benefit in the ages.

[Note]:

I was admitted to the Central South Tongji Medical College in 1951. The hospital was formed by the merger of Shanghai Tongji Medical College Qianhan and the National Wuhan University School of Medicine. After graduation, it was assigned to the surgical work of the Affiliated Hospital of Hubei College of Traditional Chinese Medicine. Therefore, they are my alma mater who studies, works, and grows.

Our cancer prevention and treatment research work has reached the forefront of the world

In the past 30 years, our scientific research achievements and scientific and technological innovation series, which have been focusing on conquering cancer research as the research direction and the following arguments are in this monograph, are first proposed internationally. All are original papers, international initiatives, and international leaders and have reached the forefront of the world.

Its main contents are as follows:

Professor Xu Ze (XZ-C) first proposed at the international level:

(1) First proposed internationally: **"Thymus atrophy, low immune function is one of the causes and pathogenesis of cancer"**

a. New findings on experimental research on the etiology and pathogenesis of cancer

b. This is the result of international leading intellectual property rights. After the investigation, this is the first time in the world.

c. See the monograph "New Concepts and New Methods for Cancer Treatment" P.13

(2) **For the first time in the world: "The theoretical basis and experimental basis of "Xu-Ze-C immune regulation and control treatment "protection of Thymus and increase of immune function"**

a. It was to propose the theoretical basis and experimental basis of cancer immune regulation therapy

b. Due to the new findings of the above experimental research, the treatment principle must be to prevent progressive atrophy of the thymus, promote thymic hyperplasia, protect bone marrow hematopoietic function, improve immune surveillance, and control immune escape of malignant cells.

c. See the monograph "New Concepts and New Methods of Cancer Treatment" P.17

(3) The first international initiative: "Cancer treatment should change the concept and establish a comprehensive treatment concept"

a. It was to propose a new concept of cancer treatment principles

b. The goal or target of cancer treatment must establish a comprehensive treatment concept for both tumor and host.

c. It should overcome the one-sided treatment concept of simply killing cancer cells

d. See the monograph "New Concepts and New Methods for Cancer Treatment" P.28

(4) The first international initiative: "A new model for the combination of multidisciplinary treatment of cancer"

a. It put forward : A new concept of multidisciplinary combination model for cancer treatment

b. The new model for multidisciplinary treatment is:

Long-term treatment mainly:

surgery + biological treatment + immunotherapy + Chinese medicine, Chinese and Western combined treatment

Short-course treatment is supplemented:

radiotherapy, chemotherapy, not long-range, not excessive

c. See the monograph "New Concepts and New Methods of Cancer Treatment" P33

Chapter 9

XZ-C proposes four major scientific contributions

In the past 30 years, I have obtained a series of research achievements and technological innovations in anti-cancer and anti-cancer metastasis research.

In the research work that has been carried out and the research work that is being carried out, it can be summarized as four major sciences dedicated to the people.

(1) It was first proposed internationally that

"To conquer cancer and launch the general attack ----to prevent cancer, to control cancer, and to treat cancer at the same attention"

—— It changed the hospital mode

  It changed treatment mode

  It proposed the general attack design, blueprint and implementation rules and plans

(2) It was first proposed internationally *"Building a Science City to Conquer Cancer"*

--- It established an overall framework for overcoming cancer

  This is the only way to overcome cancer

  It proposed the overall design, blueprint and implementing rules and plans of Science City.

(3) First it was proposed internationally

"Walked out of a new way of immune control and regulation with the combination of Chinese and Western medicine of cancer treatment"

The experimental research, Chinese medicine immunopharmacology and anti-cancer research with the combination of Chinese and Western medicine at the molecular level

a.   From the results of our laboratory experiments it was found:

After the host thymus is inoculated with cancer cells, it is acute progressive atrophy, cell proliferation is blocked, and the volume is significantly reduced.

b.   From the above experimental research findings, the inspiration is that :

Atrophy of the thymus and low immune function may be one of the causes and pathogenesis of the tumor. Therefore, tumor treatment must try to prevent thymus atrophy, promote thymocyte proliferation, and increase immunity.

c.   After 7 years of scientific research in the laboratory, it was to screen the natural drugs to form XZ-C1-10 immunomodulatory anti-cancer, anti-metastatic Chinese medicine. On the basis of the success of animal experiments, clinical verification work was carried out. After 20 years of clinical application of more than 12,000 oncology clinics, good results have been achieved.

d.   Walked out of the new path of combination of Chinese and western medicine with the traditional Chinese medicine immune regulation and control which regulates immune activity, prevents thymus atrophy, promotes thymic hyperplasia, protecst bone marrow hematopoietic function, improves immunity at the molecular level for conquering cancer.

e.   We have embarked on road of XZ-C immune regulation and control with the combination of western and Chinese medicine at the molecular level for conquering cancer------- the new path of "Chinese-style anti-cancer".

(4) "Research on Immunoregulation of Traditional Chinese Medicine - Experimental Research, Clinical Validation"

The Series products of XZ-C immunomodulation anticancer traditional Chinese medicine through the exclusive scientific research and development

a. Experimental research+clinical application+typical case list

b. XZ-C (XU ZE-China), an independently developed anti-cancer series of traditional Chinese medicine preparations, From experimental research to clinical verification, it has been applied to clinical practice on the basis of the success of animal experiments. After more than 12,000 clinical trials in more than 20 years, the curative effect is remarkable, and it is independent innovation and independent intellectual property rights.

c. XZ-C immunomodulatory Chinese medicine is screened out from more than 200 traditional Chinese herbal medicines in our country. 48 kinds of Chinese herbal medicines with good tumor inhibition rate were screened out by anti-tumor experiments in cancer-bearing mice. After forming the compound, then the anti-tumor experiment was performed again in the cancer-bearing mice, the compound inhibition rate is greater than the single-agent anti-tumor rate. Among them, XZ-C1 100% inhibits cancer cells, 100% does not kill normal cells, and has the function of strengthening the body and improving the immune function of the human body.

From our experiments on XZ-C pharmacodynamics studies it was proved:

It has a good tumor inhibition rate for Ehrlich ascites carcinoma, S180, H22 liver cancer.

Acute toxicity test in mice showed no obvious side effects. In the clinical oral administration for several years (2-6-8-10 years), no obvious side effects were observed.

In the middle and late stage cancer patients, most of them are weak and weak, tired and weak, and their appetite is weak. After taking XZ-C immunomodulation anti-cancer Chinese medicine for 4-8-12-16 weeks, it can significantly improve appetite, sleep, relieve pain, and gradually restore physical strength.

(5). The country is currently implementing the spirit of the party's "Nineteenth National Congress". It is to ensure that a well-off society is built nationwide in 2020, and rejuvenate Greater China, build an innovative country, and resolutely fight to win the three major battles, that is, pollution prevention, pollution control, smog control, to conquer cancer. This is a great pioneering work for the benefit of the country and the people. In this great situation, it is also to created good opportunities for the research work of preventing cancer, anti-cancer, and overcoming cancer. The purpose is to make people's health, to stay away from cancer, and to be a great pioneering work for future generations.

Doing a big thing, doing an unprecedented event, "to overcome cancer and launch the general attack of cancer," and "create a science city to overcome cancer" for the benefit of mankind.

How is it to implement this unprecedented event in human history?

1). Report to the government, request instructions

2). Report to the province and city, request instructions

3). Provide the suggestions to the Hubei Provincial Government and the Wuhan Municipal Government:

It is to prepare in Hubei and Wuhan:

"The first science city in the country to overcome cancer research base"

"The world's first science city to conquer cancer research base"

Site selection:

It is planning to be in the university town of Huangjiahu

Abbreviation:

"Huangjiahu Science City" Cancer Medical Research Center

It is to strive to build gradually in 5 years and to start in 2019 and completed in 2023 and it can serve cancer patients nationwide and globally.

Conquering cacer and launching the general attack of cancer is an unprecedented work of humanity. It must be created in person and must be practiced in person. This is a new cement road. Every step will leave an eternal scientific research footprint.

In the "19th National Congress of the Communist Party of China" and the work report of the current NPC government, it has been clearly stated that it is necessary to treat smog and conquer cancer as the two major scientific and technological issues of the country. To this end, our medical workers and science and technology workers must actively promote and implement them.

I am convinced that with the leadership, guidance, strong support and care of provincial and municipal leaders, under the efforts of my team, it will be completed as scheduled to benefit the majority of cancer patients.

Dr. Xu Ze, The chief designer of "Overcoming cancer and launching the general attack on cancer and building a cancer research base - Science City", the discipline, the head of the discipline to overcome cancer and to launch the general attack on cancer

Chapter 10

What research work have we carried out?

In order to conquer cancer, we have proposed the following series of research plans, overall design, planning, solutions, blueprints, master plan, the overall framework and implementation rules.

XZ-C proposes a scientific research plan to conquer cancer and launch the general attack of cancer

How to conquer cancer? I see:

Avoid empty talk, work hard, no matter how far the road to conquer cancer is, it should always start

(One)

- *It's time to "declare war on cancer" and the general attack should be launched.*

The goal of conquering cancer and launching the general attack on cancer is:

Reduce Incidence rate or morbidity, reduce mortality, improve cure rate, prolong survival, improve quality of life, and reduce complications.

- *Avoid empty talk, work hard, no matter how far the road of conquering cancer is, it should always start, the long march always has to go, and the journey of a thousand miles begins with a single step.*

- *What should it is to be done next?*

Now it is proposed to conquer cancer and to launch a general attack for cancer. It is to hope to get support from leaders at all levels. It is to be am fully aware that in order to achieve the purpose of cancer prevention, control, and treatment, it must be done by government leaders, government leaders, experts, scholars, mass participation, national mobilization, and participation of thousands of households.

- *Recognize that more than 90% of cancers are caused or closely related to environmental factors.*

Building a well-off society has great correlation with cancer prevention and cancer control. Therefore, it is proposed to overcome cancer and launch the general attack of cancer and adhere to the innovative road of cancer prevention and cancer control with Chinese characteristics.

- At present, China is implementing the spirit of the 19th National Congress of the Communist Party of China, building a well-off society in an all-round way, and ensuring the grand goal of building a well-off society nationwide by 2020. Our dreams are to conquer cancer and to build a well-off society. Everyone is healthy and away from cancer.

(Two)

- Why did I propose to launch a general attack? Why is it that there is no time to delay?

Please look at the current situation: (According to the 2012 China Cancer Registration Annual Report issued by the National Cancer Registry)

—— The current situation of cancer incidence is that the more patients are treated, the average number of new cancer patients in China is 8550, and 6 people per minute are recognized as cancer in the country.

—— The current status of cancer mortality is high, which has been the leading cause of death in urban and rural areas in China. On average, 7,500 people die of cancer every day.

—— The status quo of treatment, despite the application of traditional three major treatments for nearly a hundred years, thousands of cancer patients have been exposed to radiotherapy and chemotherapy, but what is the result? Cancer is still the leading cause of death so far.

—— The current situation of the hospital mode is to rectify or attention focused treatment with light prevent it, or only to treat cancer without prevention of cancer, the more the patient is treated, the more the patient shows up.

The status quo is:

The road that has passed in a century is to attention or to rectify the treatment with light prevention, or only to treat cancer without prevention.

<u>Cancer prevention and anti-cancer are human causes</u>, but we have only been researching cancer for many years, but we have done very little work on anti-cancer, and have done almost nothing.

- Therefore, the XZ-C proposes **a general attack plan and a general attack design** that should be used to overcome cancer, as well **as plans, routes, and blueprints** for the total attack.

To carry out an overall strategic reform of the treatment of cancer, and to reform and rectify focused treatment or heavy treatment with light prevention into both prevention and treatment at the same time and at the same level and at the same attention.

We should update our thinking, update our understanding, move forward or advance in reform, innovate in reform, and develop in reform.

It shifts from only treatment without prevention into preventing and controlling and treating at the same time and at the same level and prevention is the most important thing.

(Three)

- Cancer is the enemy of all mankind and it should evoke the common struggle of humanity around the world. The complexity of cancer is beyond human imagination. This is the hottest position in the biomedical field, bringing together the world's largest and elite research team and research elite.

- In the main direction of research on conquering cancer, conducting experimental and clinical anti-cancer research should be a key area of scientific research, and should achieve original breakthroughs.

- There are 2.7 million cancer deaths per year in the country, and an average of 7,500 people die every year from cancer. Such amazing data should be listed as a scientific research in key areas of technologically innovative countries.

- Humans should not sit still, and physicians should not do nothing. I think we should propose a general attack plan and basic design to overcome cancer, and launch a general attack on "declaring war on cancer". Avoid empty talk, work hard, build good laboratories, strengthen experimental research, basic research and clinical research.

- There are two tasks on the shoulders of our doctors. One is to treat patients and the other is to develop medicine. We should achieve leapfrog development in the strategic high-tech field of cancer, and take the innovation road of anti-cancer and anti-transfer technology innovations with our country characters and strive to enter the forefront of the world.

- Due to the increasing number of cancer patients, the incidence rate is rising and the mortality rate is high. It is recognized that cancer should not only pay attention to treatment, but also pay attention to prevention, so as to block the source, and focus on the occurrence of cancer, and develop the research on prevention and treatment during the whole process.

Xu Ze put forward the "strategic ideas and suggestions for conquering cancer" in Chapter 38 of the "New Concepts and Methods of Cancer Therapy" published by Beijing in October 2011. The book was later translated into English by Dr. Bin Wu, an American medical professional, and published in Washington, DC on March 26, 2013, and published internationally.

In June 2013, Xu Ze also proposed to "the basic idea and design of conquering cancer and launching the general attack on cancer" in an attempt to reduce the incidence of cancer, reduce mortality, improve cure rate and prolong survival.

I. "XZ-C proposes a scientific research plan to conquer cancer and launch the general attack of cancer"

The overall strategic reform and development of cancer treatment

Professor Xu Ze (XU ZE), Honorary President of Wuhan Anti-Cancer Research Association, proposed the following four feasibility reports and general design research plans for the general attack on cancer in July 2015.

(1) It is first proposed at the international level:

"Necessity and Feasibility Report on Overcoming cancer and launching the General Attack of Cancer" —— The overall strategic reform of cancer treatment shifts the focus of treatment into prevention and treatment at the same time and at the same level.

(2) It is first proposed at the international level:

"Preparing to build hospital with prevention and treatment of cancer during the whole process of cancer development and occurrence" (Global Demonstration for Cancer Prevention and Treatment Hospital)

"Implementation of the plan or preparation and feasibility report for the hospital with prevention and treatment of cancer in the whole process of anti-cance" —— Explain the necessity and feasibility of establishing a full-scale prevention and treatment hospital

(3) It is first proposed at the international level:

"The basic design and feasibility report of preparation of the general attack plan and building the Science City for conquer cancer" --- Equivalent to designing an overall framework of the design for conquering cancer with Chinese characteristics

(4) It is first proposed at the international level:

"At the same time as building a well-off society, it is recommended to the "catch or ride scientific research" - the necessity and feasibility report of carrying out the medical science research of cancer control and prevention cancer and cancer prevention and treatment work" ———— **_Adhere to the road of cancer prevention and cancer control with Chinese characteristics_**

The above four scientific research projects are all original innovations, which are all proposed for the first time in the world. They are the first in the world and the international leader, opening up a new field of anti-cancer research.

From attention of treatment with light prevention to prevention and treatment at the same time and the same level and the same attention, it is attempted to reduce the incidence of cancer and improve the cure rate of cancer.

It is possible to conquer cancer and even conquer cancer completely by opening up this new areas of research.

II. "Create the scientific research base science city that overcomes cancer multidisciplinary and cancer-related research" -- Promoting new advances in 21st century oncology medicine

XZ-C proposes:

How to overcome cancer? How can I prevent cancer?

How can I cure or treat cancer?

(1) Overview of the scientific research plans to overcome cancer and launch the general attack on cancer proposed by XZ-C.

(2) How to overcome cancer and to launch the general attack of cancer?

It must create the Innovative Molecular Oncology School and Graduate School

(3) How to overcome cancer and to launch the general attack of cancer?

The Innovative Molecular Oncology Institute and the Multidisciplinary Research Group must be created.

(4) How to overcome cancer and to launch the general attack of cancer?

It must **create "the hospital of cancer prevention and treatment with the innovative molecular tumor occurrence and development whole process"** ----- cancer prevention and control and treatment at the same time and the same attention and at the same level

(5) How to overcome cancer and to launch the general attack of cancer?

The Experimental Medicine Cancer Animal Experimental Center must be created.

(6) How to overcome cancer and to launch the general attack of cancer?

It is necessary to create **"Innovative Molecular Tumor Pharmaceuticals"** and **"To prepare the research groups and laboratories for anti-cancer, anti-cancer metastatic traditional Chinese medicine active ingredients, immunopharmacology, molecular level analysis"**

(7) How to overcome cancer and to launch the general attack of cancer?

It must create **the "Innovative Environmental Protection and Cancer Research Institute" and carry out cancer prevention system engineering**

(8) How to overcome cancer and to launch the general attack of cancer?

It **is necessary to create an innovative scientific research base for cancer multidisciplinary and cancer-related research.**

We are striving for the "Scientific City for Scientific Research Bases to Prepare Wuhan to Attack Cancer Attacks"

XZ-C's basic planning and design of launching the general attack

Professor Xu Ze (XU ZE) proposed the overall design of the Science City to overcome cancer and to launch the general attack of cancer

Dawning or Shuguang scientific research spirit

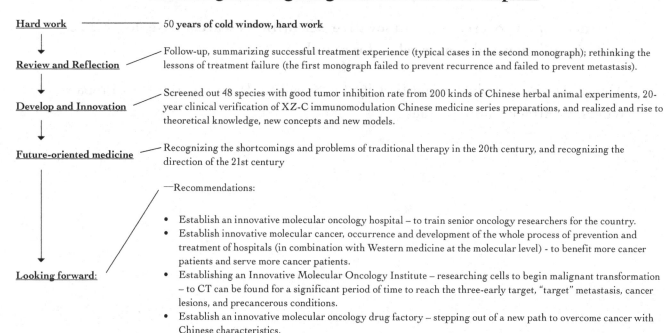

Hard work —————— 50 **years of cold window, hard work**

Review and Reflection — Follow-up, summarizing successful treatment experience (typical cases in the second monograph); rethinking the lessons of treatment failure (the first monograph failed to prevent recurrence and failed to prevent metastasis).

Develop and Innovation — Screened out 48 species with good tumor inhibition rate from 200 kinds of Chinese herbal animal experiments, 20-year clinical verification of XZ-C immunomodulation Chinese medicine series preparations, and realized and rise to theoretical knowledge, new concepts and new models.

Future-oriented medicine — Recognizing the shortcomings and problems of traditional therapy in the 20th century, and recognizing the direction of the 21st century

—Recommendations:

Looking forward:

- Establish an innovative molecular oncology hospital – to train senior oncology researchers for the country.
- Establish innovative molecular cancer, occurrence and development of the whole process of prevention and treatment of hospitals (in combination with Western medicine at the molecular level) - to benefit more cancer patients and serve more cancer patients.
- Establishing an Innovative Molecular Oncology Institute – researching cells to begin malignant transformation – to CT can be found for a significant period of time to reach the three-early target, "target" metastasis, cancer lesions, and precancerous conditions.
- Establish an innovative molecular oncology drug factory – stepping out of a new path to overcome cancer with Chinese characteristics.
- Establish an environmental protection and cancer prevention research institute and carry out anti-cancer system engineering

The theoretical system of XZ-C immunomodulation and cancer treatment has been formed.

In the book "New Concepts and New Methods of Cancer Treatment", Professor Xu Ze published a series of nearly 100 research papers summarizing the basic and clinical research results from 50 years of self-reliance and hard work which was published in the form of a new book from.

This book has formed the theoretical system of XZ-C immune regulation and control of treatment of cancer, which are the clinical basis and experimental basis for cancer treatment and are undergoing clinical application observation and verification.

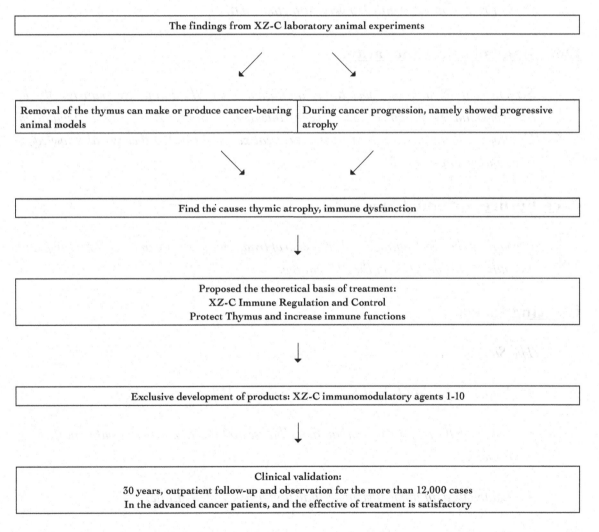

The findings from XZ-C laboratory animal experiments

Removal of the thymus can make or produce cancer-bearing animal models	During cancer progression, namely showed progressive atrophy

Find the cause: thymic atrophy, immune dysfunction

Proposed the theoretical basis of treatment:
XZ-C Immune Regulation and Control
Protect Thymus and increase immune functions

Exclusive development of products: XZ-C immunomodulatory agents 1-10

Clinical validation:
30 years, outpatient follow-up and observation for the more than 12,000 cases
In the advanced cancer patients, and the effective of treatment is satisfactory

Theoretical System of XZ-C immune regulate and control of cancer therapy

(XZ-C)(XU ZE-China)(China-Xu Ze)

III. XZ-C (XU ZE-China, Xu Ze - China) Basic idea and design for launching the general attack of cancer

Dawning or Shuguang Scientific Research Spirit

Arduous striving —— *50 years of cold window, hard work*

Look back and Reflection

↓ *Follow-up, summarizing successful experience in treatment (typical cases in the second monograph); rethinking the lessons of treatment failure (the first monograph failed to prevent recurrence and failed to prevent metastasis).*

Development and Innovation

↓ *Screened out 48 cases with good tumor inhibition rate in the animal experiments of 200 kinds of Chinese herbal medicine, 11-year clinical verification of Z-C immunomodulation Chinese medicine series preparations, and realized and rised to theoretical knowledge, new concepts, new models*

Face Future -oriented medicine

↓ *Recognized the shortcomings and problems of traditional therapy in the 20ᵗʰ century, and recognizing the direction of the 21ˢᵗ century.*

Looking forward

The Suggestions:

- *Establishing the Medical School of Innovative Molecular Oncology*

- *Establish the hospital of combination Chinese and Western with innovative molecular tumors.*

- *Established an innovative molecular tumor research institute.*

- *Establish an innovative molecular oncology drug factory.*

- *Establish an innovative environmental protection and cancer prevention research institute.*

The hospital of innovation molecular tumors and modern high tech and science talents	The hospital of creative and innovation molecular tumors with combination of chinese and western
1.The institution of Innovation molecular tumors research 2. The institution of innovation environment protection and cancer prevention	The drug factories or preparation pharmaceutics of innovation molecular tumors

Cancer animal experimental center

The science city of medical education and science research and development

The scientific base of conquering cancer and launching the general attack of cancer (Science City)

At the age of 85, the author published the medical monograph "Condense Wisdom, Conquer Cancer - Benefiting Mankind", XZ-C: How to overcome cancer? How can I prevent cancer? I see how to treat cancer.

<u>Professor Xu Ze proposed the engineering planning diagram of how to overcome of cancer</u>

<u>This medical monograph is practical, applied, and research-oriented and an outline of implementing how to overcome cancer.</u> This set of scientific research programs, scientific research design, scientific research planning, and blueprints can be used by countries, provinces, and states to implement the vision of cancer and benefit humanity.

The main project of this implementation outline is:

Conquer cancer and launch the general attack of cancer, prevention and control and treatment of cancer at the same time and at the same level and at the same attention

Create a scientific research base for multidisciplinary and cancer-related science research - Science City

The two-wing project is:

A wing - how to prevent cancer? To reduce the incidence of cancer

B wing - how to treat cancer? To improve cancer cure rate

aims:

A: Reduce the incidence of cancer

B: Improve cancer cure rate, prolong patient survival and improve quality of life

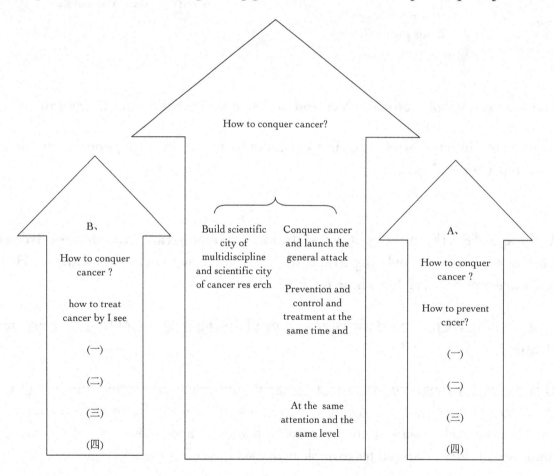

Fig. 1. Schematic diagram of XZ-C Proposed

Chapter 11

How to overcome cancer? How to treat cancer?

XZ-C proposed:

Dawning or Shuguang C-type plan No.1-6

By July 2015, we have formulated the "Dawning C-type plan", that is, Dawning is Chenguang, Chaoyang, C-type = China, that is, "Chinese-style model", a plan to overcome cancer.

How to overcome cancer? How to treat cancer?

Under the guidance of Xi Jinping's new era of socialism with Chinese characteristics, we should strive to open up a new phase of scientific research in the new era, and the scientific research work to overcome cancer should be advanced. We will strive to follow the path of independent innovation with Chinese characteristics and adhere to the road of independent innovation of Chinese and Western medicine combined with "Chinese-style anti-cancer". China will contribute more to the world's wisdom, China's programs, and China's forces to overcome cancer research, so that the sun of humanity's destiny will shine in the world.

How to overcome cancer? How to treat cancer?

XZ-C proposes Dawning C-type plan No.1-6

How to overcome cancer? How to treat cancer?

XZ-C proposed:

Dawning or Shuguang C-type plan No.1-6

Dawning C-type plan No. 1:

"Overcoming cancer and launching the general attack of cancer"

Dawning C-type plan No. 2:

"Creating a full-scale prevention and treatment hospital"

Dawning C-type plan No. 3:

"Building a science city to overcome cancer"

Dawning C-type Plan No. 4:

"Building a Multidisciplinary Research Group"

Dawning C-type plan No. 5:

"The vaccine is human hope, immunological prevention"

Dawning C-type plan No. 6:

"The prospect of immunomodulatory drugs is gratifying"

Dawning C plan

It was formulated in July 2015

(1) Dawning C-type plan No. 1:

"Conquering cancer, launching the general attack"

a. The overall strategic reform and development of cancer treatment in China

b. It was to propose a general plan, project, design, blueprint and detail rules for conquering cancer

c. Avoid empty talk, work hard, start walking

d. No matter how far the road to cancer is, you should always start.

(see separate article)

(2) Shuguang C-type plan No. 2:

"Preparing for the hospitals with prevention and treatment during the whole process"

(Global Demonstration Prevention and Treatment Hospital)

—— Strategic reform, changing the mode of running a hospital and reforming treatment mode

(3) Shuguang C-type plan No. 3:

"Building a science city to overcome cancer"

a. XZ-C proposes the overall design, planning and blueprint of Science City to overcome cancer and to launch the general attack of cancer

b. This is the only way to overcome cancer

c. This is the "high-speed rail" that conquers cancer, "high-speed" channel)

(see separate article)

(4) Shuguang C-type plan No. 4:

"Building a multidisciplinary research group and laboratory"

a. Its aim is for the cause, pathogenesis, pathophysiology, metastasis, recurrence mechanism of cancer...

To study anti-cancer, anti-recurrence, anti-metastatic measures to benefit patients by improving the overall level of medical care

b. The criteria for efficacy evaluation are:

long survival time, good quality of life, and complications no or less, each school group is a provincial key laboratory.

(see separate article)

(5) Dawning C-type plan No. 5:

"Vaccine is the hope of human beings, immunological prevention"

a. Today's immunology prevention and treatment has become an extremely important in clinical medicine and preventive medicine

Required field

b. △△学组+△△学组+△△学组→Scientific Alliance, Joint Group

(see separate article)

(6) Shuguang C-type plan No. 6: A

"The prospect of immunomodulatory drugs is gratifying"

a. Regardless of the complexity of the mechanisms behind cancer, immune suppression is the key to cancer progression

b. From the analysis of experimental results, to obtain new discoveries, new inspirations:

Thymus atrophy, immune dysfunction, decreased immune surveillance and immune escape are one of the causes and pathogenesis of cancer. Therefore, the principle of treatment should be to prevent thymus atrophy, promote thymic hyperplasia, and improve immune surveillance.

c. XZ-C immunomodulatory Chinese medicine is that 48 kinds of Chinese herbal medicines with good cancer suppression rate were screened out by in vivo anti-tumor experiments in the animal model of cancer mice, and 26 of them had better immune regulation from more than 200 kinds of traditional Chinese herbal medicines in China

(see separate article)

(6)Shuguang C-type plan No. 6: B

"The research group and laboratory of XZ-C immunomodulation anti-cancer Chinese medicine active ingredient, molecular level analysis"

a. Further research and development of Z-C immunomodulatory anti-cancer Chinese medicine active ingredients, molecular weight, structural formula, molecular level analysis

b. Method and steps:

Animal experiments; molecular level experiments; gene level experiments, first separate the active ingredients, so that the precious heritage of traditional Chinese medicine is modernized and scientific.

(see separate article)

Dawning C-type plan (China)

Hope:

Apply to incorporate the "Dawning C-type plan" into the National Cancer Program

To report the Party Central Committee and the State Council

To Hubei Provincial Party Committee and Provincial Government Report

To report Wuhan Municipal Party Committee and Municipal Government

Goal:

Conquer cancer

Mission:

Prepare a science city to overcome conquer and launch the general attack on cancer

President of Science City, General Director, President of the General Academic Committee: **Professor Xu Ze**

(Former Director of Institute of Experimental Surgery, Hubei College of Traditional Chinese Medicine)

Science City Innovative Oncology Medical   College Chief Dean
Innovative Oncology Research Institute   Leadership Team
Innovative Tumor Hospital Integrated Traditional Chinese and Western Medicine Hospital:
Innovative Cancer Prevention Research Institute

General Secretary of Science City:
Dean of the Graduate School of Science City:
The chief scientist team of Wuhan Anticancer Research Association:

Professor D. XU ZE

The chief designer of "Conquering cancer and launching the General Attack on Cancer and Creating a Science City to Fight Cancer"
Project Leader of "Overcoming the General Attack of Cancer"

In "the Science City of Conquering Cancer" it will established the following genetic testing research groups:

(1) Establish <u>genetic testing and cancer research</u> groups and laboratories

(2) Establish <u>HPV anti-cancer research</u> group and laboratory

(3) Establish <u>genetic testing and immunology and cancer research</u> groups and laboratories

(4) Establish genetic testing <u>and endocrine hormone</u> and cancer research groups and laboratories

(5) <u>Establish genetic testing and pathological sections, and related studies on immunohistochemistry</u>

(6) Establish <u>correlation analysis and research on gene detection and tumor markers</u>

(7) Establish HPV treatment, exploration research groups and laboratories

Expected results:

Using modern science and technology and analytical testing methods, the research on traditional Chinese medicine, the material basis of the efficacy of traditional Chinese medicine in clinical practice is the chemical composition contained therein. To study the anticancer effect and mechanism of traditional Chinese medicine, it is necessary to conduct in-depth research and analysis. The active ingredients in it make the precious heritage of traditional Chinese medicine more modern and scientific.

After 28 years of experimental research, basic research and clinical verification, a series of "Protection of Thymus and Increase of Immune Function" immune regulation anti-cancer Chinese medicine XZ-C1-10 has been screened. After 20 years of clinical observation, more than 12,000 cases have been verified, and the outpatient medical records are kept, a list of disease analysis, can prolong life, improve symptoms, improve the quality of life, **how to know, evaluate can extend the survival period? Some surgical explorations can not be cut down (all pathological sections confirmed diagnosis), or have been widely transferred, it is estimated that only 3-6 months, or 6-12 months of cases, after the treatment with XZ-C**

immune regulation and control medications of anti-cancer anti-metastasis and recurrence, some patients can still survive for 4 years - 5 years - 8 years - 10 years - 15 years, all of which have original data and complete data as well as follow-up data.

After a rehabilitation teacher, after a heart attack, calm down, hid in a small building, self-reliance, hard work, adhere to the animal experimental basic research and outpatient clinical validation research for anti-cancer, anti-cancer metastasis, recurrence, from the year of the flower (60 years old)→To the age of the ancients (70s)→To the age of 耄耋(80s), still perseverance, persevere in scientific research to overcome cancer, because he has retired, it failed to apply for projects, programs, so there was no research funding, however it was to fight alone, to fight alone, to be self-reliant, to work hard, no one cared, no one knew, nowhere to report, no support, hard work for more than 20 years, it has achieved a series of scientific and technological innovations, scientific research results, due to retirement In the past 20 years, no one cares, no one supports, retired professors, I don't know where to manage, where to support, so where the scientific research results are reported, I have to make the "monograph" for the benefit of mankind, but those were published as a series of monographs, and then Report to the Provincial Department of Science and Technology and the Provincial Department of Education:

1). It hopes to open an international high-end academic forum;

2). It reports to the government to apply for cancer, launch a general attack;

3). It reports to the province and the government.

It Hopes:

To Apply to establish "the first science city in the country to overcome cancer and to launch the general attack of cancer" in Hubei and Wuhan, that is, "the world's first science city to overcome the general attack of cancer."

How to implement this unprecedented event in human history?

(1) Reporting to the government, requesting instructions

(2) To Report to the province and city and to request instructions

(3) It makes recommendations to build: "The first national cancer science city" and "The world's first Science City to overcome Cancer"

in the city, Wuhan

How to overcome cancer?

XZ-C proposes: Cancer is a disaster for all mankind, and it is necessary for the people of the world to work together.

"Cancer moon shot" (US) and "Dawning C-type plan" (China)

- ------ Moving forward together, heading for the science hall to overcome cancer

Why do you want to move forward together? What common are there ?

(1) Introduction to "Chan Moon Moon Shot"

On January 12, 2016, US President Barack Obama announced in his last State of the Union address during his term of office a national plan to overcome cancer, the "Cancer moon shot", which will be under the responsibility of Biden. .

Biden will visit the Abramson Cancer Center at the University of Pennsylvania School of Medicine next week to discuss the plan. He said that the "new moon landing plan" is a commitment to overcome cancer in the world and will inspire a new generation of scientists to explore the scientific world.

Obama did not mention the specific plan of the plan in his speech, but he mentioned that the expenditure and tax bill passed by Congress in December 2015 has raised the financial budget of the National Institutes of Health (NIH).

The United States has just recently established a national immunotherapy alliance consisting of pharmaceutical companies, biotechnology companies and academic medical organizations. The alliance is trying to develop a vaccine immunotherapy before 2020 to overcome cancer and complete cancer. Monthly plan."

The American Society of Clinical Oncology (ASCO) issued a statement on its website, welcoming Obama's "New Moon Plan" and supporting Biden's leadership, saying that the "New Moon Plan" will reduce the pain and reduce the risk of cancer for humans. Death caused by cancer. The statement mentioned that "all effective treatments should be transformed from the laboratory to the clinic"; the application of "big data" technology, such as ASCO's "CancerLinQ" rapid learning system, can accelerate the pace of cancer. Enable physicians to better develop individualized treatment options for each patient and understand which areas are urgently needed to invest more research (Liu Quan).

(January 21, 2016, China Medical Tribune)

(2) Introduction to the Dawning C plan

1. Before January 12, 2016, it was put forward the progress of the scientific research plan "to overcome cancer and to launch the general attack on cancer"

2. Before January 12, 2016, we have carried out scientific research and scientific innovation series with the research direction as conquering cancer.

3. Dawning C plan

For the first time in the world it proposed that how it is to overcome cancer? XZ-C proposed "Dawning C-type plan" No.1-6

Why was it to use "Dawn"?

The dawn is the morning light, it is the dawn, it is the morning sun.

Vigorous, vigorous, original innovation, independent innovation

C=China

Type C = Chinese mode

About 8550 people in China are diagnosed with cancer every day, and 6 people are diagnosed with cancer every minute. Therefore, the research work to overcome cancer and to launch the general attack of cancer can not walk slowly, should run forward, save the wounded.

Time is money, time is money = one inch of time, one inch of gold

Time is life, time is life

Time flies, time flies

Empty talk, wrong country, hard work

Avoid talk, work hard, start walking

No matter how far the road to cancer is, you should always start.

This research plan is the original innovation, it is time to declare war on cancer, and the general attack should be launched.

Our dreams, conquer cancer, build a well-off society, everyone is healthy, stay away from cancer.

Chapter 12

How to overcome cancer? How to prevent cancer?

XZ-C proposes:

To create "Innovative Environmental Protection and Cancer Research Institute" and carry out cancer prevention system engineering

XZ-C proposes:

Dawning Cancer Prevention Program A, B, D

First

Internationally it first proposed:

XZ-C proposed Dawning cancer prevention program A, B, D for pollution prevention and pollution control and cancer prevention and anti-cancer

Dawning Type A Plan:

Goal: Prevent *Air P*ollution

Dawning B-type plan:

goal: prevention *of water* pollution

Dawning D-type plan:

goal: prevention and *control of soil* pollution

How to overcome cancer? How to prevent cancer? I see:

Professor Xu Ze proposed that the "Innovative Environmental Protection and Cancer Research Institute" should be established and cancer prevention system project should be carried out.

Where is the goal or "target" of cancer prevention? How to prevent?

The more cancer patients are treated and the more and more the patients at present, the incidence is rising, and 90% of them are related or closely related to environmental carcinogenic factors. Therefore, the goal or "target" of cancer prevention should aim to study, explore and take scientific prevention and treatment measures against the carcinogenic factors (external environment, internal environment) of the environment.

XZ-C proposes cancer prevention general design and cancer prevention system engineering:

Since the disaster of cancer covers the whole world, industrial and agricultural waste gas, waste water and waste residue also cover all over the world.

Therefore, it is necessary to establish "Innovative Environmental Protection and Cancer Research Institute" and carry out cancer prevention system engineering.

It is necessary to prevent and control the three major pollutions, and it is advisable to study the relationship between the environment and cancer.

How is it to prove the relationship between environmental pollution and cancer? There are many examples in history. In particular, environmental pollution such as air pollution, water pollution, and soil pollution has a serious impact on human carcinogenesis.

(1) Air pollution and cancer in environmental pollution:

Every minute of human life is inseparable from the air. Air pollution can cause many respiratory diseases, the most serious of which is lung cancer.

(2) Water pollution and cancer in environmental pollution:

Human beings can't live without water every time they are in production activities and life. Water pollution is mainly caused by industrial and agricultural production and urban sewage. In China, industrial pollution has intensified due to the rapid development of township and village enterprises. Water pollution is related to the high incidence of lung cancer. It is related to the occurrence of gastric cancer, intestinal cancer and esophageal cancer. Drinking unqualified water that does not meet the standard can induce or promote cancer.

(3) Soil pollution in environmental pollution and cancer:

Fertilizers, pesticides and pesticides in agricultural production can lead to soil water quality, serious soil pollution, agricultural workers exposure to a variety of pesticides, herbicides and fertilizers, some of which are known as human carcinogens.

Prevention pollution and pollution control are cancer prevention and cancer control. It can receive the effect of first-class cancer prevention. It is necessary to prevent and control the three major pollutions, to prevent pollution, to control pollution, and to overcome difficulties. It is sure to achieve the benefits of cancer prevention and cancer control and reduce the incidence of cancer.

Second

XZ-C proposed and formulated four Dawning Cancer Prevention Programs, which was first proposed internationally.

The Cancer Research Institute will carry out cancer prevention system engineering, conduct micro, ultra-micro, high-tech research, monitor and analyze carcinogenic factors, and try to eliminate it. We have developed four Dawning Cancer Prevention Programs:

1.   Dawn or Shuguang A-type plan:

Objective or aims:

To try to research the microscopic studies of carcinogenic factors of air pollution on the environment, and try to remove it to prevent air pollution leading to lung cancer.

Why is the cancer prevention system project the first to solve air pollution?

It is because the current global respiratory cancer has been the highest incidence rate, 1.295 million / 8.18 million people, both men and women are in the first place. Therefore, how to solve the problem of preventing lung cancer is a top priority.

Ways and methods:

Through monitoring and analysis for Carcinogenic factors by micro, ultra-micro, high-tech, try to detect, monitor, and try to clear it or to remove it.

2.   Dawn B-type plan

Objective or aims:

Try to study the microscopic study of the carcinogenic factors of water pollution on the environment, and try to clear or to remove or to eliminate cancers such as liver cancer, stomach cancer, and intestinal cancer caused by waterproof pollution.

Why must it pay attention to water pollution to cause cancer at present? It is because the mother rivers of the whole country and the whole world are polluted by industrial and agricultural sewage, urban sewage is discharged, river water pollution, and carcinogens increase significantly.

Professor Xu Ze (XZ-C) suggested that efforts should be made to save the nation's and global mother rivers from being seriously polluted.

Ways and methods:

"target"

To solve the pollution of industrial and agricultural sewage, the first should try to reduce fertilizer

To solve urban and rural drinking water, it must be purified

To solve drinking qualified water and drinking standard water

3.   Dawn or Shuguang C-type plan

Already mentioned above

4.   Dawn or Shuguang D type plan

Aims:

Try to study the microscopic study of the carcinogenic factors of soil pollution on the environment

Try to solve the problem of chemical fertilizers, pesticides, genetic modification and cancer ocurrence

Try to detect the presence or absence of carcinogenic factors from clothing, food, housing, and samples, and take samples of carcinogens from microscopic monitoring.

Ways and methods:

To carry or get on the microscopic detection and monitoring for prevention cancer, and put forward to prevention cancer ethical standards for cancer prevention.

Through the above-mentioned Dawning A, B, and D plans, the prevention cancer and pollution control of the atmosphere, water, and soil is a first-class prevention cancer, which can reduce the incidence of cancer, and can reach the ecological environment and the human living environment with the green hills, green water, beautiful mountains and clear waters, and bird words and fragrant flowers.

Because cancer patients cover the whole world, the pollution of industrial and agricultural wastewater, waste residue and waste gas also covers the whole world. Therefore, it is necessary to globally act together to launch the general attack and to conquer cancer.

Professor Xu Ze suggested:

1. All countries, provinces and states should establish cancer prevention research institutes (or institutions), carry out cancer prevention system projects, and carry out cancer prevention work for their own country, province and city.

2. Countries establish cancer prevention regulations and carry out comprehensively (some should be legislated)

3. I will use this project to recommend the World Health Organization to hold cancer preventioncampaign, with the goal of reducing the incidence of cancer. Conquering cancer is a frontier of science and a worldwide problem. Cancer is a human disaster, covering the whole world. People all over the world are eager to hope that one day they can overcome cancer and benefit mankind.

Third

XZ-C proposed how to overcome cancer by I see :

How to overcome cancer? In order to overcome cancer, it must create the "Innovative Environmental Cancer Research Institute"

one of the science cities to overcome cancer

(1) Why should it be to create an innovative environmental protection and cancer prevention research institute?

It is because the current cancer incidence is on the rise, 90% of which is related to the environment.

The occurrence of cancer is closely related to people's clothing, food, housing, travel and living habits.

The current environmental pollution is serious and the ecosystem is degraded, which may be related to the cancer incidence rate.

After 28 years of retrospective and reflection on the experimental research and clinical work of cancer research work, we deeply understand that cancer should not only pay attention to treatment, but also pay attention to prevention, in order to stop it at the source, and it must prevent and treat at the same attention, and the way out of anti-cancer lies on prevention cancer and prevention is the main or important thing and it is mainly for prevention.

So how is it to prevent it? What should it be to prevent? It is necessary to measure, characterize, locate, and quantify various environmental carcinogens and try to remove them.

Therefore, it is necessary to establish the cancer prevention research institute, which should conduct cancer prevention research from clothing, food, housing, and transportation, and carry out microscopic and ultra-microscopic anti-cancer research from the big environment and small environment.

How is it to conduct cancer prevention research from clothing, food, housing and transportation?

First of all, it should master the situation of clothing, food, shelter, and other carcinogens, whether it contains carcinogens, qualitative and quantitative monitoring, and then set standards and set the bottom line, in order to discuss and propose prevention and control measures.

(2) How is it to create the "Innovative Environmental Protection and Cancer Research Institute"?

Prevention cancer research is a major event. At present, there is no prevention cancer research institute in the world. It will be to apply to create the world's first environmental protection and cancer prevention research institute in the Science City of conquering cancer to monitor and to analyze macroscopic, microscopic and ultra-micro environmental carcinogens and to implement cancer prevention system engineering.

Profession Dr. XU ZE

Cadre of Innovative Molecular Level Environmental Protection Cancer Research Institute and Cancer Prevention System Engineering Leader (Secretary) Provincial Environmental Protection Department
Chief of the Institute of Innovative Cancer Research
Chairman of the Academic Committee, chief designer of the anti-cancer system engineering

Dean of the Environmental Protection and Cancer Research Institute:
Secretary General:

Forth

How to overcome cancer? In order to overcome cancer, it is necessary to launch a general attack. The general attack is to carry out the three-stage work of prevention cancer, cancer control and cancer treatment in the whole process of cancer occurrence and development, and carry out prevention and control and treatment simultaneously. It must pay attention to cancer prevention. Prevention is the top priority. How is it to prevent? What is it to prevent? What and how should it to do for prevention? This will be discussed in detail below. How to overcome cancer? In order to overcome cancer, it is necessary to create the "Innovative Cancer Prevention Research Institute" and carry out the prevention cancer research system project.

With the improvement of people's living standards, various high-tech products bring us a better life, but also bring many negative effects. Various chemical, physical, and biological environmental carcinogens appear in large numbers. Various carcinogens enter our human body or various carcinogenic factors affect our human body, leading to an increasing incidence of cancer.

Please look at the current situation:

The current situation of cancer incidence is that the more the patients are treated and the more patients, the current incidence of cancer in China is 3.12 million new cases of cancer every year, an average of 8550 new cancer patients per day, 6 people per minute nationwide was diagnosed with cancer.

Now XZ-C proposes to the scientific research plan of conquering cancer and launching the general attack of cancer, and to prevent, control and treat at the same attention and which are equally important, and the three carriages go hand in hand.

So how to prevent it? How to control? What to prevent? What to control? How much is it prevented? How much is it controlled?

The goal or "target" of the prevention or control must be clear, and the qualitative, quantitative, and localization of various environmental carcinogens must be measured.

Since cancer is thought to be caused mainly by factors such as the environment, diet, and hobbies, therefore, people will attach great importance to carcinogenic factors in the environment and strive to remove them.

In order to prevent cancer and control cancer, Professor Xu Ze proposed:

(1) Prevention cancer should be carried out from clothing, food, shelter, and transportation, and cancer prevention should be carried out from a large environment or/and a small environment.

(2) The following prevention cancer research groups should be formed, and the graduate students of each school should be invited to complete and complete this scientific research work.

Professor Xu Ze, as the chief designer, proposes the following research projects and topics. To overcome cancer, the following research work must be carried out:

(3) Understand what needs to be prevented? What needs to be controlled? How to prevent? How to control?

It must be qualitative, quantitative, and localized monitoring. There must be clear and specific data. First-hand information must be mastered in order to carry out scientific and accurate prevention cancer work. It is necessary to pay attention to the accumulation of original data so that it becomes as a scientific data and experimental basis for accurate prevention cancer.

(2) How is it to achieve this plan? How is it to carry out this scientific research work?

It can be included in the training of graduate students, and it is to be selected the research topic by Doctoral student, master student. It can not only cultivate graduate to conduct the field research, but it can also receive monitoring and analysis of prevention cancer, carcinogenic qualitative and quantitative components, further propose prevention and control measures and methods.

Method

To set the subject and to be carried out by graduate students from various schools with purposeful and task arrangement. (My graduate student is like this. The general subject of the tutor is like a table banquet. Each graduate student is a small topic, like a dish of dish, a doctoral student is a big dish, and a master student is a small dish.) It can also cultivate graduate students' scientific thinking, scientific practice ability, produce papers, produce talents, and produce results.

It must or/and is necessary to emphasize that graduate research papers are not written with pen, but also work out by scientific research work. They must pay attention to original materials, attach importance to scientific and technological innovation, and attach importance to advanced, innovative and practical. We must pay attention to scientific research and seek truth from facts.

We must pay attention to the original materials, attach importance to scientific and technological innovation, and attach importance to the advanced, innovative and practical. We must pay attention to scientific research and seek truth from facts.

How to prevent cancer from clothing, food, shelter, and transportation?

First of all, you should master and understand the situation of carcinogens such as clothing, food, housing, and transportation, whether it contains carcinogens or not? It is to do qualitative and quantitative monitoring, then set standards and set the bottom line, in order to discuss and propose prevention and control measures.

It is planned to establish the following research groups:

(1) [clothing] clothing, cosmetics and other carcinogen monitoring, prevention and control research group

purpose:

method:

technology:

Equipment conditions:

personnel:

Expected results, results:

Whether there are carcinogenic substances, qualitative, quantitative, red bottom line, microscopic, ultra-microscopic monitoring

Analysis and conclusion:

It is to propose for prevention and control measures, or further experiments, animal models

Graduate student (shuo, Bo)

tutor:

(2) [Food] Food Carcinogen Monitoring, Prevention and Control Research Group → Institute

Pickled products:

kimchi, pickles, dried salted fish, sausage, mustard, bacon, fermented bean curd, pickles, canned fish, etc., carcinogen content monitoring, qualitative and quantitative microscopic research

Frying method:

... and other carcinogen content monitoring, qualitative and quantitative microscopic research

Fry method or Fried method:

... and other carcinogen content monitoring, qualitative and quantitative microscopic research

Smoke method:

... and other carcinogen content monitoring, qualitative and quantitative microscopic research

Cooking method:

... and other carcinogen content monitoring, qualitative and quantitative microscopic research

Steaming method:

... and other carcinogen content monitoring, qualitative and quantitative microscopic research

Fume stove:

... and other carcinogen content monitoring, qualitative and quantitative microscopic research

Leftovers:

... and other carcinogen content monitoring, qualitative and quantitative microscopic research

Leftovers overnight:

... and other carcinogen content monitoring, qualitative and quantitative microscopic research

Grain:

... and other carcinogen content monitoring, qualitative and quantitative microscopic research

Oil:

... and other carcinogen content monitoring, qualitative and quantitative microscopic research

Vegetables:

... and other carcinogen content monitoring, qualitative and quantitative microscopic research

Meat:

... and other carcinogen content monitoring, qualitative and quantitative microscopic research

Fish:

... and other carcinogen content monitoring, qualitative and quantitative microscopic research

Various foods (packaged) sold by supermarkets

(3) [Living]:

Housing, decoration (painting, painting...) materials, furniture... Carcinogen monitoring, prevention, control research group

Determination of materials, air, micro, ultra-microscopic carcinogens

Whether it exceeds the standard (for several large advertising companies...)

Trace element determination and monitoring

(4) [Travel or transportation or walking]:

Vehicle Exhaust, Automotive Equipment Carcinogen Monitoring, Prevention, Control Research Group

Cars, trains, etc., equipment, air

train:

aircraft:

Battery car

(5) Water, pollution (waste water, air in each factory) carcinogen monitoring, prevention, control, research group

(6) Fertilizer, pesticide, soil, genetically modified food:

The monitoring and prevention and control research group for whether there is carcinogen or not.

(7) Monitoring, prevention, control, and research groups on whether computers or mobile phones have carcinogenic or damaging effects

(8) The monitoring, prevention, control, research group of air, air conditioning, range hood, rays, radiation, nuclear radiation to measure whether there is any carcinogen

(9) Chinese food and western food are all to be done microscopic qualitative and quantitative monitoring whether it contains carcinogenic, qualitative, quantitative, and standard

- **The goal of the study:**

to detect whether there are carcinogens and their content, qualitative, quantitative, standard

- **Method:**

arranging doctoral and master's programs, projects

Initial screening, preliminary research, to find problems → ask questions → study problems → solve problems

- **Participants:**

chefs, dieticians, mentors, postgraduate colleges, canteens, hotels, restaurants, snacks, hot dry noodles, powder

Graduate students go to the site to conduct research, experiment, practice and carry out scientific research work.

Tutor - Graduate - Nutritional Expert Trinity Monitoring, Research, Analysis

- **The overall layout** of the project, the purpose, the requirements

Can be a college, responsible for one problem

- **Arrange 100 graduate** students, ie 100 papers, preliminary on carcinogen composition, quantitative, qualitative monitoring, analysis

Funding subsidies:

- **Seek support and guidance** from the Education Department, the Science and Technology Department, the Eco-Environment Department, and the Health and Health Commission.

- **Strive for support,** guidance, and leadership from various colleges, and you will likely acquire a large number of original scientific research results in epidemiology, nutrition, preventive medicine, public health, and environmental science, and master first-hand information for cancer prevention and cancer control.

The steps, plans, programs, and general design of how to achieve the general attack on cancer have been completed, and have been published and distributed globally.

Why were there books published in English books worldwide?

It is because cancer patients cover the whole world, the pollution of industrial and agricultural wastewater, waste residue and waste gas also covers the whole world. Therefore, it is necessary to globally attack the cancer attack.

(3) The above-mentioned plan, planning, general design, and blueprint for conquering the general attack of cancer can be applied to a country, a province, a state, and a market reference application to conquer cancer and even conquer cancer.

Fifth

How to implement the creation of this prevention cancer research, XZ-C proposed the prevention cancer general design and prevention cancer system engineering

Professor Xu Ze suggested:

(1) All countries, provinces and states should establish preventioncancer research institutes (or institutions) to carry out prevention cancer system projects and carry out preventioncancer work for their own country, province, state and city. (Because there are a large number of cancer patients in various countries, provinces and cities)

(2) Countries should establish prevention cancer regulations and carry out comprehensive development (some should be legislated)

(3) I will use this project to recommend the World Health Organization to hold the prevention cancer campaign, with the goal of reducing the incidence of cancer.

Conquering cancer is at the forefront of science and a worldwide problem. Cancer is a human disaster. The whole world and the people all over the world are eager to hope that one day they can overcome cancer and benefit mankind.

(4) Research ethics should be advocated, medicine is benevolence, and ethics is the first

Research ethics:

Products, achievements, and patents should all have ethical standards.

Standard:

The bottom line should be based on standards that do not harm human health. In particular, it must not contain carcinogens.

Basic ethics:

All products, achievements, patents, goods and people are harmless and do not harm people's health, especially for children. Do not contain carcinogens.

(5) XZ-C proposes scientific research ethics. It should recommend to WHO that all products, achievements, and patents should be the bottom line of moral standards that do not harm human health, especially the carcinogens. E.g:

1). Women's cosmetics, hair dyes, children's toys... should be tested without carcinogens, without damaging human health

2). House decoration, materials ... should be tested without carcinogens

3). Food additives, preservatives, food processing packaging ... should be tested without carcinogens

4). Leather products, cloth dyes ... should be tested, no carcinogens

5). The feed of collectively fed pigs is not allowed to contain hormones, auxins, or growth hormone, or vegetarian meat, growth-promoting hormones... all should be tested without carcinogens.

6). Collective feeding of chickens and ducks should not contain hormones or auxin or growth hormones.

(6) The health administrative department shall protect life and protect health, and shall lead, master, support, and guide prevention cancer measures, prevention cancer projects, prevention cancer tests, and prevention cancer monitoring.

(7) XZ-C proposes to establish the "Prevention Cancer Research Institute" and carry out prevention cancer system engineering:

- The function methods or way in which so many carcinogens or carcinogenic factors should be studied

- These sources of pollutants should be studied and managed to stop at the source

- These carcinogenic mechanisms, their carcinogenic effects, and environmental factors leading to genetic mutations should be studied.

- It is necessary to study the "two-type society" resource-saving and environment-friendly community to prevent cancer (to achieve a beautiful green environment and living environment with beautiful flowers and birds).

To scientifically prevent pollution and control pollution

To scientifically prevent cancer prevention and control cancer

Chapter 13

The scientific research ideas and suggestions of how to lay a good job and to fight well and to win the three major pollution battles

XZ-C proposed:

How to scientifically prevent pollution and control pollution?

How to scientifically prevent cancer and control cancer?

Scientific pollution prevention and pollution control

Scientific cancer prevention and anti-cancer

Resolutely fight well and win the three major pollution battles

The scientific research ideas and suggestions of how to lay a good job and to fight well and to win the tough battles for the three big pollutions

1. How to fight well and win three major pollution battles (I see one)

2. How to fight well and win three major pollution battles (I see two)

3. How to overcome cancer? How to prevent cancer? (I see three)

4. How to scientifically prevent pollution and treat pollution (I see four)

5. How to save the mother river?

6. How to implement and realize the overall design, planning, plan and blueprint in the next step

7. How to scientifically prevent and control air pollution? water pollution?

8. The scientific research thinking routes and suggestion and advice of how to fight well and to win tough battles of three major pollutions

Advising and suggesting and contributing strategies to the World Health Organization

Note:

1. *XZ-C is Xu Ze-China, because science is borderless, but scientists have nationality and intellectual property rights.*

2. *Cancer is a disaster for all mankind, it must evoke the global people to fight with cancer, so my series of monographs, 15 are all in English, globally distributed.*

First

How to fight well and to win the tough battles of three major pollutions? (I see one)

How to scientifically prevent pollution and treat pollution? How to prevent cancer? Anti-cancer? How to overcome cancer?

XZ-C suggestion:

A "Scientific Pollution Prevention and Pollution Control Research Working Group" should be established.

An "Innovative Cancer Prevention Research Institute" should be established.

1, 金猴奋起千钧棒，玉宇澄清万里埃

(the golden monkey rises up a thousand sticks, Yuyu clarifies Wanli)

(this sentence meaning is to have the clear air to stay in our environment)

• **XZ-C proposes:**

In order to design to solve air pollution, what or where are the targets or the key aims ?

It should find a way - where is the road? This road to problem solving should be proposed.

• **XZ-C proposed:**

the establishment of the "Scientific Prevention and Control Air Pollution Research Group"

•• To aggregate wisdom and to dedicate wisdom, XZ-C proposes a series of scientific thinking, scientific research design, scientific research planning, program, designation, blueprint, scientific research process

•• The research team of conquering cancer and launching the general attack on cancer can cooperate to implement it with the Department of Chemistry of Wuhan University

• **Research team, academic committee conditions:**

Academically accomplished, fruitful, experienced experts, scholars, and senior professors

Innovative and practical research elites, academic leaders, academic leaders

Goal: results, achievements, accomplishments

2, 问渠那得清如水，为有源头活水来

(the channel is clear as water, for the active head to come to the water)

(this sentence meaning is to have clear water to drink in our environment)

• XZ-C proposes:

Designing to solve water pollution, what or where are the targets or are the key objectives of tackling the problem? It should search a way, where is the road? It should find out the way to solve the problem.

• XZ-C proposes:

"Save the mother river of the whole country and the world"

• XZ-C proposed:

the establishment of the "Scientific Prevention and Control of Water Pollution Research Group"

• XZ-C proposes a series of scientific thinking, scientific research design, scientific research planning, program, design, blueprint, scientific research products

3. XZ-C proposes:

In order to save the mother river of the whole country and the whole world, it should be proposed to the Ministry of Housing and Urban-Rural Development that due to the wrong design of the sewage discharge pipe of the high-rise building, the mother rivers of the whole country and the whole world are polluted, the mother river all are traversed, settle as sedimentation, and accumulated by manure, which will cause the mother river to become waste water and waste river after 100 years. <u>Water pollution is associated with an increased incidence of cancer.</u> (Mother River is polluted, but it is still the source of urban tap water!!)

The steps:

1. To establish "Innovative Cancer Prevention Research Institute"

To set up : "Chemical Composition Analysis Laboratory"

Quantitative analysis laboratory to analyze water quality, ingredients, trace elements

2. Equipment: a trace element analyzer, a chemical composition analyzer,

a bacterial incubator

3. Tasks are carried out by laboratories and laboratory technicians

IT can be implemented by the "Overcoming Cancer Attacks" attack team

cooperation with the Department of Chemistry of Wuhan University

and cooperation with relevant experts of the Yangtze River Water Resources Commission

It is to perform investigation and collection of water pollution and data of the Yangtze River (point, surface)

And it is to conduct analysis, forecast and evaluate the future situation

It is to collect scientific data for evaluation

The place for getting the samples:

it is set at: 1, sewage into the mouth (point); 2, water source (point)

4, in order to save the mother river of the country and the world

1) XZ-C proposes:

The letter should be written to the World Health Organization, International Cancer Center, which should propose that due to the wrong design of the Global Ministry of Housing and Urban-Rural Development, as a result, the mother river in the world is polluted by manure and dung. After a hundred years, or hundreds of years later, it will become a waste river. <u>The mother rivers of the world are the cultural birthplaces of the states. Water pollution is associated with an increase in the incidence of cancer.</u>

Why do you want to propose to the Ministry of Housing and Urban-Rural Development the wrong design of the sewage discharge pipe for high-rise buildings?

It is to awaken the people of the whole country and the whole world to recognize this serious mistake:

a. it should try to save, to remedy, and to research remedies

b. This wrong design should be terminated and changed to the correct design. This error cannot be made again.

c. The mistake of this design has caused serious consequences and should bear certain responsibilities.

(2) XZ-C proposed that X company should be set up for scientific research, and try to turn waste into treasure and recover losses.

(3) Professor Xu Ze XZ-C proposed:

a. The correct design of the mega-urban sewage drainage system in high-rise buildings should be studied.

b. It is to propose the correct design scheme, carry out the diversion draining and sub-storage, separate the sewage and digestive pipes of the domestic sewage, divert draining and separate storage, the former is decontamination treatment, the latter is to be recycling, utilization, turning waste into treasure

c. In this way, the mother rivers of the whole country and the whole world (London, New York, Tokyo, Beijing, Shanghai...) can be streamed with water. "问渠那得清如水，为有源头活水来(The English meaning is 'When the canal is clear, it is like water, and it is a source of active water.'"

5. Why should we focus on saving the mother river?

(1) XZ-C proposes:

1. For thousands of years, humans have used manure and animal manure as agricultural fertilizers to feed humans for thousands of years.

2. Nowadays, there are many high-rise buildings in the global metropolis, and the excrement of several billion people has been mistakenly designed and introduced into the mother rivers. This is a great mistake, a great loss, a great waste.

3. This is a great waste, a great historical waste, losing billions of manure and urine can not be fertilized for agriculture, is a great loss! ! This is a great mistake, a big mistake in history.

4. Not only is it a great loss, but it also causes great harm, blockage, and siltation of the river. Water pollution affects cities that are inferior.

5. and even more harmful, these polluted mother rivers are the water source of hundreds of thousands, millions, and tens of millions of people in the metropolis, and the downstream urban residents use the polluted water flowing down the upstream city.

6. Because of the loss of billions of manure and urine on the earth, it cannot be used as fertilizer. What about agricultural production? Where does the fertilizer from agricultural production come from? How to do?

7. So fertilizers came into being, and chemists, entrepreneurs, and businessmen produced large quantities of fertilizers (the world's fertilizers have been around for hundreds of years, and China's fertilizers are only 30-40 years old).

8. Fertilizers cause soil damage, and fish and shrimp also suffer.

4. Due to the wrong design of the real estate developer, the building's urination and sewer pipes were discharged into the municipal sewer pipe together with the kitchen domestic water, and finally discharged into the Yangtze River and the mother river. The consequences are: a series of serious consequences as mentioned above.

Second

How to fight well and win three major pollution battles? (I see two)

(1) XZ-C proposes:

Designing to solve air pollution, what or where is its "target" or the "aim" of tackling the problem?

The Design:

XZ-C proposes: "target" is set for air purification

1. The existing air conditioning, plus air purification network

It means: Air purification network

2. The form or sharp of product:

A. The portable air filter purification network "backpack", or "handbag"

B. The simple air filter purification network "tent"

C. The simple air filter purification network "large mask type"

D. Installed, or portable (meeting room)

E. The bedroom type night air purification net "book"

F. The Mongolia tent type application air purification filter

3. Set up a small factory, several (1-10) workshops

Hire 3-4 engineers and recruit several workers (both male and female)

4. Write a scientific research plan, list scientific research projects, production processes

a. Collect materials, materials, and literature in various countries.

b. can organize an outing inspection

XZ-C proposes:

- Indoor air conditioning purification network

- Personal backpack, portable purification filter

(2) XZ-C proposes:

Designing to solve water pollution, what or where is its "target" or the "aim" of tackling the issues?

The design:

XZ-C proposed:

"target" is defined as drinking water purification, the goal or aim is to drink the standard qualified water.

A,

1. Design small water purifier, or micro water purifier, comes with a style, very convenient to use

2. Installed on the faucet, it can be filtered and purified. It can be applied to all kinds of faucets at any time. It is very convenient to use and can be taken away.

3. Product form and shape is convenient type and suitable for the above.

B, the second form

It is to design household water purifier.

It is to Install in the kitchen water pipe, drinking water, cooking dish, cooking rice, making a meal, laundry... household water can be used

There are already manufacturers, but they are still not perfect and need further research.

C, All county and city waterworks should be qualified

It is the main and final goal to select several counties and prefecture-level cities to make tap water drinkable according to developed countries.

China is now the second largest economy in the world. It must reach the level of developed countries in Europe and America when drinking tap water that meets the standards.

You can select several county-level cities and prefecture-level cities to try first, and you can organize out-of-town inspections (it is planned to be piloted in Leping City, Jiangxi Province, Jingdezhen City).

Prevention pollution, or pollution control, and riding the car for the scientific research, can achieve the effect of first-class cancer prevention, which is aiming to study three major pollutions to prevent cancer.

Enterprises must be based on products and patents:

a, water plant produces water purification system

b, kitchen water purifier

c, drinking water faucet purifier

Third

How to overcome cancer? How to prevent cancer? (I see three)

1. **XZ-C proposes that the "Innovative Cancer Prevention Research Institute" should be established.**

Research:

Environmental factors lead to mutations in the gene R, carcinogenesis, and distortion.

It is to do the research from detecting qualitative and quantitative of clothing, food, housing, transportation, decoration, environment, small environment, micro-environment (internal environment, external environment)

Method:

macro, micro, ultra-micro, study various factors leading to R mutation

What is the big environment, small environment, internal environment, external environment, micro-environment? which factors affect the normal physiology, pathology, pathophysiological structure of cells, leading to R mutation, leading to an increase in cancer incidence?.

Established:

Component Analysis Laboratory

Personnel:

laboratory personnel, laboratory personnel, chemical personnel.

2.   How to overcome cancer? How to prevent cancer?

XZ-C proposes to create the "Innovative Environmental Protection and Cancer Research Institute" and carry out cancer prevention system engineering

XZ-C proposes:

Dawning A type anti-cancer plan

Dawning B type anti-cancer plan

Dawning D-type anti-cancer plan

How to implement this research plan to overcome cancer, I detailed the general design, master plan, specific plan, plan, bluemap.

Fourth

How to prevent pollution and pollution (I see four)

XZ-C proposed:

"Innovative Science Pollution Prevention and Pollution Control Research Institute" should be established.

Research:

What is pollution? What is dyeing?

1. What is its source? What are the consequences?

2. What is the <u>source **of air**</u> pollution? How to form?

What is the <u>source of water</u> pollution? How to form?

What is the <u>source of soil</u> pollution? How to form?

We should awaken human attention:

the residents of the global village should defend the living environment and living environment of the global village. We are all human life communities.

Do not artificially create pollution!

Do not artificially create garbage!

Do not overuse disposable items! It is rubbish after use.

3. What is the source of garbage? What are the consequences?

What is garbage?

How to form?

What are the consequences?

a, it should prevent excessive waste? Block source

(Wuhan's one-day garbage can be piled up into a hill!)

b, Minimize the use of disposable products, and use excessive packaging as little as possible.

c, it should reduce the second renovation to reduce a large amount of construction waste

Although the garbage can be recycled and used, it causes a lot of artificial air pollution, water pollution, and soil pollution.

d, it should become rich in the good methos, genuine goods, and it should reduce excessive luxury packaging. These luxury packaging is garbage after use.

e, Try to stop artificially manufacturing a large amount of garbage, and try to stop artificially large amounts of pollution.

4. How to stop a large amount of waste gas, waste residue and waste water?

How to minimize the amount of garbage and a lot of pollution?

We should improve the quality of humanities, and we should improve social ethics. We can use TV to publicize and educate and publicize socialist moral education, and strongly criticize people for creating pollution. It is to protect the living environment and life environment of human beings, everyone is responsible and always responsible, and it should be green mountains, clear and green water, and fragrant flowers and bird words. The home environment should be green hills, green water, and birds and flowers

5. Specific recommendations:

In order to implement the research work of the party's "Nineteenth National Congress" and the government work report to strengthen research on smog governance or smog management and control and the tackling research on conquering cancer.

(1) Suggestions:

1. Set up a "conquering cancer working group", and set up a "studio", which has various special topics and professional working groups.

There is a full-time staff, and it should be diligent, save, and do everything for the people, do good deeds, and seek health and welfare for future generations.

2. It involves the Provincial Department of Education, the Provincial Department of Science and Technology, the Provincial Health and Health Committee, the Provincial Department of Ecological Environment, the relevant departments of the smog scientific governance research and related conquering-cancer research.

Specially, professionally and full-time performing the scientific research with high-tech and conducting macro, micro, ultra-micro research.

3. It is recommended that the Provincial Natural Science Foundation, the Provincial Science and Technology Department, the various masters and postgraduate students choose topics, participate in scientific research on smog research and cancer prevention and treatment research, agile wisdom, technological innovation, and prosper technology.

4. Our research team first applied for the initial establishment of an "Innovative Environmental Protection and Cancer Research Institute", and invited Wu Da and Hua Ke University to participate in the guidance. It is suggested that the "Scientific Management Smog Research Group" should be established, and the first-class discipline to overcome conquer as the direction of cancer research. ".

(2) Suggestion:

It is to establish a "Scientific pollution prevention and Pollution Control Research Working Group"

There is a "studio" (or office)

It has various special topics and professional working groups.

It is based on research and scientific prevention and control of three major pollution.

Design:

a. Scientific Research Group on Prevention and Control of Air Pollution

b. Scientific Research Group on Prevention and Control of Water Pollution

c. Scientific Research Group on Prevention and Control of Soil Pollution

Wu Da, Hua Keda, and Huanong University are invited to participate in the research and guidance research, to make suggestions, to gather wisdom, to guide graduate research, to make suggestions, and to guide graduate students to choose these topics. The project topic of the tutor is combined with the topic selection of the graduate student. It is easy to regularly and on time produce scientific research results and originally innovation results.

Agglutination wisdom is to brainstorm and give wisdom.

What is wisdom? What is scientific wisdom?

It is scientific thinking, scientific research design, scientific research planning, program, design, blueprint, scientific research process.

purpose:

method:

result:

In conclusion:

Achieve results, new products, new methods, new technologies

New concept, new theory, innovation theory

Benefit the people and benefit the society

XZ-C proposes an initiative:

It is scheduled to start in Wuhan in 2019. It is planned to make academic reports on the general attack of cancer in Shanxi, Liaoning, Jiangxi and Shenzhen in 2019. These coal mines have serious air pollution and high incidence of cancer, especially lung cancer.

Why should we study antifouling and pollution control?

It is because more than 90% of cancers are related to environmental factors, these environmental factors lead to genetic mutations, cancerous changes, and distortions. Therefore, research on anti-cancer and anti-cancer must study pollution prevention and pollution control, that is, research on cancer prevention and anti-cancer, and block at the source.

Fifth,

How to save the mother river?

1. XZ-C proposes:

(1). Due to the wrong design of the sewage pipe of the housing department of the Ministry of Housing and Urban-Rural Development, the pollution of the mother river in the whole country and the whole world, the cross-flow of manure water and the sedimentation of manure deposits in the river channel will probably be a hundred years of manure and dregs. Accumulation deposits in the mother river, which will cause the mother river to become waste water and waste river.

The mother river of the whole country and the whole world is the birthplace of human culture in the whole country and the whole world. It is the blue of human culture. Today, the mother river is polluted, and the feces and feces of the metropolis are filled and accumulated in the mother river.

(2). Due to the wrong design of the sewage pipe of the house, the accumulation of manure will contaminate the mother river, and compensation should be requested to set up the X company remedy.

(3). Established company X to save the mother river, otherwise the mother river will become waste water and waste river after 100 years.

(4). For thousands of years, human agriculture on earth has human feces, urine, pigs, cattle, sheep, horses... and manure as agricultural fertilizers, which enable food production to feed humans on the earth for thousands of years and constitute human beings. society. Nowadays, there are many high-rise buildings in the metropolis. Due to the design mistakes of the sewage pipes in the houses, millions of people in the metropolis, tens of millions of people's sewage, urine and domestic sewage are discharged into the underground municipal pipeline, and finally discharged into the mother. River, Yangtze River, Yellow River, etc.

Due to design errors, large waste, historical waste, unforgivable waste, should be corrected and corrected.

It is also necessary to ring the bell to solve the problem. This is a design error of the sewage system of the house. It should be rehabilitated and corrected to set up

Company X and recycle it as fertilizer to reduce or prevent the use of fertilizer and prevent cancer.

10. XZ-C proposed:

It should promote scientific research ethics, medical is benevolence, ethics first

Research ethics:

products, patents, and results should have ethical standards

Standard: I

t should be based on the standard of not damaging human health, especially the carcinogen.

Basic ethics:

All products, achievements, patents, commodities, harmless to people, and not harmful to people's health, especially for children, must not contain carcinogens. All patents, achievements, commodities, and products must not contain sequelae or complications.

Scientists and entrepreneurs should pay attention to scientific research ethics.

Sixth

Next step is the plan or program of How to implement and achieve the overall design, planning, blueprint

1. XZ-C proposes how to overcome cancer? How to prevent cancer? How to conquer cancer? How to treat cancer?

How to carry out "to overcome cancer, launch a general attack - prevention, control, and treatment at the same attention"

How to build a scientific research base that it is to overcome cancer and launch the general attack of cancer----the science city?

(1) The general design, general plan, program, steps, and blueprints for conquering cancer, launching the general attack and preparing for the "Science City" have been completed. If it can be carried out and implemented according to the plan, it may achieve the goal of conquering cancer.

The previous general plan and design have been completed, and the next step is how to implement and implement it,

(2) Next step is the plan for carrying out and achieve the overall design, planning, and blueprint :

1). XZ-C proposes that under the leadership and guidance of the provincial and municipal departments and bureaus, it is necessary to establish a scientific research base to conquer cancer and to launch the general attack of cancer---- Science City"

-----   Cancer Research and Medical Center

Implementation, achievement of the general rules

A. How to overcome cancer? How to prevent cancer?

XZ-C proposes: to create the "Innovative Environmental Protection and Cancer Prevention Research Institute" and carry out cancer prevention system engineering

XZ-C proposes: **Dawning or Twilight anti-cancer plan A, B, D**

B. How to overcome cancer? How to treat cancer?

XZ-C proposed: Shuguang C-type plan No.1-6

Target tasks, namely implementation, carrying out, completion, and implementation of the above-mentioned Dawning C-type plan 1-6 and Dawning cancer prevention plan A, B, D

C. The attack research team of "Overcoming cancer and launching the General Attack of Cancer", set up various research groups under it, set up academic leaders in the combination of Chinese and Western medicine, anti-cancer, cancer treatment basic research and clinical research groups, academic masters, academic leaders; the research team Research objectives of the basic and clinical research groups:

The main points are:

- Basic research and clinical research to prevent postoperative recurrence and metastasis, in order to improve long-term efficacy after surgery.

The standard of efficacy evaluation:

it should be that cancer patients have long survival time, good quality of life and no complications.

- Prevent Gene mutation factors (starting cancer research from the internal environment, the external environment, and the micro-environment)

- Molecular level Chinese and Western medicine combined research, Chinese medicine immunopharmacological research, Chinese medicine anti-metastasis, recurrence clinical research, observation, verification.

Set up the Academic Research Groups under it:

A. The first academic research group:

Establish prevention, control, and treatment at the same attention, and carry out "three early" ("three early" clinics) ("three early" wards), three early diagnosis and treatment research

The hospital of the whole process of prevention, control and treatment - can be set up in the academic, academic, chain, alliance, remote clinic, publicity theory, academic.

It can be set up chain and alliance in the theory or/and academic, to do the remote clinic, to ropaganda theory, academic.

B. The second special research group:

Establish a pharmaceutical factory or preparation room to provide particles granules

To build the analytical research groups and laboratories for active ingredients, molecular levels, and gene levels of anti-cancer, anti-metastatic immune regulation and control Chinese medicine

C. The third special research group:

Establishing the cancer prevention research institute and carrying out prevention cancer system engineering

• Conducting the "toilet revolution" to establish X company to save the mother river

• Carry out the detection, monitoring, research of the big environment, small environment, clothing, food, housing, and R mutation factors; the research team set up genetic testing research group

Professor Xu Ze

The chief designer of "Collecting the General Attack on Cancer and Creating a Science City to Fight Cancer"

Head of the discipline of "Overcoming the general attack on cancer"

Seventh

How to scientifically prevent and control air pollution? Water pollution?

1. What are the three major sources of pollution? It must find the bottom, what is the source?

What causes air pollution? What is the "target" that leads to air pollution?

The solution is to filter and purify

2. What causes water pollution? What is the source?

What is the "target" of its research?

It should be set in the mistake of the sewage design of high-rise buildings. It is wrong and wrong again. It has been wrong for hundreds of years and is wrong with the global metropolis.

1). The result of the error has polluted the global mother river, and it will continue to increase the pollution of the mother river for a long time in the future. It is expected that the mother rivers of these metropolises will be abolished after a few hundred years, and it is unsuitable for human habitation.

2). The result of mistakes is big waste, historic waste, big mistakes, thousands of years of human beings using manure and urine as crop fertilizers, feeding humans on the earth for thousands of years, and our ancestors used this as agricultural fertilizer to make a living.

Nowadays, the design of the sewage system of the high-rise buildings by the sewage pipes of the houses is wrong, resulting in great waste, historical waste, and global waste.

To solve the bell, you need to ring the bell.

3). Because humans have lost manure and urine as agricultural fertilizers, chemical fertilizers have emerged as a result, and a large amount of chemical fertilizers have flooded the global farms, leading to the consequences of today. The pollution of soils by chemical fertilizers, pesticides and pesticides contains many carcinogens and damages human health. This has led to an increasing global cancer incidence today.

3.   How to solve the problem?

(1). The bell is still needed to solve the bell, and the housing design department should correct the wrong design.

Requirements:

1). National and global should correct design errors

2). How to stop polluting mother river in the next step

3). How to solve the waste of manure in the next step? How to solve the reuse?

(2)   Establishing a housing design for building a new socialist countryside should avoid repeating this mistake

Housing design in a new socialist countryside must have toilets, septic tanks, and re-farm for agriculture.

4. How to scientifically prevent and control air pollution?

a. XZ-C proposes Dawning cancer prevention A-type plan and carry out preventing pollution and pollution control and I project of cancer prevention and anti-cancer

Watt invented the steam engine. Humans have developed coal, oil and natural gas as fuel and energy in the order of 10 million tons, such as thermal power generation, smelting, steel, automobiles, airplanes, vehicles and household fuels. A large amount of harmful gases such as tar, soot, and dust are continuously discharged into the atmosphere. It is estimated that more than 80% of environmental pollutants in the atmosphere come from the combustion process of fuel. These increasing emissions, detained gas can reach 600-700 million tons, and concentrated in the city.

Air pollution can cause many diseases, especially respiratory diseases, the most serious is lung cancer.

How to do? How to solve this problem and how to solve such a serious air pollution problem?

XZ-C proposed:

Shuguang or dawning cancer prevention A-type plan, research to prevent air pollution, research, development, production of pollution prevention and pollution control, cancer prevention, anti-Ca I engineering, design shown in Figures 1, 2, 3, called dawning or Shuguang cancer prevention Type A plan, anti-pollution, cancer prevention and anti-Ca I system engineering.

B. How to scientifically prevent urban water pollution?

XZ-C proposes the Dawning cancer prevention B-type plan and II system project of preventing pollution and treating pollution and cancer prevention and anti-cancer

Modern cities, high-rise buildings, dozens of buildings, and their sewers are discharged into municipal sewage pipes, such as Beijing's 23 million people, and Wuhan's 15 million people live in high-rise buildings. Their daily toilets and toilets are discharged. ? They are all discharged into the municipal sewage pipeline, which is discharged into the river after sewage treatment. The Wuhan municipal sewage pipeline is discharged into the Yangtze River and pollutes the mother river over the years. The consequences are:

1). The waste and urine of 115 million people are wasted, which is a great waste. Why?

For 5,000 years, human beings have used manure and urine as agricultural fertilizers to feed the people of the world for five thousand years. Now they are not used, which is a huge waste of history. In the future, they will continue to waste every year and squander their sons and grandchildren. It made a great mistake in history.

Five thousand years of human survival proves that human excrement is the best fertilizer in agriculture, and now the design of high-rise buildings is wrong. The human waste is mixed with urban sewage and discharged into the mother river of the world, which is both pollution of the mother river and can not be used for human fertilization for agriculture. The loss is too great. It is a great waste of human civilization. It is a great mistake of human civilization and a great destruction of human civilization.

2). Due to the high-rise buildings in the city, human waste and domestic sewage are mixed and discharged into the municipal pipeline. After the so-called sewage treatment, they are discharged into the Yangtze River and the "Mother River". The manure that has been discharged into the Yangtze River and the waterway for many years is seriously polluted. The mother river, accumulated over the years, was deposited on the bottom of the river, seriously polluting the "mother river."

3). For five thousand years, humans have relied on human excrement as fertilizer, and the food produced has been fed by humans for thousands of years. It has produced thousands of years of human civilization and culture, but the modern high-rise buildings are big, due to the mistakes of drainage system design. The manure is lost and the natural fertilizer in the countryside is lost.

Therefore, chemical fertilizer came into being. This is caused by the design error of the high-rise drainage pipe system of the house of the Ministry of Housing and Urban Construction. It should assume responsibility, correct it, and compensate.

In short, how to resolutely fight well to win the battle for pollution prevention pollution treatment, and smog control and management?

First, to research how the three major sources of pollution comes from? What is the source and formation of smog?

It must find the bottom, conduct scientific analysis, and scientific research. Where is the source? What are the consequences?

a, How and what does produce and cause air pollution? Why and what and how leads to water pollution? Why does it cause soil pollution? What is the source? What are the consequences? How to solve?

What is the "target" of its research?

Pollution prevention and pollution control research institutes should be established to conduct scientific research and experimental research.

b, what is pollution? What is the content of the pollution? What is the damage to human health?

Prevention of pollution, pollution control, and pollutant composition analysis rooms should be established. It is with Macroscopic, microscopic, ultra-microscopic.

Equipment conditions:

trace element analyzer, chemical analyzer... It must establish a national-level advanced laboratory, our research team should cooperate with the Chemistry Department of Wuhan University to train graduate students to participate in practice.

It is to find out where the source of pollution is? It should stop at the source, try to stop. It is to solve the bell and still need to ring the bell.

What is the content of pollution?

Microscopic, ultra-micro and biochemical, molecular biology, genetic engineering research and analysis should be carried out.

c, Establish pollutant detection and monitoring

Implemented by the anti-fouling and pollution control laboratory, and the monitoring report

d, pollution prevention, pollution control and cancer prevention, cancer control research

Where should the three targets of pollution be earmarked or targeted?

How to solve? Macro, micro, and ultra-micro studies should be conducted

e, XZ-C proposed to establish the "Innovative Environmental Protection and Health Cancer Research Institute" to carry out cancer prevention system engineering, and establish a high-level laboratory.

The party's 19th National Congress decided to resolutely fight well and win the tough battles of pollution prevention and pollution treatment, and strengthen the study of smog governance. This is a great wise decision.

Where do the three major pollutions come from?

XZ-C believes that this is a complication and sequelae in the development of human science and industrial production. These complications or sequelae must be carefully studied, removed, and prevented to improve the scientific development of modern times.

This is a wise and great move to improve the development of modern science, safeguard the human living environment, defend the human living environment, and defend human health.

These modern scientific developments have brought a beautiful life and living environment to human beings, but they have also brought about some negative complications and negative effects of sequelae, which have affected the living environment and existing environment of human beings and affected human health and led some cancerous, mutation, and distortion because 90% of cancers are caused by environmental factors. Environmental factors lead to genetic mutations that lead to chromosomal deletions and abnormalities. Environmental factors can be managed and sought to find solutions. My newly published monograph "Agglutination Wisdom, Conquering Cancer - Benefiting Mankind" is a medical monograph that is more comprehensively designed and specifically planned to overcome cancer. It is a program to implement cancer, this scientific research plan, scientific research scheme, blueprint, are available for reference in various countries.

How to reduce or avoid these developmental complications and sequelae?

Solar energy, water energy and wind energy should be vigorously developed and applied. These natural energy sources, such as good collection and storage, have few complications or even sequelae after use.

Xu Ze, Xu Jie, Bin Wu

XZ-C proposes:

I hope that some universities can create this first-class discipline that focuses on cancer research and the first-class disciplines that focus on scientific pollution prevention, pollution control, and scientific prevention.

Suggestions:

The research work of Huazhong University of Science and Technology, Wuhan University, Hubei University of Traditional Chinese Medicine and other alma mater [Note] should be pushed to the forefront of the world, and the first batch of disciplines in China and the world to overcome cancer research. Under the guidance of Xi Jinping's socialism with Chinese characteristics in the new era, he strives to follow the road of innovation in anti-cancer transfer with Chinese characteristics, adheres to the road of independent innovation with Chinese characteristics, adheres to the combination of Chinese and Western medicine, and the road of independent innovation of "Chinese-style anti-cancer", hoping in Hubei, Wuhan has established this first-class discipline in the country and the world to overcome cancer, and to make new contributions to the fight against cancer. In the contemporary, it is beneficial to the future.

[Note] I was admitted to the Central South Tongji Medical College in 1951. The hospital was formed by the merger of Shanghai Tongji Medical College and Wuhan University. After graduation, I was assigned to the surgery of the Affiliated Hospital of Hubei College of Traditional Chinese Medicine. Therefore, I am the alma mater of my study, work, and growth. (Xu Ze)

164

Chapter 14

The Scientific Research Thinking Route and Suggestion Words and Contributing Strategies of how to fight well and win the three major pollution battles

(1) Professor Xu Ze (XZ-C) proposed to make suggestions to the World Health Organization:

1). Scientific ethics should be advocated, medicine is benevolence, and ethics is the first or it should promote scientific research ethics, medical is benevolence, ethics first

2). All products should have ethical standards

3). The Implementation of prevention-oriented policy:

the way out to treat cancer in the "three early", the anti-cancer way out is in cancer prevention

4). XZ-C proposes to establish the "Innovative Cancer Prevention Research Institute" and carry out cancer prevention system engineering

—— Open a new era of cancer prevention research and cancer prevention system engineering in the 21st century

(2) To advise the World Health Organization and the United Nations:

1). To save the mother river of the world (see section 12, the scientific research thinking route and recommendation words of how to fight well, win the three major pollution battles)

2). Bells need to be ringed.

(all products aircraft, trains, cars...) it should be harmless to human health, no complications, no sequelae or complications, no harm to people's health, especially the three major pollutions must not contain carcinogens. While the product is designed, it should be designed to avoid, remove, and product ethical standards should be monitored at the factory.

The scientific ethics standards:

It should be based on the standard of not damaging human health, especially the carcinogens.

The Basic ethics:

It should be that all products, achievements, patents, goods and people are harmless and do not harm people's health, especially for children, and must not contain carcinogens.

Resolutely to fight well and win three major and tough battles, scientific pollution prevention, pollution control, scientific management of smog, and to conquer cancer, which is a great pioneering work for the country and the people, and also for the scientific research work of cancer prevention, anti-cancer, and conquering cancer, creating a good opportunity for human health, the purpose is for the human health, being away from cancer, and a great initiative for the health and well-being of future generations.

The scientific research ideas and suggestions of how to lay a good job and win the three tough and major pollution battles:

XZ-C advises the World Health Organization:

1). It should promote scientific research ethics, medical is benevolence, ethics first

Physicians, nurses, scientific and technical personnel, teaching and research personnel, the first should be true knowledge and skills and talented, both ability and political or moral integrity, setting up morality and building the person, medical is benevolence, setting up moral is the first.

2). All products, achievements, and patents of science and technology should have ethical standards

a, all foods must not contain carcinogens

b, women's cosmetics must not contain carcinogens

c, food can not contain carcinogens

d, pig feed can not contain hormones, growth hormones, auxin, lean meat extraction...

e, chicken, duck feed can not contain hormones, growth hormones......

f, Catering, food, and cooked food personnel should have regular physical examinations, and there should be no infectious diseases. It should be affixed to the health card badge.

g, All kinds of snacks, meals should be food safety and should be in line with health

h, To implement the prevention-oriented policy and to reform the hospital model. Each of the top three hospitals should set up a department of cancer prevention.

i, To implement "three early" (early detection, early diagnosis, early treatment) and to research on "three early" new methods, new technologies, new drugs, and new reagents, and to block cancer in early germination stage, and all can be recovered in the early stage.

How to implement it?

To launch the general attack, and to do the prevention, control, and treatment at the same attention, the three carriages ride at the same level and attention, go hand in hand, establish a cancer prevention department, "three early" clinic, "three early" lesions and precancerous state clinic.

j, try to reduce the incidence of cancer

• To play well and win three major pollution battles. Performing pollution prevention and treatment of pollution and control in order to achieve cancer prevention and anti-cancer

- **To carry out cancer prevention monitoring system engineering from the macro environment, small or micro environment, internal environment and external environment, from clothing, food, housing and transportation.**

k, the national and global missionary scientific cancer prevention knowledge, self-early discovery of medical knowledge, the cancer prevention departments of the top three hospitals should cooperate with community training to promote the scientific knowledge and level of people's cancer prevention. <u>The cancer is blocked in the early germination state and can be completely eliminated in the early stage.</u>

3). Professor Xu Ze (XZ-C) suggested:

a. All countries, provinces and states can establish cancer prevention research institutes (or corresponding institutions) to carry out cancer prevention system projects and carry out cancer prevention work for their own country, province and city.

b. Countries establish cancer prevention regulations, and national cancer prevention (some should be legislated)

c. It is recommended that the World Health Organization convene a cancer prevention campaign. The goal is to reduce the incidence of cancer in the country.

Conquering cancer is a frontier of science and a worldwide problem. Cancer is a human disaster, covering the whole world. People all over the world are eager to overcome cancer one day and make the treasure for the benefit of mankind.

4). Professor Xu Ze (XZ-C) proposed to save the mother river by saving the mother river. It is because the mother rivers of the whole country and the world are polluted by industrial and agricultural sewage and urban sewage, the carcinogens have increased significantly.

a. In order to save the mother river of the whole country and the world, XZ-C proposed:

it is to write a letter to the World Health Organization, the International Cancer Center, it is to propose the wrong design of the sewage discharge pipe of the high-rise building of the Global Ministry of Housing and Construction, resulting in the global mother river polluted by manure water and manure stool, and it will become a waste river after 100 years. The mother rivers of the world are the cultural birthplaces of the states. Water pollution is associated with an increased incidence of cancer.

b. For thousands of years, manure and animal manure have been used as agricultural fertilizers for thousands of years to feed humans on the earth for thousands of years.

Nowadays, there are many high-rise buildings in the world's metropolises. The excrement and urine of billions of people around the world have been introduced into the mother rivers of various places by the wrong design of the sewage discharge pipes of high-rise buildings.

c. Not only is it a great loss, but it also causes great harm, blocking silted rivers, water pollution, and affecting its downstream cities.

d. and more harmful, these polluted mothers are the water source of hundreds of thousands, millions, and tens of millions of people in the metropolis. The downstream urban residents use the polluted water flowing down the upstream city.

e. Because of the loss of billions of manure and urine on the earth, it cannot be used as fertilizer. What about agricultural production? Where does the fertilizer from agricultural production come from? How to do?

f. so fertilizer came into being, chemists, entrepreneurs, businessmen mass production of fertilizer (global fertilizer for hundreds of years, China's fertilizer is only 30-40 years)

g. chemical damage caused by soil, fish and shrimp, etc. are also victimized

h. Due to the incorrect design of the sewer drainage pipe of the house, the urinal pipe of the building is discharged into the municipal sewer pipe together with the kitchen domestic water, and finally discharged into the Yangtze River and the Mother River. The consequences are as follows:

i. **Professor Xu Ze XZ-C proposed:**

*   **The correct design of the mega-urban housing drainage system with high-rise buildings should be studied**

- **Propose the correct design scheme, carry out the diversion and sub-storage, separate the domestic sewage from the excrement pipe, divert the flow, divide the storage, the former decontamination treatment, the latter recycling, use the waste to be treasure**

- **The mother rivers of the whole country and the world (London, New York, Tokyo, Beijing, Shanghai...) can be cleared.**

"Ask the channel to be as clear as water, to be a source of active water."

How to solve these problems?

5). *Professor Xu Ze (XZ-C) proposed:*

To solve the bell, you need to ring the bell. All products (aircraft, train, car) should be harmless, no sequelae, no complications, and should be designed and perfected before leaving the factory.

However, at present, the exhaust of the aircraft, a large amount of coal tar is discharged... and a large amount of pollutant gas is sprinkled into the air from the sky like a fairy flower, and the air is polluted.

The exhaust of the train discharges a large amount of coal tar... and a large amount of pollutant gas, which is sprayed into the air to pollute the air.

These are causing air pollution and leading to respiratory diseases, the most serious is lung cancer; the current global male and female lung cancer is the highest incidence of cancer.

Professor Xu Ze (XZ-C) proposed:

(1) Drafting the report to the Ministry of Real Estate - the wrong design of the real estate developer due to the design of the sewage system of the sewage discharge pipe of the new high-rise building.

a. The result of the error has polluted the mother river of the world, and it will continue to pollute for a long time in the future. It is expected that the mother rivers of these metropolises will be abolished after 100 years, and it is unsuitable for human habitation. This is a historical mistake.

b. The result of the mistake is a big waste, a historic waste. For thousands of years, humans have used manure as a crop fertilizer to feed humans on the earth for thousands of years. Our ancestors used this as agricultural fertilizer to survive. .

Nowadays, the design of the sewage system of high-rise buildings is wrong, which leads to historical waste and global waste.

The Housing Department, the housing design department should be responsible for, should be compensated, and the bell must be ringed. To solve the bell, you need to ring the bell.

c. Since the earth's manure and urine are lost on the earth and cannot be used as agricultural fertilizer, where does the fertilizer needed for agricultural production come from? How to do? So fertilizer came into being, and chemists, entrepreneurs, and businessmen produced large quantities of fertilizers (the world's fertilizers have been around for hundreds of years, and China's fertilizers are only 30-40 years). **A large amount of fertilizer is flooding the world's farms, leading to today's consequences, pollution of soil by fertilizers, pesticides and pesticides.**

Fertilizers cause soil damage, fish and shrimps are also affected. The pollution of soil by chemical fertilizers, pesticides and pesticides contains many carcinogens, which damages human health and leads to an increasing global cancer incidence today.

Due to the wrong design of the sewage discharge pipe of the house, the urination and manure pipes of the building were discharged into the municipal sewer pipe together with the domestic sewage pipe, and finally discharged into the Yangtze River and the mother river. The consequences are as follows: a series of serious consequences as mentioned above.

(2) What should I do? how to solve this problem?

XZ-C proposes:

Drafting the letter to sue the wrong design of the Housing Department's housing system for real estate developers

Requirements:

1). National and global should correct the wrong design of the housing sewage system

2). How to stop polluting mother river in the next step

3). How to solve the waste of manure (agricultural fertilizer) of hundreds of millions of people in high-rise buildings in metropolis? How to solve the reuse?

4). Building a new socialist countryside design should avoid repeating this mistake

Why does it need to make suggestions to the World Health Organization?

It is because cancer patients cover the whole world, the pollution of industrial and agricultural wastewater, waste residue and waste gas also covers the whole world. Therefore, the world must be able to overcome cancer and launch the general attack of cancer; prevention cancer, anti-cancer, cancer treatment, especially cancer prevention is the top priority; it is to study these sources of pollution, design to stop at the source, and strive to prevent cancer safety hazards, block it in the budding state.

At present, the hospital model of the global cancer hospital or the oncology center is all focused on treating patients with advanced and middle-aged patients with poor efficacy, exhausting human and financial resources, failing to improve the cure rate and reducing the incidence rate, but only attention to treatment with Light prevention, or only have treatment without prevention, the more patients are treated, the more the patients become.

The current status quo is:

the road that has passed in a century is to rectify and to focus on treatment with ignore the prevention, or only to treat without prevention. For many years we have only been doing research on cancer treatment, but we have done very little work on cancer prevention and have done almost nothing. As a result, the incidence of cancer continues to rise.

At present, the global hospitals or cancer centers are fully committed to treatment, attention to treatment and light prevention, or just treatment without prevention. XZ-C believes that this mode of hospitalization, or cancer treatment, is unlikely to overcome cancer and it is impossible to reduce the incidence. **The global cancer hospital or cancer center must carry out an overall strategic reform of cancer treatment, shifting focusing on treatment-oriented and attention to treatment without prevention into prevention, control, and treatment at the same time.**

Looking back and reflecting on it, for a century, cancer prevention research has not paid attention to it, prevention has not paid attention to, prevention-oriented health work policy has not been paid attention to, and has not been implemented. As a result, the more patients are treated and the more the patients with cancer, the more morbidity, the higher the mortality rate and the higher the mortality rate.

Chapter 15

To adhere to take the innovation road of cancer prevention and cancer control in a well-off society with Chinese characteristics

While building a well-off society, it is recommended to carry out medical scientific research and cancer prevention and treatment work for cancer prevention and cancer control.

How to do? How to reduce the incidence of cancer? How to improve the cure rate of cancer? How to reduce cancer mortality? How to prolong the patient's survival? How to improve the quality of life?

XZ-C believes that the general attack of overcoming cancer should be launched and prevention and treatment should be carried out at the same time and at the same attention.

XZ-C proposes to overcome cancer and to launch the general attack of cancer, namely, the three stages of cancer prevention, cancer control and cancer treatment are at the same time, the three carriages go hand in hand to achieve the goal of reducing cancer incidence, improving cancer cure rate, reducing cancer mortality and prolonging cancer patient survival term. If you only treat cancer without prevention, or heavy treatment with light prevention, you can never overcome cancer because it can't reduce the cancer rate, and the more patients are treated, the more the new patients show up.

Therefore:

XZ-C proposed: "Overcoming cancer and launching the general attack of cancer – cancer prevention, cancer control, cancer treatment at the same attention"

XZ-C proposes to establish an initiative: "Creating an Environmental Protection and Cancer Research Institute" and carrying out a cancer prevention system project

—— *Opening a new era of cancer prevention research and cancer prevention system engineering in the 21st century, conquering cancer is the frontier of science and a worldwide tough problem. Cancer is a human disaster, covering the whole world. People all over the world are eager to hope that one day they can overcome cancer and benefit humanity.*

How to do? How to reduce the incidence of cancer? How to improve the cure rate of cancer? How to reduce cancer mortality? How to prolong the survival of cancer patients? How to improve the quality of life?

Looking back and reflecting on it, for a century, cancer prevention has not paid attention to it, prevention has not paid attention to it, and prevention-oriented health work policy has not been taken seriously and has not been implemented. As a result, the more cancer patients are treated, the higher the incidence rate and the higher the mortality rate are.

At present, the country is implementing the spirit of the 19th National Congress of the Communist Party of China and ensuring the realization of the grand goal of building a well-off society nationwide by 2020. The country is building an innovative country and prospering technological innovation. The National Science and Technology Innovation Conference deepened the institutional reform and decided to enter the ranks of innovative countries in 2020. Its goal is to achieve a major breakthrough in scientific research in key areas, and new achievements in several fields have entered the forefront of the world. The scientific quality of the whole nation has generally improved and entered an innovative country.

This great situation has also created a major opportunity for us to be "conquer cancer" as the direction for our scientific research work, and deeply encouraged me to actively participate and innovate. **I deeply understand that cancer should not only pay attention to treatment, but also pay attention to prevention, in order to stop at the source. The way out for cancer treatment is "three early" (early detection, early diagnosis, early treatment), and the way to fight cancer is prevention.**

What is "ride research"?

This is what I thought, and no one in the literature mentioned it. It is a historic and great pioneering work to build an ecological civilization, protect an ecological environment, build a well-off society, and build an innovative country. It is a great initiative in the present, benefiting the future, seeking health and welfare for hundreds of millions of people, and seeking health and welfare for future generations. . Under this great situation and great opportunities, it has also created good opportunities for research work on cancer prevention and cancer prevention. Bringing up anti-cancer, anti-cancer and cancer-fighting research work, we will surely receive fruitful results, and strive to achieve new achievements in the basics and clinical research of cancer treatment in China, and strive to overcome the key to cancer. Field scientific research has achieved a major breakthrough in originality.

Under the current situation of energy saving, pollution prevention and pollution control, it is conducive to the scientific research and prevention and control of cancer prevention and cancer control. The environment has a great relationship with cancer, energy conservation and emission reduction, pollution reduction and pollution control, and the construction of environmentally friendly society is closely related to the prevention of environmental carcinogenesis. As early as the 1980s, many experts and scholars at home and abroad believed that more than 90% of cancers were caused by environmental factors. Protecting and restoring a good environment is an important part of preventing cancer.

I have been engaged in experimental basic research and clinical medical practice in oncology surgery for half a century. Deeply aware of the purpose of achieving cancer prevention and control, it must be done by the government, experts, scholars, the masses to participate, the mobilization of the whole people, and the participation of thousands of families. At present, China is building an innovative country and building a well-off society. It is precisely the work of the government, the masses, the mobilization of the whole people, and the participation of thousands of families. It will certainly improve the awareness of cancer prevention among the people and achieve the role of cancer prevention and cancer control. Our province and our city have significantly reduced the incidence of cancer.

I would like to suggest:

in the construction of a well-off society and rural urbanization work, it is to formulate cancer prevention and anti-cancer programs, formulate cancer prevention and anti-cancer measures, and formulate plans and measures for cancer prevention and control in the new towns and the new rural areas. It is to carry out cancer prevention and cancer control work. It is to adhere to the road of innovation in cancer prevention and cancer control with Chinese

characteristics, overcome cancer, build a well-off society, and be healthy and healthy.

It is to conduct research work and measures of cancer control and cancer prevention and cancer control. The purpose is to make people's health, stay away from cancer, and reduce the incidence of cancer in China, our province and our city.

First

Building a well-off society is conducive to the scientific research on cancer prevention and cancer control and its prevention and control work.

In order to build a well-off society, while building a new social countryside and the new towns, it should simultaneously carry out cancer prevention work, so that in the well-off society, everyone can improve their knowledge of cancer prevention and anti-cancer, and everyone is healthy and far from cancer. *How can a well-off society, a new social countryside, and a new town carry out cancer prevention and anti-cancer? Cancer prevention should be carried out from the aspects of clothing, food, housing and transportation and from improving the living environment and improving the living habits, there is basic knowledge in this area. Most cancers can be avoided and can be prevented.*

In order to carry out cancer prevention and cancer control work, we should first understand and study the relationship between environment and cancer:

(1) Relationship between the environment and cancer

1). Air pollution and cancer

Humans have developed tons of tons of coal, oil and natural gas as fuel and energy, such as thermal power or firepower generation, smelting steel, automobiles and aircraft, constantly polluting a large amount of tar, kerosene, dust and other harmful gases into the atmosphere to pollute the environment. Air pollution can cause many diseases, the most serious is lung cancer.

2). water pollution and cancer

The pollution of water quality is mainly caused by industrial and agricultural production and urban sewage.

3). Soil pollution, food chain and cancer

Large-scale industrial and agricultural production activities of human beings have injected a large amount of industrial waste water slag and pesticides and fertilizers into the soil, which has deteriorated soil quality and threatened human health. It is also a carcinogenic factor.

China's industrial development has made great contributions to China's economic development. However, while industrial development has brought about environmental pollution problems, it is necessary to actively take measures to strictly control pollution control.

Building a resource-saving and environment-friendly society are placed in a prominent position in the industrialization and modernization development strategy, are implemented to each unit, each family. Building an environment-friendly society is an important action to highlight environmental protection and is a top priority for curbing environmental degradation.

At present, we are conducting a comprehensive supporting experiment for resource-saving and environment-friendly society construction to save energy, reduce emissions, and discharge sewage. This policy has a great correlation with work and cancer prevention and control work because:

(1). **In the process of searching for the cause and occurrence of cancer, human beings have conducted extensive exploration and accumulated a wealth of knowledge. <u>The most prominent of these is the discovery that more than 90% of cancers are caused or closely related to environmental factors</u>.**

At present, our province and our city are carrying out energy conservation and emission reduction, pollution reduction and pollution control, and environmental pollution control. It will greatly reduce pollutants and carcinogens in air, water and food. Therefore, it has a great correlation with prevention cancer and cancer control.

(2). The United Nations Health Organization proposes **that 1/3 of cancers can be prevented; one third of cancers can be cured by early treatment; one third of cancers can alleviate symptoms and prolong life through effective treatment. Therefore, cancer can be considered preventable.**

The importance of cancer prevention must be fully understood. Environmental factors and inappropriate social behavior are the most important pathogenic factors that can be avoided or interfered with.

Through energy conservation, pollution prevention, pollution control, people have improved their health knowledge, and the effective interventions for carcinogenic factors such as environmental pollution will definitely reduce the incidence of related cancers.

(3).Environmental pollution can increase the incidence of cancer:

I deeply understand:

Why should we engage in energy-saving and emission-reduction and environmentally friendly "two-type society"?

It is because with the development of modern industrialization, a large amount of energy consumption, a large number of production, in the course of life, a large amount of harmful gases such as tar, soot, dust, etc. are discharged into the atmosphere around the clock, atmospheric pollution, water pollution, soil pollution, Food pollution and occupational carcinogens have soared. The incidence and mortality of lung cancer in western developed countries have increased rapidly in recent decades. For example, the mortality rate of lung cancer in the United Kingdom was 10/10 million in 1930, and it was as high as 120.3/100,000 in 1975, a 12-fold increase in 45 years. In the United States from 1934 to 1974, the mortality rate of **male lung cancer** increased from 3.0/100,000 to 54.5/100,000, an increase of 17 times. The above data is amazing. If energy conservation and emission reduction are not carried out, a large amount of emissions will be polluted, which will greatly damage human health and promote the rapid growth of cancer incidence and mortality. <u>Energy conservation and emission reduction is for the healthy development of industrialization and continues to leap.</u>

It is because environmental pollution is harmful to society and harmful to human life. Improving the environment, preventing pollution, and safeguarding health will help build a healthy, happy, harmonious and environment-friendly society.

So, what is the danger of environmental pollution?

What is most fearful is that environmental pollutants contain many carcinogens, which promotes the rise of cancer incidence. For example, the damage of nuclear power plants in Japan has led to a significant increase in the concentration of nuclear radioactive materials in the surrounding air, water, soil, and food, which has led to an increase in the incidence of leukemia and cancer, which not only jeopardizes contemporary but also jeopardizes future generations.

(4). The Harm of environmental pollution:

As it is all known, the harmfulness of environmental pollution is:

1)), it damages to people's lives; radiation, nuclear radiation, bacteria, viruses, harmful chemical poisons, air pollution, water pollution, soil pollution, food pollution not only damage people's lives and health, but also lead to an increasing incidence of human cancer;

2)), it is causing epidemic spread of infectious diseases;

3)), A large number of polluting chemicals, harmful gases, harmful water sources, fertilizers, and pesticides can cause cancer and mutation, causing high risk of cancer and high incidence.

Therefore, to reduce the incidence of cancer, we must improve the environment, prevent and control pollution, and build an environment-friendly society and a harmonious society.

The anti-cancer strategy should be cancer prevention and cancer control, using Class I prevention, Class II prevention, and Class III prevention. I deeply believe that the current pollution prevention and pollution control is a level I prevention, and it is a fundamental cancer prevention measure. Under the leadership of the government, the masses have mobilized the mass prevention measures.

Second

It is recommended to carry out the medical scientific research and cancer prevention and treatment work for cancer prevention and cancer control while creating a well-off society.

1). It is believed that the current energy-saving emission reduction, pollution prevention and pollution **control is a level I prevention cancer prevention and cancer control**. Its purpose and effect can achieve the level I prevention of cancer. This is a great opportunity for a once-in-a-lifetime event. It is imperative to seize this great opportunity that is once in a lifetime. I have been engaged in experimental basic research and clinical medical practice of oncology surgery for half a century. I know that in order to achieve the goal of cancer prevention and control, it must be led by the government, experts, scholars, the masses, the mobilization of the whole people, and the work of thousands of households. It will definitely improve the awareness of cancer prevention among the people, achieve the effect of preventing cancer and cancer, and receive the effect of reducing the incidence of cancer in our province and the city.

2). Carrying out cancer prevention and cancer control. At present, there is no practical and feasible way. We must not only proceed from the technical and tactical aspects, but must focus on the strategy and implement the people-oriented principle, and fundamentally emphasize the harmony between people and the environment. Scientific research must be carried out to explore and innovate. Science is an endless frontier, and scientific research is endless. With the vision of development, looking forward, under the guidance of the scientific concept of development, conducting scientific research on energy conservation, pollution prevention, treatment and prevention of cancer, cancer control, and reduction of cancer incidence, there will be many that are still unknown. New knowledge, even original innovative research results and the creation of new disciplines, new industries.

I deeply understand this policy and work: energy saving, pollution prevention, pollution control, which itself contains the significance and effect of anti-cancer and cancer control. However, it is not really pointed out. I would like to make a suggestion. I suggest that the province and the city clearly point out that while building a well-off society, we will carry out some research on cancer control and prevention and formulate cancer control plans and measures. Raising people's awareness of cancer prevention is also an innovation, and it is also a pioneering work for the benefit of the country and the people.

To raise people's awareness of cancer prevention, it must have a purpose to build a well-off society. This is the vital interest in caring for the health of the people. It will surely be supported and grateful by the people of the province, and will be more serious and active in energy conservation and emission reduction and in

the prevention of pollution and pollution control, cancer prevention and cancer control work.

Cancer prevention and anti-cancer work is a tough hard bone, but it should continue to linger. **Because cancer is a major hazard to humans, cancer prevention and anti-cancer are human careers and responsibility.** It is deeply understood that if it would like to do this work well, it is impossible to rely on the personal efforts of experts and scholars. It must be mobilized by the government and mobilized by the whole people before it can be done. It is necessary to get out of the innovation road of cancer prevention and anti-cancer with Chinese characteristics. I am convinced that while building a well-off society, we will carry out prevention and treatment plans of cancer prevention and anti-cancer as well as cancer prevention measures for group prevention and group control. The cancer incidence and mortality rate of our province and my Wuhan city circle (8+1) will definitely drop significantly.

Third

To adhere to Chinese characteristics to build a well-off society and at the same time to explore the innovative roads to prevent cancer and to control cancer

China's energy conservation and emission reduction, pollution prevention and pollution control, building a well-off society, through efforts, will inevitably achieve great results in reducing the incidence of cancer. This is the characteristic of prevention cancer and cancer control in socialist countries. This is an innovative road for building a well-off society with Chinese characteristics to prevent cancer and control cancer. After 3-5 years of successful work experience, it can expand and introduce this innovation road of that building a well-off society in our province and the city combines the prevention of cancer and cancer control with Chinese characteristics to the whole country and pushed to the world.

Why is it cancer prevention and cancer control here? It is because more than 90% of cancers are related to environmental pollution. It can effectively prevent the cancer occurrence and control the cancer development if it is to improve environmental pollution. If pollution is controlled, it may prevent or control carcinogens from entering the body. Both the improvement of the environment and the improvement of the small environment can reduce, prevent or control the effects of environmental carcinogens entering the human body or environmental carcinogens on the human body.

At present, it is a great situation to carry out energy conservation and emission reduction. It is also a great opportunity to carry out research on anti-cancer and cancer control by "taking a ride on scientific research". It is a great opportunity for a rare event. In the past, it was also realized that anti-cancer is important, but I can only talk about it on paper and make publicity. Now, under the concrete practice of building a well-off society, prevention of cancer and cancer control can make a big difference. It can be achieved to reduce the incidence of cancer in our province and the city.

It is everyone's responsibility to prevent cancer and control cancer. Medical workers should recognize the burden of their shoulders. Under this great situation, we will do a good job in preventing cancer, improve people's awareness of cancer prevention, change some living habits, improve some living environment, be environmentally friendly, and live in harmony. People will be healthy, happy, long-lived and far from cancer.

In order to do this work, we have created the Wuhan Anti-Cancer Research Society, and established a professional committee for anti-cancer metastasis and recurrence, and organized more experts, scholars and people with lofty ideals to carry out medical scientific research on cancer prevention and control. Every effort will be made to open up the work of benefiting the country and the people.

Therefore, while doing a good job in energy conservation and emission reduction, pollution prevention and pollution control, and building a well-off society, I would like to make the following recommendations:

To carry out "riding in research", carry out research on cancer prevention and control, and formulate cancer planning and measures (see Annex 2); to improve environmental pollution, and to eliminate or avoid some environmental carcinogenic risk factors, to strengthen publicity education on cancer prevention, to popularize cancer prevention knowledge, to establish a sound monitoring system, to monitor high-risk groups, and the government-led and the experts and the scholars and the national participate. The whole people improve their awareness of cancer prevention. It is convinced that the great results of the double harvest with being environmentally friendly and reducing the incidence of cancer in the Wuhan metropolitan area will be achieved.

How to build a well-off society and how to implement specific measures, strategies, policies, steps and programs of conquering cancer in building a well-off society. **Government guidance is the key. The development of personnel training is also key.**

Talent must *have modern life science knowledge. There must be modern scientific knowledge and technology for the prevention and treatment of cancer occurrence and development; it must have cancer prevention, anti-cancer knowledge and technology; it must also have environmental science knowledge and technology.* At present, universities have environmental colleges and life sciences colleges. But it needs to have modern high-tech high-level talents with life science knowledge and skills and knowledge and skills in environmental science **make vigorously growth or development or establishment or flourish of the well-off society cancer prevention, anti-cancer, pollution prevention, pollution control, the experimental research on science and technology innovation into the laboratories of colleges and universities. The experimental talents with strong hands-on ability can make the laboratory of colleges and universities in China develop vigorously.**

It is deeply understood that while building a well-off society, it will be to engage in a "ride-taking scientific research" which is to prevent cancer and to control cancer while it is building a well-off society and carrying out preventing cancer and controlling cancer.

It may be a new breakthrough in building a well-off society, and it will also add new content for innovating Wuhan, innovating Hubei, and innovating China for the construction of a national central city.

Chapter 16

The great correlation between building a resource-saving and environment-friendly society and cancer prevention and cancer control

First

Building environmentally friendly enterprises and strengthening social responsibility are important measures to curb environmental degradation, Is "bottleneck" to crack the resource environment, and is imperative to curb environmental degradation.

Three major far-reaching changes have taken place in the world since the industrial revolution. Or there have been three major and far-reaching changes in the world:

1. **It is a tremendous increase in social productivity and an unprecedented expansion of the scale of the economy. The economy has grown nearly a hundredfold, creating unprecedented material wealth, and thus rapidly advancing the process of human civilization;**

2. The population is exploding. The world's population has quadrupled in the 20th century. It has reached 6.3 billion and continues to increase at an annual rate of about 90 million;

3. **Due** to the excessive development and consumption of natural resources, massive emissions of pollutants, lead to global resource shortages, environmental pollution and ecological damage. The environmental problems brought about by industrialization have not only become problems of a region and a country but also become global problems, such as climate warming, destruction of the ozone layer, sharp decline in biodiversity, land degradation and desertification, acid

rain and so on. These problems have forced humans to reflect on the traditional development model at the expense of special resources and the environment, and explore new development and management models.

At present, due to the long-term inheritance of traditional industrial civilization, in some places, the wealth of material and wealth has been brought about by the rapid economic growth. **But indiscriminately consume natural resources and pollute the environment, has greatly restricted the economic and social development, Environment and resources and scarcity as the basic elements of production, it has become a "bottleneck" for many local developments. Or some places have brought wealth of material and wealth due to rapid economic growth, but the production methods that consume natural resources and pollute the environment unrestrained have already made the economy and society Development has been greatly constrained, and the environment and resources and scarcity as the basic elements of production have become the "bottleneck" for development in many places.**

The report of the 17th National Congress of the Communist Party of China or the report of the Party's 17th National Congress pointed out: "It is necessary or imperative to place to put a resource-conserving and environment-friendly society in a prominent position in the industrialization and modernization development strategy and implement it in every unit and every family." Building environmentally-friendly enterprises is an important action to implement the scientific development concept, build an environment-friendly society, and realize the historic transformation of environmental protection from each unit and from the micro level. It is an inevitable choice for enterprises to enhance their social responsibilities and maximize their value. It is an urgent task to crack the "bottleneck" of the resource environment and curb the deterioration of the environment.

The national environmental protection department attaches great importance to the creation of environmentally friendly enterprises. Since 2003, the establishment of national environmentally friendly enterprises has been carried out. Local environmental protection departments at all levels and many enterprises have responded positively. On November 12, 2004, the first batch of national environmentally friendly enterprises awarding ceremony were organized. Vice Premier Zeng Peiyan sent a congratulatory letter: "Creating a 'national environmentally friendly enterprise' is a concrete action to implement the scientific development concept. It has positive significance for promoting harmony or promoting the harmonious development between man and nature." On December 9, 2006, the **"National Environmentally Friendly Enterprise" naming conf**erence was held in Beijing.

After more than three years of establishment, after strict examination, from the more than 400 enterprises recommended by the provinces, the former State Environmental Protection Administration named 44 national environmentally friendly enterprises, distributed in 18 provinces, municipalities and autonomous regions across the country involving more than a dozen industries such as chemical, petroleum, building materials, energy, steel and automobiles. Practice has proved that the national environmentally friendly enterprises are becoming the model and example/ excellent demonstration for China's industrial enterprises to implement the scientific development concept, **the leader of taking the new industrialization roads and practicing circular economy, the shepherd of building the resource-saving and environment-friendly society, and promoting society and the pioneer or/and vanguard that promotes the sound and rapid or good and fast development of the social economy.**

In order to deeply recommend the creation of environmentally friendly companies, since December 2006, the former State Environmental Protection Administration and the Swedish Environmental Protection Agency jointly launched the "Promoting China's Environmentally Friendly Enterprise Capacity Building Project". The project management and implementation parties respectively are the former State Environmental Protection Administration and the Swedish Environmental Protection Agency. The project office is located in Project 2 of the Office of Foreign Economic Cooperation of the Ministry of Environmental Protection (formerly the State Environmental Protection Administration). The technical support units of the project are the Environmental Planning Institute of the Ministry of Environmental Protection, the Environmental Development Center of the Ministry of Environmental Protection, and the Environmental Impact Assessment Research Center. The Chinese experts of the project include personnel from the Environmental Planning Institute and the Environmental Development Center of the Ministry of Environmental Protection and experts from provincial environmental research institutions.

During the two-year period, through research, investigation, organizing seminars, developing training, and other forms, learning Swedish's advanced experience and technical methods in corporate environmental management, understanding the effective environmental incentives and instruments used in the industrialization process in Sweden and Europe, it has been completion of the revision of the indicators for the creation of environmentally friendly enterprises suitable for China's national conditions, and it has formulated and improved various preferential policies and incentive policies, strengthened the capacity of the national environmental protection department and its related technical departments to use various policy instruments and control of industrial environmental pollution. Through related work, it has been training a group of researchers who have mastered new environmental management techniques and researchers in corporate environmental management policies, and with a point to bring the area, the realization of the concept of environmental friendliness is mainly focused on the main unemployed, Strengthen the technical support ability for enterprise creation work.

After more than two years of research, investigation and practice, the project team completed various tasks. In the end, good results were achieved and the expected goals were achieved. In order to sum up experience and strengthen communication, the project team based on research, study and discussion during the two-year period has been refining and writing the Research Report on Promoting China's Environmentally Friendly Enterprise Capacity Building Project.

On this basis, in order to better enable the readers to understand and share the project results, **we have written this report into the book "Industrial Pollution Control and Environmentally Friendly Enterprises".**

The book is divided into six chapters. There are:

Chapter 1, China's industrial development and environmental pollution, introduces China's industrial development and pollution emissions.

Chapter 2, China's existing industrial pollution prevention measures and assessments, reviews and summarizes China's industrial pollution control processes and means, and evaluates major industrial pollution control methods.

Chapter 3, China's environmentally friendly enterprise evaluation index system, describes and analyzes the environmentally friendly enterprise evaluation index system implemented at that time, and finds out the existing problems.

Chapter 4, China Environmental Friendly Enterprise Creation Practice, conducted a simple analysis of China's environmental management system, introduced China's environmentally friendly enterprise creation project, conducted an in-depth analysis of its management system, and identified existing problems.

Chapter 5, Swedish Experience in Industrial Pollution Control, introduces the main experience of industrial pollution control in Sweden, focusing on environmental legislation, economic instruments, green procurement and public participation.

Chapter 6, conclusions and policy recommendations, draws conclusions on China's industrial pollution control, environmentally friendly enterprise creation and Swedish experience, and proposed policy recommendations from two aspects of China's industrial pollution control and environmentally friendly enterprises.

The meaning or connotation of the Environmentally friendly enterprise is the following:

"Environmentally friendly enterprises" are enterprises that are friendly to the natural ecological environment and develop harmoniously with the society. The environmentally friendly companies should achieve excellent environmental performance, which is manifested in three aspects:

1). **The environment is law-abiding and does not cause obvious damage to the surrounding natural ecology and social environment;**

2). **Continuously improve environmental management to maximize the reduction of environmental pollution while developing the economy;**

3). **Further assume the social responsibility of environmental protection and promote the improvement of regional environmental quality.**

The environmentally friendly companies is the core component of "harmonious and friendly society". That is to say, the enterprise realizes the mutual benefit and common development of man and nature, industrial development and environmental protection, and the enterprise and surrounding communities in the development.

The environmentally friendly companies are the core component of an environmentally friendly society. National environmentally friendly enterprises are the highest affirmation of China's environmental performance. Creating a national environmentally friendly company is China's corporate incentive mechanism based on international advanced experience and focusing on national conditions, or the establishment of a national environmentally friendly enterprise is the industry incentive mechanism of China with reference to international advanced experience and focusing on national conditions. Its purpose is to establish a new industrialization path by setting up outstanding enterprises and driving more enterprises **to take** advantage of high technology content, good economic returns, low resource consumption, less environmental pollution, and full utilization of human resources. In short, the creation work adopts the form of government guidance and enterprise voluntary, stimulating excellent enterprises to achieve better environmental performance.

In order to promote the "three historic changes" in environmental protection and achieve sound and rapid economic development, China should also comprehensively adopt various means and measures in industrial pollution control and the creation of environmentally friendly enterprises, not only must there be laws and regulations and administrative means, but also the application of market economic means and voluntary means should be increased. At the same time, Chinese companies should learn from Swedish companies' social responsibility. While gaining economic benefits, we should pursue the maximization of social and environmental benefits, and even start with the pursuit of social responsibility, develop and expand enterprises in the service society, and improve economic efficiency. l pollution control and the creation of environmentally friendly enterprises, not only with laws and regulations. Administrative means, but also should increase the application of market economy means and voluntary means.

Second

The suggestions on accelerating the construction of environmentally friendly enterprises in our country

At present or currently, due to the long-term adherence to the traditional industrial civilization, although some places have brought wealth of material and wealth due to the rapid economic growth. However, the unconstrained consumption of natural resources and pollution of the environment has greatly restricted the development of the economy and society. **The lack of environment and resources as the basic elements of production has become a "bottleneck" for many local developments. The report of the 17th National Congress indicated:**

"It is imperative to put a resource-conserving and environment-friendly society in a prominent position in the industrialization and modernization development strategy and implement it in every unit and every family." It is the implementation of science from each unit and micro level. The development

concept, the construction of an environment-friendly society, and the important actions to realize the historical transformation of environmental protection are the inevitable choices for enterprises to enhance their social responsibilities and maximize their value. They are the urgent task of cracking the bottleneck of the resource environment and curbing the deterioration of the environment.

The State Environmental Protection Administration attaches great importance to the creation of environmentally friendly enterprises. Since 2003, the establishment of national environmentally friendly enterprises has been carried out, and local environmental protection departments and many enterprises have responded positively. On November 12, 2004, the first batch of national environmentally friendly enterprises awarding ceremony was held. Vice Premier Zeng Peiyan sent a congratulatory letter: "Creating a 'national environmentally friendly enterprise' is a concrete action to implement the scientific development concept and has positive significance for promoting the harmonious development of man and nature."

On December 9, 2006, the "National Environmentally Friendly Enterprise" naming conference was held in Beijing. Through more than three years of creation work, the economy has been strictly examined. Among the more than 400 enterprises recommended by the provinces, the former State Environmental Protection Administration has named 38 national environmentally friendly enterprises, which are distributed in 18 provinces, municipalities and districts across the country, involving chemical industry including more than a dozen industries such as petroleum, building materials, energy, steel and automobiles.

In order to further promote the creation of environmentally friendly enterprises, since December 2006, the State Environmental Protection Administration and the Swedish Environmental Protection Agency have jointly launched the "Recommended Environmentally Friendly Enterprise Capacity Building Project." During the two-year project period through the study and investigation seminars and other forms, learning Swedish advanced experience in business management, and understanding the effective environmental incentives and means adopted by Sweden and even Europe in the process of industrialization, <u>it was to complete the revision of environmentally friendly enterprises that are suitable for China's national conditions, and improve each Preferential policies and incentives to strengthen the ability of the State Environmental Protection Administration and its related technical departments to use various policy instruments and control of industrial environmental pollution.</u>

The project will also through the pilot work or experimental work to train a group of technical personnel who have mastered the new environmental management techniques, and to achieve or to realize the key points of environmentally friendly concepts in many major industries and to strengthen the technical support for the creation of enterprises.

Third

To adhere to take the innovative road of prevention cancer and cancer control with Chinese characteristics

Through the efforts China's energy conservation and emission reduction, pollution prevention and pollution control, building a well-off society will inevitably achieve great results in reducing the incidence of cancer. This is the characteristic of prevention cancer and cancer control in socialist countries. This is an innovative road for building a well-off society with Chinese characteristics to prevent cancer and control cancer. After 3-5 years of successful work experience, we pushed the new road of building the energy-saving emission reduction, pollution prevention and treatment pollution combined with prevention and control, cancer control, which it is Chinese characteristics of cancer prevention, cancer control into the whole country and pushed to the world.

Why is it to put forward "cancer prevention and cancer control" here?

Because more than 90% of cancers are related to environmental pollution and improve environmental pollution, there may be a role in preventing cancer and controlling cancer.

If pollution is controlled, it may prevent or control carcinogens from entering the body. Both the improvement of the environment and the improvement of the small environment can reduce, prevent or control the effects of environmental carcinogens entering the human body or environmental carcinogens on the human body.

At present, it is a great situation for energy conservation and emission reduction, and a great opportunity to carry out research work on cancer prevention and cancer control is a golden opportunity. In the past, I also realized that prevention cancer is important, but I can only talk about it on paper and make publicity.

Now, under the specific practice of energy saving, pollution prevention and pollution control, prevention cancer and cancer control can make a big difference. It can be achieved to reduce the incidence of cancer in our province and city. It is everyone's responsibility to prevent cancer and control cancer. Medical workers should recognize the burden of their shoulders. Under this great situation, we will do a good job in preventing cancer, improve people's awareness of cancer prevention, change some living habits, improve some living environment, be environmentally friendly, and live in harmony. People will be healthy, happy, long-lived and far from cancer.

In order to do this work, we have created the Wuhan anti-Cancer Research Society, and established a professional committee for anti-cancer metastasis and recurrence, and organized more experts, scholars and people with lofty ideals to carry out medical scientific research on cancer prevention and control. Every effort will be made to open up the work of benefiting the country and the people.

Appendix A

The Major Progress in Cancer Research in the Past 100 Years

In April 2007, the American Association for Cancer Research (AACR) invited the famous oncologists around the world to review the history of cancer research. The summary is as follows:

A Great Progress in Study on Tumor over 100 Years

In Apr. 2007, American Association for Cancer Research (AACR) invited the famous tumor scholars all over the world to review the history of study on tumor, which is now briefly extracted as follows:

1907	It was discovered that the solar exposure was related to skin cancer and later it was proven by the animal model that sunlight and ultraviolet radiation could lead to skin cancer.
1908	The tumor was successfully transferred to another animal from one animal with cell-free concentrate. Fowl leukosis, lymphadenoma and sarcomata model was established and this discovery was later deemed as the evidence that the filterable taddecheese would lead to tumor.
1915	The first animal model of chemical-induced tumor was established. Repeated painting of tar could produce skin tumor on rabbit.
1916	It was discovered that the incidence of breast carcinoma on mice could be reduced after removal of the ovary, indicating ovarian hormone may lead to breast carcinoma.
1924	It was discovered by the study on metabolism that the tumor was manifested as anoxia metabolism.
1928	It was deemed that "gene mutation was the basic reason of producing the carcinoma".

1928   The cells of cervical carcinoma were observed through the exuviation smear of vagina. The method of detecting the <u>suspected</u> patient with cervical carcinoma with smear method was widely accepted by the people step by step and used as the effective detection and prevention method of the cancer until Pap smear method was applied in 1960.

1928   It was discovered that X-ray could lead to mutation. X–ray could lead to the gene mutation of common fruit fly, which was the theoretical basis of the carcinogen participation in tumorigensis.

1930   Benzopyrene, the first chemical carcinogen was separated form the coal tar and the carcinogenesis of these chemical constituents was made clear through the animal model experiment.

1932   The artificial hormone was injected to induce the breast carcinoma of mice.

1937   The leucocythemia of the mouse was transfected through transplantation of the single leukemic cell.

1938   It was discovered through study that chemical carcinogenesis process was divided into two different stages including excitation stage and promotion stage.

1939   The transplanted animal tumor could produce the blood vessel. The tumor transplanted on the ears of the rabbit could produce the vascular net, which was the early evidence of formation of the blood vessel, later the anti- angiogenesis became one target of the treatment of tumor.

1940   The heat control could reduce the incidence of tumor on the mice.

1941   The hormone dependence of prostatic carcinoma was proven. Physical castration therapy and estrogen chemical castration therapy could reduce tumor load of the metastatic prostatic carcinoma while the androgen injected could promote the metastasis.

1946   The nitrogen mustard was firstly used for tumor chemotherapy. It was observed that after contacting the nitrogen mustard, the soldiers in time of war could meet with reduction of white blood cells, enlightening the people on using the nitrogen mustard for tumor chemotherapy and the intravenously injected nitrogen mustard for treating the lymphadenoma and leukemia that could not be controlled by radiotherapy, in this way, the disease was remitted for several months. The nitrogen mustard was used for tumor treatment initially in 1949.

1948   The first chemotherapy on leukemia of children was successful. The artificial folic acid antagonist was applied to 16 children with leukemia among which 10 patients got a relieving course of 3 months.

1950   It was discovered by the study on epidemiology that smoking was related to pulmonary carcinoma.

1951   The virus spread the leucocythemia of mice. It was discovered by the study that the leucocythemia could be spread through virus from one mouse of one germ line to another mouse of another germ line and spread from one generation to the next generation vertically. Before this, it was deemed by the people that the tumor was a hereditary disease, which laid a foundation for the study on other tumor viruses and of the mice and other species in the future.

1951	Co-60 (^{60} Co) radiation equipment came out.
1951	The ultrasonic detection was firstly used for diagnosis of tumor.
1958	It was proven that the food additive prohibited by the food additive modification organ could induce the occurrence of carcinoma on human or animal.
1959	The leucocythemia induced by the food additive was related to the radioactive dose. It was proven that the radiation could induce the human carcinoma and the natural characteristics of the relation between radioactive dose and effect were also illuminated.
1963	Hodgkin lymphoma was treated with chemical method. In 1960, Hodgkin lymphoma was reported in the Sahara in Africa, which was featured in regional distribution. In those days, it was deemed that it was induced by the virus and the tumor induced by the virus was firstly successfully cured and later it was proven as Epstein virus.
1964	Luther L. Terry, an American surgeon proposed that the smoking was related to the pulmonary carcinoma.
1969	The tumor was successfully transplanted to the nude mice of different germ line.
1970	The multi-drug resistance of cell line was proposed. The multi-drug resistance of cell toxicant was the main reason of failure of chemotherapy.
1971	The growth of tumor depended on the regenerative blood vessel. Since the discovery of the tumor metastasis, it had been known that the tumor could not grow in the tissue without blood vessel. It was shown by the continuous experiments that the tumor growth factor could promote the generation of the new blood vessel and the growth of the tumor. Finally, these gene factors offered the basis for the molecular-targeted therapy of tumor.
1971	President Nixon presented an anti-cancer slogan in the address in UN.
1972	The paclitaxel, the extract from the natural vegetables could be used for chemotherapy.
1976	The virus oncogene existed in the related proto-oncogene in the normal cells. Through hybridzation technique (before DNA precedence ordering), it was discovered by the researcher that the virus oncogene existed in the chicken's cells, and so did in other families (such as mice and human kind) through study.
1977	Tamoxifen was approved for the clinical treatment of breast carcinoma.
1978	Nitrosamine in the tobacco leaf was proven as the cancerogenous substance in the cigarette. The nitrosamine derived from nicotia in the cigarette was discovered in the animal model that it was cancerogenous and soon later it was proven to be related to pulmonary carcinoma and oral carcinoma of human being.
1979	p53 gene was discovered, which was initially deemed as a kind of oncogene and finally proven as a kind of anti-oncogene by the subsequent study.

1979   Discovery of protein-tyrosine kinase (PTK) and illumination of the tyrosine phosphorylation process. One new kind of protein-tyrosine kinase (PTK) was discovered, which was related to gene products of T antigenic conversion protein and rous sarcoma virus in the polyoma virus. This discovery told us that the maladjustment of tyrosine phosphorylation process catalyzed by activated protein-tyrosine kinase could result in the malignant transformation of cells. In the following several years, the pathogenic protein-tyrosine kinase depressant was approved for clinical treatment.

1980   The degradation of peripheral collagen of the tumor impelled the metastasis of tumor. In the tumor metastasis process, it was necessary for the cancer cells to break through the epithelial layer and the true skin layer so as to invade the circulating system. It was proven by the study that tumor cells could excrete collagenase so as to degrade the peripheral collagen while the cell strains with relatively high excretion level of collagenase would be metastatic more easily.

1980   The prostate specific antigen (PSA) was discovered. Detection of PSA level in the body is the first kind of routine detection method to screen and prevent the carcinoma of prostate with tumor markers through assessing the risks of suffering the carcinoma of prostate.

1980   The importance of DNA methylation in the occurrence and development of carcinoma was revealed.

1982   The primary oncogene concept was launched. The conclusion that the oncogene in the normal cell genome could meet with variance and carcinomatosis was made through combination of the previous findings.

1982   The helicobacter pylori (Hp) was separated from the gastric ulcer of human. It was indicated by the findings over the past 10 years that the virus was cancerogenous, however, it was accepted by the people after several years that the infection of Hp would lead to the gastric ulcer while the continual Hp infection and inflammation would result in canceration.

1983   Papilloma viral infection of human was one of the pathogenic factors of cervical carcinoma. Type 16 and 18 papillomavirus of human separated from the biopsy specimen was proven to be related to the height of cervical carcinoma. This discovery would encourage the people to research, develop and use the corresponding bacterin to prevent the cervical carcinoma.

1983   American Academy of Science issued the report named "Diet, Nutrition and Carcinoma" and proposed American Association of Carcinoma to guide the healthy diet of the public so as to reduce the incidence of the carcinoma.

1990   National Institutes of Health and Department of Energy officially launched the human genome project.

1991   The specific variance of p53 gene in the hepatic carcinoma was related to the environmental carcinogen, namely aflatoxin.

1994   The carcinoma originated from the normal cells that could be transformed into cancer cells and it was shown by the survey that the stem cells in the normal tissue with clear source was most possible to develop into the cancer cells in the process of renovation.

2004   The bacterin for anti human papillomavirus (HPV) could prevent the cervical carcinoma. The type of the most common carcinogenic human papillomavirus that the bacterin can prevent mainly included HPV16 and HPV18, which could prevent 70% of the cervical carcinoma all over the world.

Chapter 17

XZ-C proposes:

Cancer is a human disaster, the scientific research work of cancer prevention cannot walk slowly, and it should run forward to save the dead and help wounded

XZ-C proposed: the scientific research work for cancer prevention can not walk slowly and it should run ahead and go forward, save the dead and help the wounded

The White Paper on the Status of Cancer Treatment

- Worldwide cancer incidence

- Worldwide cancer mortality

- Status of 5-year survival rates of cancer in all of the world

White paper on the status of cancer treatment

(1) Cancer incidence worldwide

(2) Death rate of cancer patients worldwide

(3) The current status of cancer 5-year survival rate in all of the world

White paper on the status of cancer treatment

XZ-C

Cancer is a disaster for all mankind. It must fight globally and the people of the world will work together.

Conquering cancer and launching a general attack is an unprecedented event for the benefit of mankind.

First

XZ-C proposed:

Cancer scientific research work cannot walk slowly, should run ahead, save the wounded

Why did I propose to overcome cancer and launch a general attack?

It is that I have been working on the series of ideas and design research for cancer for 5-6 years because. We have made a whole set of basic ideas and designs, plans and blueprints to overcome cancer. In the 38th chapter of the monograph "New Concepts and New Methods of Cancer Treatment" published in 2011, the chapter "The strategic thinking and recommendations for cancer prevention" is proposed in this chapter, and the "Total Attack on Cancer Attack" is proposed.

Later, in 2013, it was proposed "To build a comprehensive design for the Cancer Science City." In August 2013, it was first proposed internationally: "XZ-C Scientific Research Plan for Overcoming the General Attack of Cancer." In July 2015, it was proposed and named "Dawning C-type Plan", which proposed "to overcome the general attack of cancer" and "to build a science city to overcome cancer." This work is being reported and requested to be implemented.

Conquering cancer and launching the general attack of cancer is an unprecedented work of humanity. It is necessary to personally create experience and practice it personally.

About 8550 people in China are diagnosed with cancer every day, and 6 people are diagnosed with cancer every minute. Therefore, research and research work to overcome the general attack of cancer, can not walk slowly, should run forward, save the wounded.

Second

XZ-C proposes:

Cancer is a disaster for all mankind, it must fight with the world, and the people of the world will work together.

1. The disaster of cancer covers the whole world (Figure 1.1)

Worldwide cancer incidence

Publication on the incidence of cancer in five continents. The 2002 volume of the publication, co-published by the International Agency for Research on Cancer (IARC) and the International Association for Cancer Registration, contains data on 50 cancers from 215 populations in 55 countries.

The IARC Special Report brings together findings from a cross-disciplinary panel of experts from different regions of the world on retrospective analysis of different potential carcinogenic risk factors. These panels evaluated a number of factors (including chemical factors, complex mixtures, occupational exposure factors, physical and biological factors, and lifestyle habits) to increase the risk of cancer risk.

Since 1971, the panel has evaluated more than 900 factors, of which nearly 400 have been identified as carcinogenic or potential carcinogenic factors. The full catalogue and classification of these factors is regularly updated and can be found at http://monographs.iarc.fr/. This catalogue is the scientific basis for public health, other disciplines, and national health authorities to take steps to avoid exposure to potential carcinogenic factors.

Worldwide cancer incidence

Cancers around the world, as well as morbidity and mortality in some special organ parts, vary widely. The WHO Cancer Mortality Database and the GLOBOCAN 2002 database provide data on the incidence, prevalence and mortality of 27 different cancers in each country in 2002.

In 2002, there were an estimated 10.9 million new cancer patients (53% male and 47% female), of which 5.1 million occurred in developed countries and 5.8 million occurred in less developed countries.

The number of cancer deaths was 6.7 million (57% male and 43% female), 2.7 million in developed countries and 4 million in less developed countries. An estimated 24.5 million patients are still alive with various cancers (not including skin non-melanoma cancer within 5 years after diagnosis).

According to population standardization, cancer incidence and mortality in different regions of the world are shown in Figure 1.1.

2. The mortality rate and current status of cancer patients worldwide

2017.2.5 Reference message

[Effie, Geneva, February 3rd] The World Health Organization released data on the occasion of the "World Cancer Day" on February 4, saying that 8.8 million people die of cancer every year in the world, and the highest number of deaths from respiratory cancer, up to 1.695 million people a year.

The latest published data is based on 2015 statistics, increasing the number of people dying from cancer each year from an estimated 8.1 million in 2010 to 8.8 million.

The deadliest cancers that are second only to respiratory cancer are liver cancer (788,000 deaths per year), colorectal cancer (774,000), stomach cancer (753,300) and breast cancer (571,000).

The global mortality rate of cancers such as esophageal cancer (415,000), pancreatic cancer (358,000), prostate cancer (334,800), and lymphoma (334,300) are also high.

In terms of gender, there are nearly 5 million male deaths among 8.8 million cancer deaths. For men, the most common types of cancers are respiratory cancer and liver cancer.

For women, the cancer with the highest mortality rate is breast cancer and respiratory cancer.

In terms of regional distribution, the most common cancer cases are in the western Pacific, with respiratory cancer and liver cancer accounting for the highest proportion.

Second only to the Western Pacific is Southeast Asia, where respiratory cancer, oral cancer and throat cancer account for the highest proportion.

In Europe, the most deadly cancer is also respiratory cancer, followed by colorectal cancer.

The disaster of cancer covers the whole world. People all over the world are eager to hope to overcome cancer one day. It is hoped that the state, government, experts, scholars and scientists can find out anti-cancer measures so that people can stay away from cancer.

3. Current status of global cancer 5-year survival rate

Today, the current state of global cancer 5-year survival rate is still at a lower level.

It can be said that there are more and more methods and means available to clinicians today in the clinical diagnosis and treatment of tumors. However, we have to face up to a reality. A large number of clinical epidemiological analysis shows that the maturity and development of the ability and means of diagnosis and treatment, and the improvement of the overall treatment effect of the tumor do not seem to be completely synchronized. According to the data distributed by The American Cancer Society (pictured), the diagnosis and treatment of various malignant tumors has been greatly improved over the past decade, But its 5-year survival rate is still at a lower level.

For example, the 5-year survival rate of global colon cancer in 2004 was 62%. Although the diagnostic techniques and surgical treatment of colon cancer have made great progress, it has only increased to 65% and no breakthrough has been made. The etiology, epidemiological studies and various treatment techniques of liver cancer have been greatly improved, but the current 5-year survival rate is only 18%, which is only 11% higher than 10 years ago. How to improve the prognosis of patients is still a problem that plagues hepatobiliary surgeons. The mortality rate of gastric cancer has been high. Despite the continuous improvement of surgical techniques, the 5-year survival rate of gastric cancer has only increased from 23% 10 years ago to 29%. In addition, the 5-year survival rate of pancreatic cancer is not much changed from 10 years ago, and it is 5%; the 5-year survival rate of esophageal cancer has been maintained at 14%; the 5-year survival rate of breast cancer has been 87% from 10 years ago. Down to the current 79%, cervical cancer has dropped from 71% to 69%, and the 5-year survival rate of lung cancer has dropped from 15% to the current 14%.

Chapter 18

XZ-C proposed:

It should promote scientific research ethics and medicine is benevolence, Setting up the moral is first

XZ-C proposes: It should promote scientific research ethics and medicine is benevolence, Setting up the moral is first

- Scientific Research ethics

- standard

- Basic ethics

XZ-C proposes: scientific research ethics should be advocated, medicine is benevolence, and ethics is the first

"How to achieve the steps, plans, plans, and overall design of conquering cancer and launching the general attack to cancer" which XZ-C has been completed has been published in a book and distributed worldwide.

Why publish English books worldwide? It is because cancer patients cover the whole world, the pollution of industrial and agricultural wastewater, waste residue and waste gas also covers the whole world. Therefore, it is necessary for us to work together globally to conquer cancer and launch the total cancer attack.

The above-mentioned plan, planning, general design, and blueprint for the general attack of cancer can be applied to a country, a province, a state, and a market reference application to conquer cancer and even conquer cancer.

First

How to implement the creation of this anti-cancer research, XZ-C proposed the anti-cancer general design and anti-cancer system engineering

Professor Xu Ze suggested:

(1) All countries, provinces and states should establish anti-cancer research institutes (or institutions) to carry out anti-cancer system projects and carry out

anti-cancer work for their own country, province, state and city. (Because there are a large number of cancer patients in various countries, provinces and cities)

(2) Countries should establish anti-cancer regulations and carry out comprehensive development (some should be legislated)

(3) I will use this project to recommend the World Health Organization to hold an anti-cancer campaign, with the goal of reducing the incidence of cancer. Conquering cancer is a frontier of science and a worldwide problem. Cancer is a human disaster, covering the whole world. People all over the world are eager to hope that one day they can overcome cancer and benefit mankind.

Professor Xu Ze XZ-C proposed:

(4) Research ethics should be advocated, medicine is benevolence, and ethics is the first

Research ethics:

Products, achievements, and patents should all have ethical standards.

Standard:

The bottom line should be based on standards that do not harm human health. In particular, it must not contain carcinogens.

Basic ethics:

All products, achievements, patents, goods and people are harmless and do not harm people's health, especially for children. Do not contain carcinogens.

(5) XZ-C proposes scientific ethics, and should recommend to WHO that all products, achievements, and patents should be the bottom line of moral standards that do not harm human health, especially the carcinogens. E.g:

1 Women's cosmetics, hair dyes, children's toys... should be tested without carcinogens, without damaging human health

2 house decoration, materials ... should be tested without carcinogens

3 food additives, preservatives, food processing packaging ... should be tested without carcinogens

4 leather products, cloth dyes ... should be tested, no carcinogens

5 The feed of collectively fed pigs is not allowed to contain hormones, auxins, vegetarian meat, growth-promoting hormones... all should be tested without carcinogens.

6 group feed chicken, duck feed must not contain hormones, auxin ... should be tested without carcinogens

(6) The health administrative department shall protect and protect health, and shall lead, lead, support, and guide anti-cancer measures, anti-cancer projects, anti-cancer tests, and anti-cancer monitoring.

(7) XZ-C proposes to establish the "Anti-Cancer Research Institute" and carry out anti-cancer system engineering:

• The way in which so many carcinogens or carcinogenic factors should be studied

• These sources of pollutants should be studied and managed to stop at the source

• These carcinogenic mechanisms should be studied, their carcinogenic effects, and environmental factors leading to genetic mutations.

• It is necessary to study the "two-type society" resource-saving and environment-friendly community to prevent cancer (to achieve a beautiful green environment and living environment with beautiful flowers and birds).

Chapter 19

The past and future of oncology development

The past and future of oncology development

- **Prospects and Predictive Assessment for Cancer Treatment**

- **The Past and Future of Cancer Science Development**

First

Analysis of the next research prospects and the prospective assessment of cancer treatment

—— Molecular targeted drugs attract people's attention

—— The prospect of immunomodulatory drugs is gratifying

—— Immunotherapy opens a new era of cancer treatment

—— Biological therapy and combination of Chinese and Western medicine are two effective ways to fight cancer metastasis

- Applying vaccine therapy is human hope

—— The way out for cancer treatment is "three early"

—— The way to fight cancer is prevention

1. Molecular targeted drug therapy attracts attention

The Philadelphia chromosome opened the door to targeted therapy. In 1960 the researchers in Philadelphia, USA found a chromosomal abnormality in patients with chronic myeloid leukemia (CML). A few years later, the researchers found that this was the result of the long arm translocation of chromosomes 9 and 22. Since this chromosomal abnormality was first discovered in Philadelphia (Phiadelphia), it was named the Philadelphia (Ph) chromosome. This chromosome has also become a target for CML targeted therapy marketed 40 years later. In 2001, the first drug that was proven to be resistant to Philadelphia molecular chromosome defects - imatinib.

The target drug trastuzumab, which targets human epidermal growth factor receptor 2 (HER2), is then used to treat HER2-positive breast cancer.

Bevacizumab, which targets VEGF, and cetuximab, which targets EGFR, treats colorectal cancer.

Gefitinib and erlotinib targeting EGFR are used for the treatment of non-small cell lung cancer.

Molecular targeting drugs are cell stabilizers, and most patients cannot achieve complete remission (CR) or partial remission (PR), but rather stable disease and improved quality of life. In addition to gefitinib, erlotinib, imatinib, more need to be combined with chemotherapy drugs.

Molecularly targeted drugs represent a new class of anticancer drugs, and Gleevec is a classic example ***of controlling cancer by inhibiting abnormal molecules that cause cancer without damaging other normal nuclear tissues.*** More and more molecularly targeted drugs have been used in cancer treatment. For example, Rituximab for the treatment of B cell lymphoma, treatment of trastuzumab (Trastuzumab) in the breast, and gefitinib, erlotinib, etc. for treating lung cancer. Targeted therapy brings anti-tumor hope.

2.   The prospect of immunomodulatory drugs is gratifying

Regardless of the complexity of the mechanisms behind cancer, immune suppression is the key to cancer progression. By removing immunosuppressive factors and restoring the recognition of cancer cells by immune system cells, it is effective against cancer.

More and more research evidence shows that by regulating the body's immune system, it is possible to achieve cancer control. Treating tumors by activating the body's anti-tumor immune system is an area that is currently exciting for researchers. The next major breakthrough in cancer is likely to stem from this.

In order to explore the etiology, pathogenesis and pathophysiology of cancer, our laboratory has carried out a series of animal experiments in the laboratory for 4 years, and obtained new findings from the experimental results. New inspirations: thymus atrophy, low immune function is cancer One of the causes and pathogenesis, Xu Ze (Zu Ze) proposed at the International Society of Oncology in 2013: one of the causes of cancer, one of which is thymocyte atrophy, immune function is low, immune surveillance ability is reduced, and immune escape.

Therefore, the treatment principle must be to prevent progressive atrophy of the thymus, promote thymic hyperplasia, protect bone marrow hematopoietic function, improve immune surveillance, and provide experimental basis and theoretical basis for cancer immune regulation treatment.

Through the above four years to explore the basic experimental research on the mechanism of recurrence and metastasis, after three years from the natural medicine Chinese herbal medicine internal laboratory through the cancer-bearing animal experiment

Through the above four years to explore the basic experimental research on the mechanism of recurrence and metastasis, after 3 years from the natural medicine Chinese herbal medicine internal laboratory through the cancer-bearing animal experiment screening, 48 kinds of Chinese medicines were screened out to have a better tumor inhibition rate, and then the cancer-bearing animals were screened to form XZ-C1-10 anti-cancer immune regulation Chinese medicine.

After 20 years of clinical application of more than 12,000 patients with advanced cancer in the oncology clinic, the clinical observation and verification confirmed that the principle of immune regulation and treatment of "protection of Thymus and increase of immune" is reasonable and the curative effect is satisfactory. The application of immunomodulatory Chinese medicine has achieved good results, improved the quality of life, and significantly prolonged the survival period.

3.   ASCO Announces Major Progress in Clinical Oncology in 2015

Immunotherapy opens a new era of cancer treatment

On February 4, 2016, the American Society of Clinical Oncology (ASCO) announced the "2016 Annual Report: ASCO Clinical Oncology Progress" at Capitol Hill, Washington, DC. The report details the global clinical oncology in 2015. The research is summarized and at the same time, the future research direction is forecasted. ASCO rated the 2015 progress as "tumor immunotherapy."

ASCO President Julie M. Vose believes that the most important development in 2015 is the discovery of immunotherapy. She wrote in the foreword: "We are no longer determined by tumor type and staging as we have in the past. Treatment, in the era of precision medicine, we select or exclude treatment based on each patient and tumor genetic data. No other major advances, like immunology can be translated into clinical practice, so ASCO decided that the biggest progress in 2015 is immunotherapy."

The chairman of the committee, Professor Don Dizon, also believes that the annual research results are increasing, but from the perspective of being able to benefit patients, <u>the most important development this year should be immunotherapy.</u>

Second

The past and future of oncology development

(1) Two leap in the treatment of malignant tumors in the last two centuries

Looking back over the past 100 years, human beings have been deeply worried about cancer. So far, there is still no essential understanding of cancer formation, that is, what factors are controlled by normal cell proliferation, and how they lose the control of proliferation and become malignant cells.

In the last two centuries, there have been two leaps in the treatment of malignant tumors:

The first was in 1890, Hals tad proposed the concept of tumor radicalization.

The second time was the integration of chemotherapy into radical surgery (adjuvant chemotherapy or neoadjuvant chemotherapy) in the 1970s.

Since then, malignant tumor treatment has been faltering

Fish is a systemic intravenous route. After half a century, it has not been able to reduce mortality, and it has not stopped recurrence, metastasis, and mortality.

Now we have questioned and reformed the traditional doctrine of the traditional method of administration, and changed the opinions of the traditional methods into intravascular administration of target organs, and combined with the establishment of XZ-C comprehensive treatment and XZ-C immunomodulatory therapy (ie, immunization). Chemotherapy) may help to promote the current state of the past.

(2) <u>In 1971, President Nixon issued the "Anti-Cancer Declaration" and proposed anti-cancer slogans in the UN speech.</u>

In 1971, the US Congress passed a "National Cancer Regulations" and President Nixon issued the "Anti-Cancer Declaration", so he invested a considerable amount of human and financial resources to overcome cancer in one fell swoop.

In December 1971, President Richard Nixon presented an anti-cancer slogan in a message from the United Nations.

42 years have passed, and now Nixon has made a lot of progress, and has made many significant advances in cancer research, such as the discovery of tumor suppressor genes, the advent of monoclonal antibodies, the use of CT and magnetic resonance imaging, and ultrasound and endoscopic techniques. Improvement, innovation of various treatments.

However, in the second decade of the 21st century, the mortality rates of lung cancer and colon cancer that constitute the greatest threat to human beings are basically the same as those of 50 years ago. Cancer deaths are still the leading cause of death for urban and rural residents in China.

Experts in medicine, biology, and related disciplines began to reflect. Most scientists believe that the prevention and treatment of tumors should start with the most basic problems, namely, the nature of cancer cells, the mechanism of disease, the metabolic characteristics of cancer cells, and their signal transduction. To understand the "face of the mountain" of cancer, the only way to prevent cancer is to be effective.

Conduct interdisciplinary collaborative research, promote cooperation between basic research and clinical medical research, and attach importance to clinical research.

Clinical basic research must be carried out, and without breakthroughs in basic research, clinical efficacy is difficult to improve.

(3) **In 1982, Oldham founded the theory of biological response regulation**. On this basis, he proposed the fourth model of cancer treatment in 1984. According to the theory of biological response regulation, under normal circumstances, the dynamic balance between tumor and body defense, tumor occurrence and even invasion, metastasis, is completely caused by this imbalance of dynamic balance. **If the state of the disorder has been artificially adjusted to a normal level, the growth of the tumor can be controlled and allowed to subside.**

Biotherapeutic treatment is to modulate this biological response by supplementing, inducing or activating, in vitro, the cell-active virulence, biological cell (or) factors inherent in the biological response system of the body.

Biotherapy differs from the previous three treatment modes, namely surgery, radiation therapy and chemotherapy, with the goal of directly attacking tumors. The scope of biotherapeutics clearly exceeds the traditional concept of immunotherapy because the dynamic balance between the body and the tumor is not limited to immune responses, **but also involves various regulatory genes and cytokines involved in tumor proliferation**.

Biological response modifiers (BRMs) have opened up new areas of cancer biotherapy. At present, BRM is widely regarded in the medical community as the fourth program of tumors.

(4) **Due to the increasing number of cancer patients, the incidence rate is rising and the mortality rate stays high and doesn't go down, it is recognized that cancer should not only pay attention to treatment, but also pay attention to prevention to stop the source. The research aims to focus on the prevention and treatment of the whole process of cancer occurrence and development.**

Xu Ze put forward the "Strategic of walking Out and Suggestions for conquering Cancer" in the "New Concepts and New Methods of Cancer Treatment" published in October 2011. In June 2013, XZ-C proposed again to "the basic idea and design of conquering cancer and launching the general attack on cancer" in an attempt to reduce the incidence of cancer, reduce mortality, improve cure rate and prolong survival.

The total attack is cancer prevention + cancer control + cancer treatment at the same time and the same level and same attention

Prevention of cancer:

Class I prevention of cancer can be achieved by building a "two-oriented society" and building a well-off society to conduct "ride research".

Control cancer:

through the "three early" clinic, precancerous lesion treatment, screening.

Treatment of cancer:

surgery + immune regulation + biological therapy + differentiation induction therapy + integrated Chinese and Western medicine treatment, supplemented by release and chemotherapy.

The near-term goal:

to curb the momentum of cancer development, reduce its incidence, and gradually improve the cure rate, gradually realizing three thirds.

Four leap or progression in the treatment of malignant tumors in the last two centuries

First leap

In 1890 Halstad proposed the concept of radical tumor surgery

Second leap

In the 1970s, Fish integrated chemotherapy into radical surgery.

(adjuvant chemotherapy or neoadjuvant chemotherapy)

After that, the treatment of malignant tumors was wondering there; since then, malignant tumor treatment has been faltering

In 1982, oldhan founded the theory of biological response regulation. On this basis, in 1984, the fourth model of BRM biotherapy was proposed and received extensive attention.

Third leap or progress

Molecular targeted therapy attracts attention

In 1960, Philadelphia researchers in the United States found chromosomal abnormalities in CMC

In the 1940s, this chromosome also became a target for CML targeted therapy.

Fourth leap or progress

The prospect of immunomodulatory drugs is gratifying

ASCO Announces Major Progress in Clinical Oncology in 2015

Immunotherapy opens a new era of cancer treatment

XZ-C Publishing Medical Monograph

It is to propose:

overcome cancer, launch a general attack -------- cancer prevention, cancer control, treatment at the same level and at the same attention and at the same time.

Reforming the mode of running a hospital, changing only the rule of only treatment without prevention into prevention, control, and treatment.

Reforming the treatment model, the way out for cancer treatment is in three early, pre-cancer, prevention is the most important

It is to propose:

Create cancer prevention research and carry out cancer prevention research system engineering - open a new era of cancer prevention research and cancer preventionsystem engineering in the 21st century

Prevent cancer from the big environment and small environment

Prevent cancer from clothing, food, shelter, and walk

Chapter 20

How to overcome cancer?

XZ-C proposes:

Cancer is a disaster for all mankind. It is necessary for the people all over the world to work together. China and US joint together to do research or to attack cancer

Cancer Prevention and Anti-cancer

Conquer cancer and launch a general attack

Moon Plan (USA) and Dawning C Plan (China)

--------------- Moving forward together, heading for the science hall to conquer cancer

1. In the past 100 years the history record of the "conquering cancer" program which has been raised internationally.

2. To do an unprecedented event for the benefit of mankind

3. To move forward together and to head to the science hall to overcome cancer

4. Dawn or Shuguang C-type plan

5. Situation analysis (1)

—— Analysis of their respective technological advantages (US, China)

6. Situation analysis (2)

—— Analysis of why not take the lead from the oncology department, cancer center or provincial cancer hospital of some famous university affiliated hospitals in China and our province? They have superior equipment and superb medical technology

—— Analysis of why it is led by the University of Chinese Medicine?

7. Situation analysis (3)

—— Analysis of what is the prospect of the current three major treatments (surgery, radiotherapy, chemotherapy)? What is the future?

8. Situation analysis (4)

The goal of Conquering cancer

The routes to overcome cancer

How to carry out cancer prevention and anti-cancer in Wuhan?

How to prevent cancer and to control cancer in the community?

First

In the past 100 years the history record of the "conquering cancer" program which has been raised internationally.

The two presidents have proposed the National Plan for Conquering Cancer. A Chinese doctor XZ-C proposed the designing, solutions, and a series of planning blueprint for conquering cancers. He also wrote books, published a monograph (a full English version, global distribution).

(1). In 1971, the US Congress passed a "National Cancer Regulations" and President Nixon issued the "Anti-Cancer Declaration." So he invested a lot of manpower and financial resources to overcome cancer in one fell swoop.

In December 1971, President Richard Nixon presented an anti-cancer slogan in a message from the United Nations.

(2). On January 12, 2016, US President Barack Obama announced a national plan to "conquer cancer" in his annual State of the Union address speech, which was under the responsibility of Vice President Biden.

The name of the program:

"Cancer moon Shot"

Goal:

Conquer cancer

On June 29, 2016, US Vice President Vice President Biden convened a summit to broadcast the National Cancer Month Plan to the United States from 9 am to 6 pm in the White House. Dozens of cancer centers and community organizations across the country, including doctors, nurses, scientists, volunteers, patients, families, cancer survivors, and rehabilitators, participate in this mission to overcome cancer and encourage scientists to focus on cancer.

The White House called on Americans to join them to host community events.

Immunotherapy opens a new era of cancer treatment and announces $1 billion a year to be used to overcome cancer research.

(3). In 2011, Chinese physician Xu Ze put forward "strategic ideas and suggestions for conquering cancer" in his monograph. In August 2013, at the International Congress of Oncology, it was first proposed: "XZ-C research plan to overcome cancer and launch the general attack of cancer." In July 2015, it was to put forward the "Dawning C-type plan" to overcome conquer and launch the general attack of cancer.

- **Chapter 38 of "New Concepts and New Methods for Cancer Therapy" in Xu Ze's third monograph**

In this monograph, with a chapter it made "strategic ideas and suggestions for conquering cancer."

How to overcome cancer I see one:

the road of scientific research road lies in exploring the experimental basis of cancer etiology, pathogenesis and pathophysiology

How to overcome cancer I see two:

the road to scientific research lies in the scientific research on the prevention and treatment of cancer during the whole process of cancer occurrence and development

How to overcome cancer I see three:

the road to scientific research lies in the development of multidisciplinary research, the establishment of cancer-related research groups, special in-depth clinical basic and clinical research

This book was translated into English in 2013 under the title "New Concept and New Way of Treatment of Cancer".

The full English version was published in Washington, DC in March 2013 and is distributed worldwide.

- Xu Ze's fourth book "On Innovation of Treatment of Cancer"

—— (Cancer treatment innovation theory)

Full English version, published in Washington, DC in December 2015, with electronic version, global distribution

Brief introduction to this book:

The experimental research; Chinese medicine immunopharmacology and anti-cancer research of the combination with Chinese and Western medicine at the molecular level; it has formed the theoretical system of XZ-C immune regulation and control of treatment of cancer.

Walked Out of a new way to use immunomodulatory Chinese medicine, regulate and control immune activity, prevent thymus atrophy, promote thymic hyperplasia, protect bone marrow hematopoietic function, improve immune surveillance, and combine Western medicine at the molecular level to overcome cancer.

• Xu Ze's fifth monograph "The Road To Overcome Cancer"

Full English version, published in Washington, DC on December 6, 2016, with electronic version, global distribution

Chapter 11 of this book is "an initiative to overcome the general attack on cancer"

— The overall strategic reform of cancer treatment

Section 1 is "the necessary to launch the general attack

Section 2 is "the feasibility of launching the general attack

Section 3 is "XZ-C Plan of conquering cancer and launching the General Attack of Cancer

Chapter 12 is "Strengthening research on anti-cancer and cancer prevention and treatment and changing the status of heavy treatment and ignoring prevention"

The first section is "it must recognize the current problems and clarify the research direction".

The second quarter is "in order to overcome conquer, it pays attention to cancer prevention and treatment and the results or the effects of cancer lie on "three early"."

Chapter 13 is "Suggestions on the Cultivation of Scientific and Technological Innovation Talents and the Transformation of Scientific Research Achievements"

Section 1 is "in order to overcome cancer, technology talent is the key

Section 2 is "Establishing a good laboratory"

Chapter 14 is "Adhere to the new road of anti-cancer with Chinese characteristics"

This book has been published in English for more than half a year. Therefore, China, Hubei, and Wuhan should catch up with cancer research. Because the general attack on cancer has been proposed by professors in China and Wuhan, and has published a monograph, it should be carried out in the domestic work to overcome the general attack on cancer, and should report to the province and city.

Contemporarily, now, the research work of overcoming cancer, Chinese has been done by Chinese physician the most, the earliest, who published monographs. There are the experimental research, theory, and clinical practice.

It was originally hoped that our country's leadership reported to the United Nations that it would overcome cancer and launch a general attack. However, the President of the United States has announced plans to overcome the cancer national plan, calling on all American and global scientists to unite wisdom to overcome cancer.

I should remember the story of smallpox and cowpea in the Ming Dynasty of China! The kind of cowpea was invented by Chinese doctors, but after being passed to France, it was reported by French doctors.

How to do? It should apply to open an international oncology conference in Wuhan: "To overcome the peak of the cancer attack general academic forum, the first batch of scientific research results have been achieved by the international announcement that China has overcome the general attack on cancer."

How to do? It should apply to open an international cancer conference in Wuhan:

The Summit Academic Forum of "Overcoming cancer and launching the general attack on cancer" which is going to announce to the international that China has achieved the first batch of scientific research results in the overall attack on cancer."

Second

Why do you say that you can move forward together? What are you together?

(1) Chapter 38 of "Strategic ideas and suggestions for conquering cancer" was Published in Xu Ze's third book of "New Concepts and Methods of Cancer Treatment" in Beijing in 2011 (Chinese version), and later published in Washington in 2013 (English version) and proposed: "conquering cancer"

How to overcome cancer I see one:

the road to scientific research lies in exploring the etiology, pathogenesis, pathophysiology of cancer

How to overcome cancer I see two:

the road to scientific research lies in the study of cancer prevention and treatment during the whole process of cancer occurrence and development.

How to overcome cancer I see three:

the road to scientific research lies in the development of multidisciplinary research, the establishment of relevant specialist groups, special in-depth basic and clinical research

The book was translated into English by Dr. Bin Wu, an American medical scientist. The English book titled "New Concept and New Way of Treatment of Cancer" was published in Washington in June 2013 and distributed in Europe and America.

This book focuses on: conquering cancer and attacking the general attack of cancer

(2) Xu Ze's fourth monograph "On Innovation of Treatment of Cancer" - (English version of cancer treatment innovation) published in Washington, DC in December 2015, electronic version, global distribution

This book focuses on: immune regulation and control of treatment of cancer

The Experimental research, Chinese medicine immunopharmacology and the anti-cancer research with the combination of Chinese and Western medicine at the molecular level which has formed a theoretical system of immune regulation and control of treatment of cancer.

Step out of the new road with the traditional Chinese medicine immune regulation and control which is to regulate immune activity, prevent thymus atrophy, promote thymic hyperplasia, protect bone marrow hematopoietic function, improve immune surveillance, and combine Western medicine with Chinese medicine at the molecular level to overcome cancer.

The above two books were that

The former focuses on: conquering cancer

The latter focuses on: immune regulation and control of treatment of cancer

(3) On January 12, 2016, US President Barack Obama proposed a national cancer plan to overcome cancer in his State of the Union address:

Conquering cancer.

The name of the program is:

"Cancer moon shot", which is administered by Vice President Biden. Biden proposes to focus on immunotherapy, immune prevention, and immunotherapy to open a new era of cancer treatment.

On June 29, 2016, Vice President Vice President convened a summit to broadcast the National Cancer Lunar Plan to the United States from 9 am to 6 pm in the White House to encourage scientists to concentrate on conquering cancer and announce that 10 billions of dollars per year are used to overcome cancer research.

The above goal:

Overcome cancer

Methods and pathways:

The immune method treats cancer and prevents cancer

In short, the 39 chapter of the above-mentioned Xu Ze's third monograph puts forward:

To overcome cancer and how to overcome cancer;

The fourth monograph of the whole book focuses on:

immune regulation and control of treatment of cancer, walked out of a new path to overcome cancer.

The goal of "Cancer Moon Shot" with the United States is to overcome cancer, and the method and route are immunotherapy.

Both of the above goals are to overcome cancer, and the methods and routes are immunotherapy, immune regulation and control, and immune prevention. The goals, methods, and approaches of the two are the same.

Therefore, it is proposed to move forward together and to go to the science hall to conquer cancer.

A.

How to overcome cancer?

XZ-C's recommendation of that needs/ requires two wheels, A wheel, B wheel

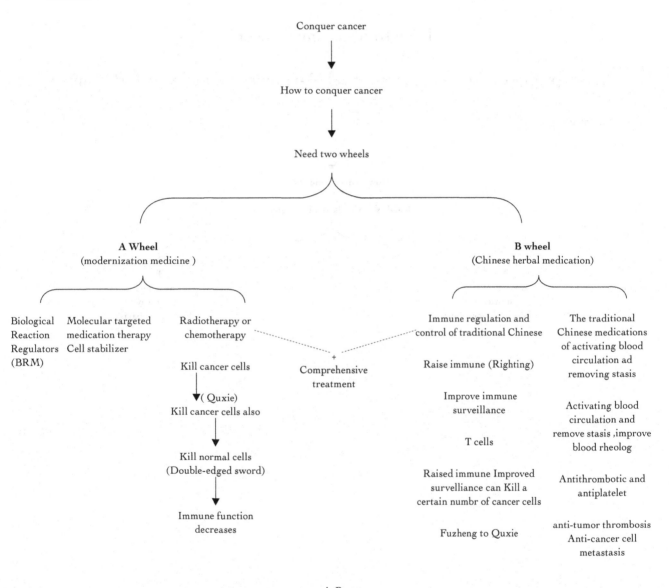

B.

How to overcome cancer?

XZ-C put forward to require A wheel and A runway, and B wheel and B runway

How to overcome cancer?

XZ-C proposes the need for A-wheel, A-runway and B-wheel, B-runway

runway

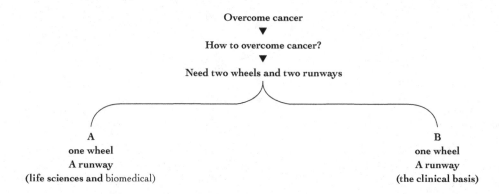

Overcome cancer
▼
How to overcome cancer?
▼
Need two wheels and two runways

A
one wheel
A runway
(life sciences and biomedical)

B
one wheel
A runway
(the clinical basis)

The A wheel and A runway are :

a. the DNA found

Under a variety of internal and external factors the body occurs the mutation or error, causing DNA structure and function changes, resulting in cancer.

b. the gene mutation

1928 it was considered that gene mutation is the root cause of cancer and tumor occurrence and the development is involved in genes and the basic life activities such as the cell proliferation, differentiation, apoptosis and other etc, therefore, it is now recognized as a disease of the tumor.

c. the Philadelphia chromosome opens targeted therapy

In 1960, the researchers in Philadelphia found that there was a chromosomal abnormality in patients with chronic myeloid leukemia (CML), and that years later it was found to be the result of chromosomes of chromosome 9 and chromosome 22. The chromosome became the target of CML targeted therapy for 40 years. In 2001 it was the first time confirmed to the drug of being against Philadelphia chromosome molecular defects - imatinib.

Etiology, pathogenesis, pathophysiology and related factors
The B wheel and B runway are :

a. The virus

- 1951 it was found that virus can transmit the mice leukemia.

- In 1960 the African sub-Saharan region reported that Hodgkin's lymphoma was thought to be caused by a virus and later confirmed as an AIDS virus.

- 1983 human papillomavirus infection is one of the factors of cervical cancer.

- Preventive vaccines for cervical cancer in 2006 were approved by the US FDA.

b. the immune

- in 2001 in the Animal experiments it was found that removal of thymus can produce a mouse model of mice.

Mouse thymus had the acute progressive atrophy after inoculated with cancer cells and cell proliferation was blocked and the immune function was low, the volume was significantly reduced, thymus atrophy, immune function was slow and it could promote cancer metastasis.

c. the hormones

- in 1916 it was found that removal of ovaries can reduce the incidence of breast cancer, suggesting that ovarian can promote the occurrence of breast cancer.

- in 1941 the hormone dependence of the prostate cancer was confirmed and the injection of androgen could promote metastasis.

d. the environmental pollution

- In 1907, the sun exposure was associated with skin cancer

- in 1978 the nitrosamines in tobacco leaves were confirmed to be carcinogens in cigarettes and were found to be carcinogenic in animal models

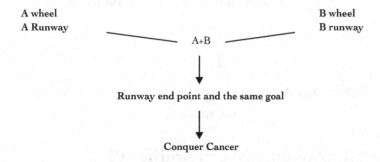

C.

How to overcome cancer?

For the first time in the world XZ-C proposed to aim at the three targets A, B and C to conquer cancer

Treatment must be based on the etiology, pathogenesis, pathophysiology.

Prevention cancer and cancer treatment must also prevent and treat the cause, pathogenesis and cancer metastasis mechanism.

How does the tumor happen?

Research should be carried out according to each goal or "target" in the process of tumorigenesis.

The occurrence of tumors is caused by genetic and environmental factors, gene mutations, abnormal expression or deletion, resulting in a common feature of tumor cells-----uncontrolled infinite reproduction.

1.   The occurrence of tumor is in

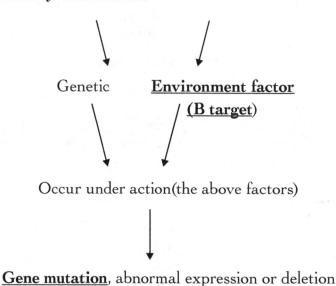

Genetic   **Environment factor**
                 (B target)

Occur under action(the above factors)

Gene mutation, abnormal expression or deletion
(A target)

Finally, the result of abnormal cell proliferation

1. *The occurrence of tumor is in*

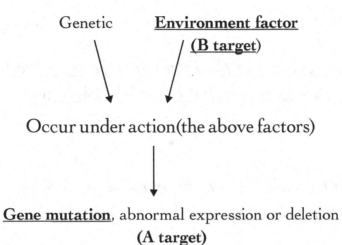

Genetic   **Environment factor**
(B target)

Occur under action(the above factors)

Gene mutation, abnormal expression or deletion
(A target)

Finally the result of abnormal cell proliferation is led

2. *The normal immune system of the body*

Our body has the ability to detect, identify, and remove tumor cells

(C target)

(The immune system should be adjusted so as to identify and remove the tumor cells)

2. *The normal immune system of the body*

The body has the ability to detect, identify, and remove tumor cells

(C target) (The immune system should be adjusted so as to identify and remove tumor cells)

3. *However, the process of interaction tumor cells and immune system is subjected to or controlled by*

The regulation and control by massive immune activation/or inhibition of molecular (C target)

(C target) (the application of up-regulated immune activator

thereby is to inhibit immune escape or evasion and inhibit tumor growth)

3. *However, the process of the interaction between the tumor cells and immune system* **is controlled by or is subject to**

$$\downarrow$$

The control and regulation of the massive molecular of the immune activation/or inhibition

(C target)

(C target) (the application of up-regulated immune activator is inhibiting immune evasion and inhibiting tumor growth)

4. **Tumor cells is through** *Downregulating immune activator or/and upregulating immunosuppressive molecules*

$$\downarrow$$

To Inhibit the body's anti-tumor immune response

$$\downarrow$$

To achieve immune escape and overgrowth

4. **The Tumor cells** by upregulating immunosuppressive molecules or downregulating immune activator

$$\downarrow$$

Inhibition of the body's anti-tumor immune response

$$\downarrow$$

To achieve immune escape and overgrowth

D.

As outlined above, according to the theory of occurrence of tumors,

XZ-C proposes:

The aim or target for conquering cancer should be:

A target:

It should be directed or aimed to genetic mutations, abnormal expression or deletion.

However:

Are gene mutations, abnormal expression or deletions the cause of cancer? Or is it the result or the fruit?

Why does cancer mutation occur? What reason or causes leads gene to mutate? What are the consequences of the gene mutation?

It is an environmental factor that causes genetic mutation.

B target

It should be for environmental factors.

B target is the goal of cancer prevention

Environmental factors:

The external environment - air, water, soil, physical, chemical, biological factors, clothing, food, housing, travel

The Internal environment - micro, ultra-micro, immune, endocrine, neurohumoral

It is the environment (internal and external) → causing genetic mutation.

Therefore, it is necessary to create the "Cancer Prevention Research Institute" to carry out cancer prevention system engineering.

C target:

It should be:

- *adjust the normal immune system to remove tumor cells,*

- a large number of immune activations, up-regulation and activation, balancing the interaction between the tumor and the immune system

- Immune activating molecules should be up-regulated to suppress immune escape and inhibit tumor growth

- *Perform Immunization prevention and immunotherapy; vaccines are human expectations*

E.

XZ-C proposed that several rules of Chinese medicine can be applied to the treatment of tumors

Professor Xu Ze (XZ-C) proposed several rules for Chinese medicine, which can be applied to the treatment of tumors and conduction the combination of Chinese and Western medicine. Experimental research and clinical basic research on the combination of Chinese and Western medicine should be carried out, as well as clinical application verification observation should be carried out.

A	A'
The treatment rules of TCM	**The treatment rules of Western medicine**
Fuzheng Guben support Righting and firm Essence)	• **Improve immunity function, immune regulation and control, and immunity function reconstruction** • **The anti-cancer immunological pharmacology of traditional Chinese medicine and the mechanism of action of anti-cancer traditional Chinese medicine for immune regulation should be studied.** • **Experimental study on the combination of Chinese and Western medicine at the molecular level**
To activate the blood circulation and remove the blood stasis	To be anti-cancer metastasis, anti-cancer thrombosis, anti-micro-transfer and anti-formation of cancer plugs or thrombosis so that it must resist blood clots and improve blood circulation; To be activating blood circulation can remove the blood stasis and can paralyze and avoid the formation of cancerous plugs; To eliminate cancer cells on the way to metastasis must resolve cancerous plugs and micro-cancers thrombosis so as to prevent cancer cell metastasis
To removing inflammation and detoxification	some cancers may be related to chronic inflammation, stubborn ulcers such as chronic atrophic gastritis, chronic pelvic inflammatory disease, cervicitis, chronic hepatitis, etc., some are cancer pre-lesion which can be treated with heat-clearing(inflammation) and detoxifying Chinese medicine to control

soften solids and firm and dissolving the nodules	In the current examination CT, sometimes reported that there are multiple small nodules, small, only a few millimeters in the certain organ, which can not be operated by chemotherapy and radiotherapy, can be treated by these softening Chinese medicine, and have the dynamic observation, **often have a good effect**

Prevention cancer and anti-cancer

Conquer cancer and launch a general attack

"New Moon Plan" (USA) and Dawning C Plan (China)

- Moving forward together, heading for the science hall to overcome cancer

1. Do an unprecedented event for the benefit of mankind

2. go forward together, head to the science hall to overcome cancer

3. Dawn or Shuguang C-type plan

4. Situation analysis (1)

5. Situation analysis (2)

6. Situation analysis (3)

7. Situation analysis (4)

Conquer cancer and launch a general attack

(One)

"New Moon Plan" (US) and "Dawning C Plan" (China)

- Moving forward together, heading for the science hall to overcome cancer

I.   Introduction to the "moon shot"

On January 12, 2016, US President Barack Obama announced in his last State of the Union address during his term of office a national plan to conquer cancer, namely, the new moon landing plan that Vice President Biden called in 2015. ", the plan will be handled by Biden. In May 2015, the son of Biden died of brain cancer, only 46 years old. Since then, Biden has announced that he will not participate in the 2016 presidential election and will join the anti-cancer career during the remaining vice presidential term.

Biden will visit the Abramson Cancer Center at the University of Pennsylvania School of Medicine next week to discuss the plan. He said that the "new moon landing plan" is a commitment to overcome cancer in the world and will inspire a new generation of scientists to explore the scientific world.

Obama did not mention the specific plan of the plan in his speech, but he mentioned that the expenditure and tax bill passed by Congress in December 2015 has raised the financial budget of the National Institutes of Health (NIH).

The United States has just recently established a national immunotherapy alliance consisting of pharmaceutical companies, biotechnology companies and academic medical organizations. The alliance is trying to develop a vaccine immunotherapy before 2020 to overcome cancer and complete "New Moon landing plan."

The American Society of Clinical Oncology (ASCO) issued a statement on its website, welcoming Obama's "New Moon landing Plan" and supporting Biden's leadership, saying that the "New Moon Landing Plan" will reduce the pain and reduce the risk of cancer for humans and reduce Death caused by cancer. The statement mentioned that "all effective treatments should be transformed from the laboratory to the clinic"; the application of "big data" technology, such as ASCO's "CancerLinQ" rapid learning system, can accelerate the pace of cancer and enable physicians to better develop individualized treatment options for each patient and understand which areas are urgently needed to invest more research.

2. Introduction to the Dawning C Plan

1. Before January 12, 2016, it was advanced or proposed the progress of the scientific research plan "to overcome cancer and to launch the general attack of cancer"

2. Before January 12, 2016, we have taken research on conquering cancer as a research direction, and have carried out scientific research achievements and technological innovation series.

3. Shuguang C-type plan

"New Moon Plan" (US) and "Dawning C Plan" (China)

New moon landing plan	Dawning C plan
United States	China
Plan Name:	Plan name:
"New Moon Plan"	"Dawning C-type plan"
Goal:	Goal:
Conquer cancer	Conquer cancer
Nation:	Nature:
National Plan to Conquer Cancer	Advocate and
Announcement:	The total designer:
Announced in the State of the Union Address	Professor Xu Ze proposed in 2011 to "conquer cancer, launch a general attack", and in 2013 proposed "to build a comprehensive design for cancer science city", in 2013 proposed "XZ-C to overcome the general research plan for cancer attack" In July 2015, the "Dawning C-type plan" was proposed. In July 2015, four application reports for the feasibility report of the general attack on cancer were proposed. In August 2015, the application for the government was established in Hubei and Wuhan. Conquer the initial vision and design of the cancer working group test area.
Announcer:	
President Obama	
Announced:	
January 12, 2016	
The person in charge of the plan:	Racing with moon shot
Vice President Biden	1. Before January 12, 2016, we proposed the research work that has been carried out to "conquer the general attack of cancer." Proposing "to overcome the general attack of cancer", this is unprecedented work, XZ-C (Xu Ze-China, Xu Ze - China).
The specific plan of the plan: unknown	
National Institutes of Health: increased financial budget	
(NIH)	Dawning C plan
Recently formed: pharmaceutical company	China
Biotechnology company	

Academic medical organization The alliance is trying to develop a vaccine therapy by 2020 to overcome cancer and complete a new cancer landing program. New moon landing plan United States	(1) Chapter 38 of the monograph "New Concepts and New Methods of Cancer Treatment" published by Xu Ze in October 2011 uses a chapter to propose "strategic ideas and suggestions for conquering cancer." (2) In June 2013, Xu Ze proposed to "conquer the basic concept and design of the general attack on cancer" in an attempt to reduce the incidence of cancer, reduce cancer mortality, improve the cure rate, and prolong the survival period. The total attack is anti-cancer + cancer control + Governing cancer, the three carriages go hand in hand (3) Xu Ze first proposed in the international exhibition in August 2013: "XZ-C Scientific Research Plan for Overcoming the General Attack of Cancer" - The overall strategy and development of cancer treatment in China (4) In July 2015, Professor Xu Ze proposed the following four feasibility reports for the general attack on cancer. "XZ-C proposes a research plan to overcome the general attack of cancer" —— The overall strategic reform and development of cancer treatment in China 1 first proposed at the international level: "Necessity and Feasibility Report on Overcoming the General Attack of Cancer" 2 first proposed at the international level: "Preparing to build cancer, develop and prevent the whole hospital" (Global Demonstration Prevention and Treatment Hospital)

"Implementation of the plan for the prevention and treatment of cancer in the whole process of anti-cancer and feasibility report"

—— Explain the necessity and feasibility of establishing a full-scale prevention and treatment hospital

3   first proposed at the international level:

"To build a general plan to overcome cancer and the basic vision and feasibility report of Science City"

-    Equivalent to designing an overall framework for Chinese characteristics to overcome cancer design

4   first proposed at the international level:

"In the construction of a well-off society, it is recommended to "catch the research" - the necessity and feasibility report of medical research and cancer prevention and treatment for cancer prevention and cancer control - adhere to the road of anti-cancer and cancer control with Chinese characteristics

Dawning C Plan

China

•   Our dreams, conquer cancer, build a well-off society, everyone is healthy, stay away from cancer

•   These four scientific research projects were first proposed internationally. They are the first international initiative and internationally leading. They have opened up new fields of anti-cancer research and will open up a new era of anti-cancer research.

•   Putting a general attack on cancer, this is an unprecedented job

(5) Professor Xu Ze's fourth book, "Only The Book of Innovation", published in Washington, DC, December, 2015, published in English, published globally, and distributed electronically. Edition, introduce new book

Introduction to the new book: experimental research, Chinese medicine immunopharmacology and molecular level Chinese and Western medicine combined with anti-cancer research, has initially formed the theoretical system of XZ-C immune regulation and treatment of cancer.

Step out of a traditional Chinese medicine immune regulation, regulate immune activity, prevent thymus atrophy, promote thymic hyperplasia, protect bone marrow hematopoietic function, improve immune surveillance, and combine Western medicine at the molecular level to overcome the new path of cancer.

Dawning C Plan

China

(9) Xu Ze's fifth "Monograph" new book: "The Road to Over Cancer"

—— Reform, innovation and development of cancer treatment

Published in Washington, DC in December 2016, published in English, distributed worldwide

2 Before January 12, 2016, we have carried out research and development of science and technology innovation series with the focus on cancer research.

(1) New findings from experimental research:

In January 2001, Xu Ze published a new discovery from laboratory experimental tumor research in his monograph "New Understanding and New Models of Cancer Therapy":

1 Excision of the thymus (Thymus) can be used to create a model of cancer-bearing animals. Injection of immunosuppressive agents can help establish animal models of cancer.

2 After the host thymus was inoculated with cancer cells, it showed acute progressive atrophy, cell proliferation was blocked, and the volume was significantly reduced. The laboratory was observed in a laboratory model of more than 6,000 cancers in 7 years. The experimental results showed that the tumor progressed even if the thymus Progressive atrophy.

Dawning C Plan

China

(2) In the second chapter of "New Concepts and Methods of Cancer Treatment" published by Xu Ze in October 2011, the new findings of experimental research on cancer etiology, pathogenesis and pathophysiology are proposed:

"Thymus atrophy, immune dysfunction is one of the causes and pathogenesis of cancer", and in Chapter 3, based on the enlightenment of animal experiments, the principle of treatment should protect, regulate, and activate the anti-cancer immune system in the human body. Put forward: "The theoretical basis and experimental basis of the "Zhang-Climb-up" of XZ-C immunomodulation therapy.

(3)　Report cancer research papers at the American Society of International Oncology:

1　Received an invitation letter from the American Association for Cancer Research AACR to Xu Ze, and reported "XZ-C immunomodulation anticancer therapy" at the International Cancer Society in Washington, USA in September 2013, which has aroused extensive attention in the international oncology community. And highly valued.

2　From October 27 to 30, 2013, attending the 12th International Conference on Cancer Research of the American Association for Cancer Research (AACR) in Washington, DC, and reported: "Thymus atrophy, low immune function is the cause of cancer, one of the pathogenesis", and The academic report on the theoretical basis and experimental basis of the principle of "protecting the thymus and protecting the thymus (improving the thymus, improving immunity), "protecting the marrow and producing blood" (protecting bone marrow blood stem cells), was warmly welcomed and highly valued by the participants.

Dawning C Plan

China

(4)　Monographs published before 2016

In the above experimental research, basic research, and clinical verification to overcome cancer research, we have gone through 28 years and obtained a series of scientific research achievements and scientific and technological innovation series of anti-cancer, anti-cancer metastasis and recurrence research. The research papers on innovation or independent innovation are published in my series of monographs.

	1 In January 2001, the first monograph "New Understanding and New Model of Cancer Treatment" was published. Hubei Science and Technology Press, Xu Ze 2 In January 2006, the second monograph "New Concepts and New Methods for Cancer Metastasis Treatment" was published. Beijing People's Military Medical Publishing House, Xu Ze In April 2007, the General Administration of Press of the People's Republic of China issued a certificate for the "Three Hundreds" original book publishing project. 3 In October 2011, the third monograph "New Concepts and New Methods for Cancer Treatment" was published. Beijing People's Military Medical Publishing House, Xu Ze, Xu Jie / Zhu 4 The fourth monograph was published in December 2015. The English version of "On Innovation Of Treatment Of Cancer" (the first volume of cancer treatment innovation) was published in Washington, DC, and distributed worldwide. Ze, Xu Jie 5 December 2016 published the fifth monograph "The Road to Cancer", the English version of "The Road To Over Come Cancer", published in Washington, DC, global distribution Dawning C Plan China

These five monographs are the results of four different levels of research, four difficult stages of scientific research, and four different levels of research. (I published my first monograph at the age of 67, the second monograph at the age of 73, the third monograph at the age of 78, the third monograph in English and the English version at the age of 80, Washington Publishing, International Distribution, At the age of 82, he published the fourth monograph, the full English version, published in Washington, and distributed globally. At the age of 83, the fifth monograph was published in the first quarter of 2016.)

(These five monographs will be a reference for the compulsory courses of the Innovative Molecular Oncology School)

(5)   Visiting the Stirling Cancer Institute in Houston, USA

In order to strengthen the exchanges and cooperation between international scientific and technological organizations, on December 10, 2009, we were invited to visit the Stirling Cancer Institute in the United States. We were warmly welcomed and warmly treated by the colleagues of the Institute. The 86-year-old professor and A number of professors, researchers, nude animal model laboratories, and anti-cancer drug analysis laboratories participated in the discussion and exchanges, and reported the latest scientific research results with slides.

Dawning C Plan

China

We presented a color map of the Institute of Cancer Metastasis and Recurrence in our Institute to the Institute of Oncology, and introduced the research on tumor-free technology in radical surgery and the experiment of removing the thymus to produce cancer-bearing animal models. Research, as well as the exclusive development of ZC immunomodulation anti-cancer, anti-metastatic Chinese medicine series Z-C1-10. I also presented the monograph "New Concepts and New Methods for Cancer Metastasis Treatment" published by me. It is the three hundred original books that won the book award in China, and was warmly welcomed and appreciated by the researchers.

(6)   Innovation - The basic and clinical research on anti-cancer and anti-cancer metastasis in the past 28 years has preliminarily embarked on a "Chinese-style anti-cancer", Chinese and Western medicine combined with immune regulation and treatment of cancer, we have accumulated more than 12,000 cases in 20 years The clinical application experience can be pushed to the whole country, can go to the world, can connect with the "Belt and Road", make Chinese medicine to the world, make "Chinese-style anti-cancer", Chinese and Western medicine combined with immune regulation and treatment of cancer, not only develops and enriches immunity The content of studying cancer has brought China's medical modernization into line with the international market and is at the forefront of the world.

Prevention cancer and anti-cancer

Conquer cancer and launch a general attack

(Two)

Dawning C-type plan (China)

"New Moon Plan" (USA) and "Dawning C Plan" (China)

Moving forward together, heading for the science hall to overcome cancer

Dawning or Shuguang C-type plan No. 1 - No. 6

Why use the word "Dawn"?

The dawn is the morning light, it is the dawn, it is the morning sun.

Vigorous, vigorous, original innovation, independent innovation

C=China

Type C = Chinese mode

About 8550 people in China are diagnosed with cancer every day, and 6 people are diagnosed with cancer every minute. Therefore, the research work to overcome cancer and launch the general attack of cancer, can not walk slowly, should run forward, save the wounded.

Time is money, time is money = one inch of time, one inch of gold

Time is life, time is life

Time flies, time flies

Empty talk can lead wrong country, hard work can flourish country

Avoid empty talk, attention to work hard, start off to walk

No matter how far the road to conquer cancer is, you should always start.

This scientific research plan is the original innovation, it is time to declare war on cancer, and the general attack should be launched.

Our dreams, conquer cancer, build a well-off society, everyone is healthy, stay away from cancer

Dawning C plan

Formulated in July 2015

1. Dawning C-type plan No. 1:

"Conquering cancer and launching the general attack"

—— The overall strategic reform and development of cancer treatment in China

It was to propose a general plan, scheme, design, blueprint and rules for conquering cancer

Avoid empty talk, attention to work hard, start off to walk

No matter how far the road to conquer cancer is, you should always start.

(see the detail in the separate article)

2. Dawning or Shuguang C-type plan No. 2:

"Preparation of the hospitals with prevention and treatment during the whole process"

(Global Demonstration Prevention and Treatment Hospital)

—— Strategic reform, changing the mode of running a hospital

Reforming treatment mode

3. Dawning C-type plan No. 3:

"Building a science city to overcome cancer"

—— XZ-C proposes the overall design, planning and blueprint of Science City to overcome cancer and to launch the general attack of cancer

- This is the only way to overcome cancer

This is the "high-speed rail" that conquers cancer, "high-speed" channel)

(see the detail in the separate article)

4. Dawning or Shuguang C-type plan No. 4:

"Building a multidisciplinary research group and laboratory"

- aiming for the cause, pathogenesis, pathophysiology, metastasis, recurrence mechanism of cancer...

It is to study anti-cancer, anti-recurrence, anti-metastatic measures to improve the overall level of medical care

Benefit

—— The criteria for efficacy evaluation are:

long survival time, good quality of life, and complications

No or less, each school group is a provincial key laboratory.

(see separate article)

5. Dawning C-type plan No. 5:

"The vaccine is the hope of human beings, immunological prevention"

—— Today's immunology prevention and treatment has become an extremely important in clinical medicine and preventive medicine

Required field

—— △△study group+△△study group+△△study group→Scientific Alliance, Joint Group

(see separate article)

6. **Dawning C-type plan No. 6: A**

"The prospect of immunomodulatory drugs is gratifying"

-   Regardless of the complexity of the mechanisms behind cancer, immune suppression is the progression of cancer

The essential

-   From the analysis of experimental results, to obtain new discoveries, new inspirations:

Thymus atrophy, immune dysfunction, decreased immune surveillance and immune escape are one of the causes and pathogenesis of cancer. Therefore, the principle of treatment should be to prevent thymus atrophy, promote thymic hyperplasia, and improve immune surveillance.

—— XZ-C immunomodulatory Chinese medicine, is more than 200 kinds of traditional Chinese herbal medicines from China

In the animal model of cancer mice, 48 kinds of Chinese herbal medicines with good cancer suppression rate were screened by in vivo anti-tumor experiments, and 26 of them had better immune regulation.

(see separate article)

Dawning or Shuguang C-type plan No. 6: B

"the research group and laboratory XZ-C immunomodulation anti-cancer Chinese medicine active ingredient, molecular level analysis"

—— Further research and development of XZ-C immunomodulation anti-cancer Chinese medicine active ingredient, molecular weight, knot

Construction, molecular level analysis

—— Methods, steps: animal experiment, molecular level experiment; gene level experiment, first

Separating the active ingredients first makes the precious heritage of traditional Chinese medicine modern and scientific.

(see separate article)

"The Science City o f Conquering Cancer" established the following genetic testing research groups:

(1) Establish genetic testing and cancer research groups and laboratories

(2) Establish HPV anti-cancer research group and laboratory

(3) Establish genetic testing and immunology and cancer research groups and laboratories

(4) Establish genetic testing and endocrine hormone and cancer research groups and laboratories

(5) Establish genetic testing and pathological sections, and related studies on immunohistochemistry

(6) Establish correlation analysis and research on gene detection and tumor markers

(7) Establish HPV treatment, exploration research groups and laboratories

The Expected Results:

Using modern science and technology and analytical testing methods, the study of traditional Chinese medicine, the material basis of the efficacy of traditional Chinese medicine in clinical practice is the chemical composition contained therein. To study the anti-cancer work of traditional Chinese medicine and its mechanism, it is necessary to conduct in-depth research and analysis. The active ingredients in it make the precious heritage of traditional Chinese medicine more modern and scientific.

After 28 years of experimental research, basic research and clinical verification, a series of "Chest Enhancement" immunomodulatory anticancer Chinese medicine XZ-C1-10 has been screened. After 20 years of clinical observation, more than 12,000 cases have been verified. Prolong life, improve symptoms, improve quality of life, how to know, evaluate can prolong survival? Some surgical explorations can not be cut down (all pathological sections confirmed diagnosis), or have been widely transferred, it is estimated that only 3-6 months, or 6-12 months of cases, XZ-C immune regulation and anti-cancer, For patients with anti-metastasis and recurrence, some patients can still survive for 4 to 5 years to 8 years, with original data and complete data as well as follow-up data.

After a rehabilitation teacher, after a heart attack, calm down, hide in a small building, self-reliance, hard work, adhere to anti-cancer, anti-cancer metastasis, recurrence of animal experimental basic research and outpatient clinical validation research, from the year of the flower (60 years old)→To the age of the ancients (70s)→To the age of older and older(80s), still perseverance, persevere in scientific research to overcome cancer, because he has retired, failed to apply for projects, projects, so no research Funding is to fight alone, to fight alone, to be self-reliant, to work hard, no one cares, no one knows, nowhere to report, no support, hard work for more than 20 years, has achieved a series of scientific and technological innovations, scientific research results, due to retirement In the past 20 years, no one cares, no one supports, retired professors, I don't know where to manage, where to support, so where the scientific research results are reported, I have to make a "monograph" for the benefit of mankind, but published a series of monographs, and then Report to the Provincial Department of Science and Technology and the Provincial Department of Education: 1 hope to open an international high-end academic forum; 2 report to the government to apply for cancer, launch a general attack; 3 report to the province, the provincial government The city has conquered the cancer test area (station) and tried it first. Hope: Apply to establish "the first science city in the country to overcome the general attack of cancer" in Hubei and Wuhan, that is, "the world's first science city to overcome the general attack of cancer."

How to implement this unprecedented event in human history?

(1) Reporting to the government, requesting instructions

(2) Report to the province and city, request instructions

(3) Make recommendations to the city to build in Wuhan:

"The first national cancer science city"

"The world's first to overcome Cancer Science City"

Annex 2

Briefly describes the research environment and recent international research situation:

"Cancer moon shot" (US)	"Dawning C-type plan" (middle)
1. "Cancer moon shot" (US)	"Dawning C-type plan" (middle)
(Introduction)	(Introduction)
On January 12, 2016, US President Barack Obama announced a national plan to overcome cancer in his annual State of the Union speech. The plan is under the responsibility of Vice President Biden.	Plan name: "Dawning C-type plan"
	The main content of the plan is:
The name of the program: "New Moon Plan"	"Overcoming the general attack on cancer" and
	"Building a science city to overcome cancer"
Goal: Conquer cancer	Goal: Conquer cancer nature:
Nature: National plan to overcome cancer	Advocate and chief designer:
Announced: announced in the President's State of the Union address	(1) Chapter 38 of the monograph "New Concepts and New Methods of Cancer Treatment" published by Xu Ze in October 2011 uses a chapter to propose "strategic ideas and suggestions for conquering cancer."
Announcer: President Obama	
Announced: January 12, 2016	
The person in charge of the plan: Vice President Biden	(2) In June 2013, at the International Academic Conference, "Basic Ideas and Designs for Overcoming the General Attack of Cancer Attack"
The specific plan of the plan is unknown	
National Institutes of Health: increased financial budget	(3) In August 2013, the first international XZ-C research plan to overcome the general attack of cancer was put forward in the world. The overall strategy and development of cancer treatment in China
Recently formed:	
Pharmaceutical company	

Biotechnology company

Academic medical organization

The alliance is trying to develop a vaccine therapy by 2020 to complete the new cancer landing program.

New moon landing plan

United States

1. On January 12, 2016, President Obama announced in the State of the Union address a national plan to overcome cancer, which was under the responsibility of Vice President Biden.

The name of the program: "New Moon Plan"

Goal: Conquer cancer

Nature: National plan to overcome cancer

2. In the second week of the program's announcement, Vice President Biden visited the Abramson Cancer Center at the University of Pennsylvania School of Medicine and discussed the plan. He said that the "new moon landing plan" is a commitment to overcome cancer in the world and will inspire a new generation of scientists to explore the scientific world.

(4) Xu Ze proposed in July 2015 "four reports on the feasibility of attacking the general attack on cancer"

"Xu Ze proposes a scientific research plan to overcome the general attack of cancer"

—— The overall strategic reform and development of cancer treatment in China

1 first proposed at the international level:

"Necessity and Feasibility Report on Overcoming the General Attack of Cancer"

2 first proposed at the international level:

"Preparing to build cancer, develop and prevent the whole hospital"

(Global Demonstration Prevention and Treatment Hospital)

"Implementation of the plan for the prevention and treatment of cancer in the whole process of anti-cancer and feasibility report"

—— Explain the necessity and feasibility of establishing a full-scale prevention and treatment hospital

3 first proposed at the international level:

"To build a general plan to overcome cancer and the basic vision and feasibility report of Science City"

3. On February 4, 2016, the American Society of Clinical Oncology (ASCO) announced the "2016 Annual Report: ASCO Clinical Oncology Progress" on Capitol Hill, Washington, and reviewed the 2015 progress, "Tumor Immunotherapy". ASCO Chairman Julie M. Vose believes that the most important development in 2015 is the discovery of immunotherapy. She said in the foreword: "We no longer decide treatment based on tumor type and stage as in the past. In the era of precision medicine, we select or exclude treatment based on each patient and tumor genetic data. No other major advances can be translated into clinical practice like immunology, so the biggest advance in 2015 is immunotherapy." Immunotherapy opens tumor treatment New Era.

4. On April 28, 2016, a policy luncheon was held at the US Capitol to discuss Vice President Biden's "Cancer Moon Shot", "Cancer Moon Plan" and the price structure of the drug. Presided over by former US Senator Tom Coburn. The fourth author of the fourth book "On Imovation of Treatment of Cancer" and translator Bin Wu was invited to attend the meeting and discuss.

(Note: Xu Ze's fourth monograph: "On Inmovation of Treatment of Cancer" - published on December 25, 2015 in Washington, English, globally distributed, and electronically distributed Introduce a new book.

- Equivalent to designing an overall framework for Chinese characteristics to overcome cancer design

4 first proposed at the international level:

"In the construction of a well-off society, it is recommended to "catch the research" - the necessity and feasibility report of medical research and cancer prevention and treatment for cancer prevention and cancer control - adhere to the road of anti-cancer and cancer control with Chinese characteristics

(5) Before January 12, 2016, we have been conducting research work for "to overcome the general attack on cancer" for 3-4 years. It is unprecedented to propose scientific research work to "conquer the general attack of cancer."

Dawning C plan

China

Before January 12, 2016, we have carried out research and development of science and technology innovation series with the focus on cancer research.

(1) New findings from experimental research:

In January 2001, Xu Ze published a new discovery from laboratory experimental tumor research in his monograph "New Understanding and New Models of Cancer Therapy":

1 Excision of the thymus (Thymus) can be used to create a model of cancer-bearing animals. Injection of immunosuppressive agents can help establish animal models of cancer.

New moon landing plan

United States

Introduction to the new book:

Experimental research, Chinese medicine immunopharmacological research and molecular level Chinese and Western medicine combined with anti-cancer research have initially formed the theoretical system of XZ-C immunomodulation and cancer treatment.

Step out of a traditional Chinese medicine immune regulation, regulate immune activity, prevent thymus atrophy, promote thymic hyperplasia, protect bone marrow hematopoietic function, improve immune surveillance, and combine Western medicine at the molecular level to overcome the new path of cancer.

Xu Ze, Xu Jie (China)

Bin Wu (United States)

(The former senator Tom and many members of the conference have an electronic version of our new book, all of which read our book.

5. On June 3, 2016, the American Society of Clinical Oncology Annual Meeting was held in Chicago, one of the highest level clinical cancer conferences in the world. The theme of the conference focused on "concentrating wisdom and conquering cancer." Vice President Biden reported on the US's anti-cancer "moon Shot" plan at the conference. A total of 50,000 people attended the conference, which was unprecedented and attracted worldwide attention.

2 After the host thymus was inoculated with cancer cells, it showed acute progressive atrophy, cell proliferation was blocked, and the volume was significantly reduced. The laboratory was observed in a laboratory model of more than 6,000 cancers in 7 years. The experimental results showed that the tumor progressed even if the thymus Progressive atrophy.

(2) In the second chapter of "New Concepts and Methods of Cancer Treatment" published by Xu Ze in October 2011, the new findings of experimental research on cancer etiology, pathogenesis and pathophysiology are proposed:

"Thymus atrophy, immune dysfunction is one of the causes and pathogenesis of cancer", and in Chapter 3, based on the enlightenment of animal experiments, the principle of treatment should protect, regulate, and activate the anti-cancer immune system in the human body. Put forward: "The theoretical basis and experimental basis of the "Zhang-Climb-up" of XZ-C immunomodulation therapy.

(3) Report cancer research papers at the American Society of International Oncology:

1 Received an invitation letter from the American Association for Cancer Research AACR to Xu Ze, and reported "XZ-C immunomodulation anticancer therapy" at the International Cancer Society in Washington, USA in September 2013, which has aroused extensive attention in the international oncology community. And highly valued.

6. On May 25, 2016, Vice President Biden visited Hopkins University and Cancer Research Journal to report the "New Moon Plan", saying that in the future, mainly immunotherapy will conquer cancer, and immunotherapy will control cancer. This new discovery strongly supports immunotherapy and has a research funding of $1 million for Hopkins University. The cover of the magazine featured photos of Vice President Biden's visit.

7. On June 29, 2016, US Vice President Vice President Biden convened a summit to broadcast the National Cancer Month Plan to the United States from 9 am to 6 pm in the White House. Dozens of cancer centers and community organizations across the country, including doctors, nurses, scientists, volunteers, patients, families, cancer survivors, and rehabilitators, participate in this mission to overcome cancer and encourage scientists to focus on cancer.

The American Cancer Society's Cancer Action Network and the Chief Cancer Officer and Chief Medical Officer and President of the American Cancer Society (ACS) are present at this historic summit event.

The White House called on Americans to join them to host community events.

Immunotherapy opens a new era of cancer treatment and announces $1 billion a year to tackle cancer research.

2 From October 27 to 30, 2013, attending the 12th International Conference on Cancer Research of the American Association for Cancer Research (AACR) in Washington, DC, and reported: "Thymus atrophy, low immune function is the cause of cancer, one of the pathogenesis", and The academic report on the theoretical basis and experimental basis of the principle of "protecting the thymus and protecting the thymus (improving the thymus, improving immunity), "protecting the marrow and producing blood" (protecting bone marrow blood stem cells), was warmly welcomed and highly valued by the participants.

Dawning C plan

China

(4) Publishing monographs

In the above experimental research, basic research, and clinical verification to overcome cancer research, we have gone through 28 years and obtained a series of scientific research achievements and scientific and technological innovation series of anti-cancer, anti-cancer metastasis and recurrence research. The research papers on innovation or independent innovation are published in my series of monographs.

1 In January 2001, the first monograph "New Understanding and New Model of Cancer Treatment" was published.

Hubei Science and Technology Press, Xu Ze

	2 In January 2006, the second monograph "New Concepts and New Methods for Cancer Metastasis Treatment" was published. Beijing People's Military Medical Publishing House, Xu Ze In April 2007, the General Administration of Press of the People's Republic of China issued a certificate for the "Three Hundreds" original book publishing project. 3 In October 2011, the third monograph "New Concepts and New Methods for Cancer Treatment" was published. Beijing People's Military Medical Publishing House, Xu Ze, Xu Jie / Zhu 4 The fourth monograph was published in December 2015. The English version of "On Innovation Of Treatment Of Cancer" (the first volume of cancer treatment innovation) was published in Washington, DC, and distributed worldwide. Ze, Xu Jie 5 The fifth monograph "The Road To Overcome Cancer" <Overcoming Cancer Road> The English version was published in Washington in December and distributed worldwide.

	(5) Innovation - The basic and clinical research on anti-cancer and anti-cancer metastasis for 28 years has preliminarily embarked on a "Chinese-style anti-cancer", Chinese and Western medicine combined with immune regulation and treatment of cancer, we have accumulated more than 12,000 cases in 20 years The clinical application experience can be pushed to the whole country, can go to the world, can connect with the "Belt and Road", make Chinese medicine to the world, make "Chinese-style anti-cancer", Chinese and Western medicine combined with immune regulation and treatment of cancer, not only develops and enriches immunity The content of studying cancer has brought China's medical modernization into line with the international market and is at the forefront of the world.

Cancer research plan

Original innovation

Secret level: Class A

Prevention cancer and anti-cancer

Conquer cancer and launch a general attack

(Three)

"New landing Moon Plan or Cancer Moon Shot" (US) and "Dawning C Plan" (China)

- Moving forward together, heading for the science hall to overcome cancer

Situation analysis (1)

First, analyze their respective technological advantages

Second, analyze the current status

Third, analyze the next research prospects

Fourth, "Dawning C-type plan" scientific technology innovation, the outline of the implemention

"New landing Moon Plan or Cancer Moon Shot" (US) and "Dawning C Plan" (China)

- Moving forward together, heading for the science hall to overcome cancer

Situation analysis (1)

First

To analyze their respective technological advantages

Modern medicine originated from Europe and the United States. In the past 100 years, the modern American medicine has developed and advanced, and it has been far ahead. It has developed into microscopic → ultra-micro → precision medicine, nanotechnology, however, modern medicine in China is still far behind and depends on imported medicine, follow the learning behind. There are 39 cancer research centers in the United States, and the Anderson Cancer Center is one of the first three comprehensive cancer treatment centers designated by the US National Cancer Action Program in 1971. It is also one of the 39 comprehensive cancer treatment centers designated by the Oncology Medical Association. The Anderson Cancer Center is recognized as the best cancer hospital in the world, ranking first in the field of cancer treatment and scientific research. The MD Anderson Cancer Center has more than 20,000 employees, including nearly 2,000 doctors and more than 500 beds. Each year, more than 19,000 inpatients in the United States and other countries are admitted, and the number of outpatients per day is 1,800.

As mentioned above, China's modern medicine is still far behind the United States. In cancer treatment, it relies more on imported medicine, and its own inventions, patents, and intellectual property rights are small.

While race against people, What is it to race about ?What is better than running a man? Is there any comparison? What do you want to compare?

Because China's advantages are:

1. Traditional Chinese medicine, anti-cancer traditional Chinese medicine, immune-regulating and controlling traditional Chinese medicine, promoting blood circulation and removing blood stasis

2. Combination of Chinese and Western medicine, combined with innovation

The advantages of the United States are:

Modern medicine, advanced diagnosis and treatment technology, targeted medicine.

We should give full play to China's advantages and potentials, and we should increase efforts to develop and explore the advantages of Chinese herbal medicine.

Situation Analysis:

Western medicine:

USA > China

Traditional Chinese Medicine:

China >USA

Surgery:

USA and China are the same (operations that the United States can do, China can do, and there are many cases)

Diagnostic technology equipment:

The United States and China are the same (large hospitals have equipment)

Radiotherapy and chemotherapy:

the United States and China are the same

Traditional Chinese medicine:

Chinese> USA [Most can improve symptoms, improve physical fitness, prolong survival, increase immunity (lesion cannot become shrunk, but can survive with tumor, live for a long time), can be used as an auxiliary treatment for surgery, can be developed, excavated]

Experimental research, innovation, patents, inventions, new drugs, targeted drugs:

USA>China

Second

To analyze the current status

1. Status:

Please look at the current situation: ((Today is the 1920s or currently the 21st century)

(1) Status of cancer incidence rate

The more patients are treated and the more patients are, the 3.32 million new cases of cancer in China each year, with an average of 8550 new cancer patients per day, and 6 people diagnosed with cancer every minute in the country.

(2) Status of cancer mortality:

It is the highest cause of death in urban and rural areas in China. The number of deaths due to cancer is 2.7 million per year, and an average of 7,500 people die every day from cancer.

(3) Status of treatment:

Despite the application of traditional three major treatments for nearly a hundred years, thousands of cancer patients have been exposed to radiotherapy and chemotherapy, but what is the result? So far, cancer is still the leading cause of death. Although regular, systematic radiotherapy and/or chemotherapy, or detoxification, has not stopped cancer metastasis and recurrence, the results have been minimal.

(4) Current status of the hospital model of the oncology hospital or oncology department:

1). Fully focused on treatment, focusing on the middle and late stages, poor efficacy, exhausted human and financial resources, and failed to achieve lower mortality, improve cure rate and reduce morbidity.

2). Only treatment, or attaching treatment with light prevention, the more treatment and the more patients.

3). ignored the "three early" and ignored precancerous lesions.

4). Many large-scale cancer hospitals and university affiliated hospital oncology departments (or centers) have not established laboratories, and can not carry out basic research or clinical basic research of cancer because without the breakthrough of basic research, clinical efficacy is difficult to improve. "Oncology" is still the most backward discipline in the current medical sciences. Why? It is because the etiology, pathogenesis, pathophysiology of oncology are still unclear, people still lack sufficient understanding of its pathogenesis and cancer cell metastasis mechanism, and still lack sufficient understanding of the complex biological behavior of cancer cells, so the current treatment plan is still It is quite blind, so it is necessary to establish a laboratory for basic research and clinical basic research.

5). The road that has passed in a century is to attention or to rectify the treatment with light prevention, or to treat without prevention. Prevention cancer and anti-cancer are human causes, but over the years we have only been working on cancer treatment, doing very little on prevention cancer work, and almost never doing it.

2. What to do?

(1) Conducting cancer research is an urgent need of the current oncology discipline.

1). It must know the current problems of oncology.

2). It must know the problems in the current treatment.

(2) How can we reduce the incidence, improve the cure rate, and reduce the mortality rate?

1). How to improve cancer cure rate and reduce mortality

—— The way out for cancer treatment is "three early" (early detection, early diagnosis, early treatment), early cancer treatment is effective and can be cured.

In particular, precancerous lesions are well treated and can be cured. One-third of cancers can be cured by early treatment.

2). How to reduce the incidence of cancer

—— The way out to fight cancer is prevention, and more than 1/3 of cancer can be prevented.

Third

To analyze the next research prospects

1. The analysis of we should give play to our advantages in areas where China has advantages.

However, China also has our advantages. We should give full play to our advantages in areas where our country has advantages. In the field of cancer research, traditional Chinese medicine is an advantage of China. To play the role of this advantage in the field of cancer research, to explore and develop prevention cancer, anti-cancer herbal agents, and the research of playing this advantage should be a strategic vision of international significance.

The combination of Chinese and Western medicine is the characteristics and advantages of Chinese medicine. The goal of combining Chinese and Western medicine should be to combine innovation, and the goal of combining innovation should be to improve the treatment effect. The standard of efficacy for cancer patients should be: The patient has a long survival time, good quality of life and few complications.

The combination of Chinese and Western medicine, it comes from Chinese medicine, higher than Chinese medicine; It comes from Western medicine, higher than Western medicine. The goal of combining is to combine innovation, and the result of innovation should be innovation "Chinese medicine" and innovation "Chinese style anti-cancer".

At present, in addition to research on synthetic drugs, countries all over the world are also studying herbs in the region and the country. Scientists have returned to nature to find new anticancer drugs and study the immunotherapeutic capabilities of biological response modifiers. China has a lot of natural medicines in this field, such as lentinan, ginseng polysaccharide, ganoderma lucidum polysaccharide, Hericium erinaceus polysaccharide and many other natural plant herbs etc, which contain a variety of histones, polysaccharides, have a better role of biological response modifiers, have immunomodulatory effects.

All the experiments in the experimental conditions of experimental tumors should be further studied in depth, scientifically, objectively, and realistically, with modern science and technology, and carry out in-depth and modern research on traditional Chinese medicine immunopharmacology.

Many Chinese herbal medicines are immune enhancers, biological response modifiers, and tonics. Many of them can strengthen the body's immunity and anti-cancer power. Trying to improve the body's immunity is an important measure to prevent cancer and cancer. How to improve immunity? Chinese herbal medicine is an extremely important advantage.

2. The research work we have carried out in the past 28 years:

(1) New findings in anti-cancer and anti-cancer metastasis research

1). from the results of follow-up it was found:

a. postoperative recurrence, metastasis is the key to affect the long-term efficacy of surgery

b. Prompt clinicians must pay attention to and study the prevention and treatment measures for postoperative recurrence and metastasis

2). from experimental tumor research it was found:

a. the experimental results suggest that the removal of the thymus can create a cancer-bearing animal model

b. The experimental results suggest that the immune system is low first, and then the cancer is likely to occur and develop.

c. Experimental results suggest that metastasis is related to immunity, and immune function is low, which may promote cancer metastasis.

d. The experimental results suggest that the host thymus is acute progressive atrophy immediately after inoculation of cancer cells, cell proliferation is blocked, and the volume is significantly reduced.

e. The experimental results suggest that some experimental rats are not inoculated, or the tumor is small, the thymus does not shrink significantly. In order to study the relationship between tumor and thymus atrophy, the tumor is resected when the tumor grows with a large finger after inoculation of the cancer cells. After anatomy, the thymus was not atrophied again after one month.

f. The above experimental results prove that: the progress of the tumor makes the thymus progressively atrophy. Then, can we adopt some methods to prevent the thymus atrophy of the host, and adopt the mouse for fetal liver, fetal spleen and fetal thymocyte transplantation? The experimental study of immune function showed that: S, T, L three groups of cells combined transplantation, the recent complete tumor regression rate was 40%, the long-term tumor complete regression rate was 46.6%, the tumor completely disappeared long-term survival.

In summary, from the above series of experimental studies, it is found that thymus atrophy and immune dysfunction may be one of the causes and pathogenesis of cancer.

3). XZ presented in this monograph and at the International Oncology Society: **"One of the causes and pathogenesis of cancer may be thymus atrophy and immune dysfunction"**. After the investigation, this is the first time in the world.

4). XZ presented in this monograph and at the International Oncology Society: "Theoretical Basis and Experimental Basis of XZ-C Immunomodulation Therapy -" protection of Thymus and Increase of immune function "(protecting the thymus, raising immunity) and protecting the marrow to produce blood (protecting bone Hematopoietic stem cells), this is the first time internationally presented.

5). XZ puts forward the initiative in this monograph: "The aim or target of cancer treatment must simultaneously establish a comprehensive treatment concept for both tumor and host." At present, hospitals at home and abroad put chemotherapy and chemotherapy to kill cancer cells. We think this is one-sided. The treatment concept not only does not protect the patient's immunity, but also kills the host's immune cells and bone hematopoietic cells in a large amount, resulting in the lower the immune function of the chemotherapy, and the transfer of chemotherapy.

6). XZ proposes in this monograph:

Establish a multidisciplinary comprehensive treatment plan The whole process of treatment is the main axis:

surgery-based + biological therapy, immunotherapy, integrated Chinese and Western medicine treatment, XZ-C immunomodulation treatment......

The Short-course treatment is the auxiliary axis:

mainly for radiotherapy and chemotherapy. It should not be treated for a long time, and should not be excessive. It should change the current status of over-treatment in some hospitals.

7). XZ proposed a new concept of cancer anti-metastasis treatment in this monograph. It is believed that there are three manifestations of cancer in the human body:

the first is primary cancer; the second is metastatic cancer; and the third is cancer cell group on the way to metastasis.

__The new treatment model of which it is to carry out cofferdams, block or interfere, cut off the transfer route or cancer cell group on the way to transfer is the key to anti-cancer metastasis__.

8). The theoretical system of XZ-C cancer treatment was formed:

immune regulation and controlling treatment.

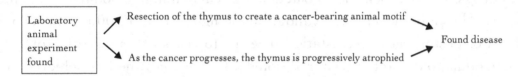

It is because:

thymus atrophy, immune function is low → the theoretical basis for the proposed treatment: XZ-C immune regulation and control "protection of Thymus an increase of immune function" → exclusive development products: XZ-C1-10 → clinical verification: 16 years of outpatient observation and follow-up of advanced cancer patients More than 12,000 cases can improve the quality of life and prolong survival.

(2). Research Overview XZ-C immunomodulation of anticancer Chinese medicine

1). Looking for new anti-cancer and anti-transfer anti-recurrence new research from natural medicine, the existing anti-cancer drugs kill both cancer cells and normal cells, and have large adverse reactions. We used anti-tumor experiments in cancer-bearing mice to find new drugs that only inhibit cancer cells without affecting normal cells.

a. Using the method of in vitro culture of cancer cells to conduct screening experiments on the rate of inhibition of cancer in Chinese herbal medicine - in vitro screening test

b. Manufacture of animal models and experimental study on the rate of cancer suppression in Chinese-female animals in vivo - in vivo anti-tumor screening test

We spent a full three years on the anti-tumor screening experiments of cancer-bearing animals in 200 kinds of Chinese herbal medicines used in traditional anti-cancer prescriptions and anti-cancer agents reported in various places. A total of nearly 6000 tumor-bearing animal models were made, and the liver, spleen, lung, thymus, and kidney were dissected after death. Results 48 kinds of traditional Chinese medicines with good anti-tumor effect and good regulation and exemption were screened out.

2). Clinical validation work

Through the above four years to explore the basic experimental research of recurrence and metastasis, and after three years of experimental research from natural drugs, we have identified a batch of XZ-C1-10 immunomodulatory Chinese medicine. Through the clinical validation of more than 12,000 patients with advanced or postoperative metastatic cancer in 16 years, the application of XZ-C immunomodulation of anticancer traditional Chinese medicine has achieved good results, which can improve the quality of life of patients, improve the symptoms of patients, and significantly prolong the survival of patients.

(3) Experimental study and clinical efficacy of XZ-C immunomodulation anticancer Chinese medicine in the treatment of malignant tumors

1). XZ-C immunomodulation anticancer Chinese medicine is the result of modernization of traditional Chinese medicine

2). XZ-C immunomodulation anticancer Chinese medicine treatment of cancer cases list and typical cases

(4). To study the anti-cancer effect of traditional Chinese medicine, it is necessary to carry out modern scientific research, analysis and purification of effective components and modern immunopharmacological experiments and research. Although we should give full play to China's advantages in areas where China has advantages, in the field of cancer research, the combination of traditional

Chinese medicine and Chinese and Western medicine is China's advantage. To play the role of this advantage in the field of cancer research, scientific research, experimental research, effective component analysis, purification and modern pharmacological experiments should be carried out to study the anticancer effects and mechanisms of traditional Chinese medicine, and modernize and make Chinese medicine modernization and scientific.

However, it is necessary to recognize the advantages of Chinese medicine, what are the shortcomings, and whether it is toxic or not. The application should consider the "long", "short", "de", and "missing" of the patient. It is necessary to carry out modern scientific research, "should be going to be crude and fine" and "to falsify the truth", scientific research, analysis, clinical verification, and it should be scientific, authenticity, safety. During doctors are conducting scientific research and clinical application, it must have both ability and moral or political integrity, medicine is benevolence, the ethics is the first.

(5). TO analyze the next research prospects, the prospective assessment of cancer treatment:

- Molecular targeted drug therapy attracts attention

- The outlook for immunomodulatory drugs is gratifying

- Immunotherapy opens a new era of cancer treatment

- Applying vaccines to treat cancer is a human hope

- The way out for cancer treatment is in three early mornings

- The way out to conquer cancer is prevention

3. Our initial work in conquering cancer:

(1). Chapter 38 of the monograph "New Concepts and New Methods of Cancer Therapy" published by Xu Ze in October 2011 uses a chapter to propose "strategic ideas and suggestions for conquering cancer."

(2). In June 2013, Xu Ze proposed to "conquer the basic concept and design of the general attack on cancer" in an attempt to reduce the incidence of cancer, reduce cancer mortality, improve the cure rate, and prolong the survival period. The total attack is prevention cancer + cancer control + cancer treatment, the three carriages go hand in hand.

(3). Xu Ze first proposed in the international exhibition in August 2013:

"XZ-C Scientific Research Plan to conquer cancer and to launch the General Attack of Cancer" - The overall strategy and development of cancer treatment in China

(4). Xu Ze proposed the following four feasibility reports for conquering cancer and launching the general attack on cancer in July 2015.

"XZ-C proposes a scientific research plan to overcome cancer and to conquer cancer and launch the general attack of cancer" - the overall strategic reform and development of cancer treatment in China

1), it was first proposed at the international level:

"Necessity and Feasibility Report on overcoming cancer and launching the General Attack of Cancer"

2), it first proposed at the international level:

"Preparing to build the hospital with the prevention and treatment during the whole process of cancer occurrence and development"

(Global Demonstration Prevention and Treatment Hospital)

Imagine and Feasibility report of preparation of the hospital with the full-scale prevention and treatment

—— Explain the necessity and feasibility of establishing a full-scale prevention and treatment hospital"

3), it is first proposed at the international level:

"To build a general plan to overcome cancer and the basic vision and feasibility report of Science City"

- Equivalent to designing an overall framework for Chinese characteristics to overcome cancer design

4), it is first proposed at the international level:

"In the construction of a well-off society, it is recommended to "catch the research" - the necessity and feasibility report of medical research and cancer prevention and treatment for cancer prevention and cancer control - adhere to the road of prevention cancer and cancer control with Chinese characteristics

These four scientific research projects were first proposed internationally, opening up new areas of anti-cancer research.

It is unprecedented work to propose a general attack to overcome cancer.

(5). Xu Ze's fourth "Monograph" new book:

"On Innovation Of Treatment Of Cancer" - published in Washington, December 2015, published in English, globally, and distributed electronically Introducing a new book

Introduction to the new book:

Experimental research, Chinese medicine immunopharmacology and molecular level Chinese and Western medicine combined with anti-cancer research, has initially formed the theoretical system of XZ-C immune regulation and treatment of cancer.

Step out of a traditional Chinese medicine immune regulation, regulate immune activity, prevent thymus atrophy, promote thymic hyperplasia, protect bone marrow hematopoietic function, improve immune surveillance, and combine Western medicine at the molecular level to overcome the new path of cancer.

How to overcome cancer, I see:

- Avoid empty talk, work hard, no matter how far the road to cancer is, you should always start.

- To overcome cancer, the general attack should be launched. What is the total attack on cancer?

The general attack is to carry out the three-stage work of anti-cancer, cancer control and cancer treatment in the whole process of cancer occurrence and development, and carry out simultaneously.

That is:

Prevention of cancer - before cancer formation

Cancer control - precancerous lesions with a tendency to malignant

Treating cancer - has formed a lesion or metastasis

The goal of the total attack:

Reduce cancer lesions, reduce cancer mortality, improve cure rate, prolong survival, improve quality of life, and reduce complications.

- What should I do next?

Now it is proposed to overcome cancer and launch a general attack.

I hope to get support from leaders at all levels.

I am fully aware that in order to achieve the purpose of cancer prevention, control, and treatment, it must be done by government leaders, government leaders, experts, scholars, mass participation, national mobilization, and participation of thousands of households.

- Due to the increasing number of cancer patients, the incidence rate is rising and the mortality rate is high. It is recognized that cancer should not only pay attention to treatment, but also pay attention to prevention, so as to block the source, and focus on the occurrence of cancer and the research aims to focus on the prevention and treatment of cancer occurrence and development.

Fourth

"Dawning C-type plan" scientific and technological innovation, realization of outlines, avoiding empty talk, heavy work, starting

1. Combination of Chinese and Western medicine

Comprehensive (Chinese and Western) anti-cancer strength

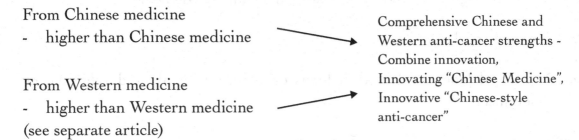

From Chinese medicine
- higher than Chinese medicine

From Western medicine
- higher than Western medicine
(see separate article)

Comprehensive Chinese and Western anti-cancer strengths -
Combine innovation,
Innovating "Chinese Medicine",
Innovative "Chinese-style anti-cancer"

2. I would like to invite Hubei University of Traditional Chinese Medicine,

Wuhan Association for Science and Technology ⟶ Take the lead

initiate

Co-organized by Wuhan Anticancer Research Association under the leadership of the province and city

(see separate article)

3. Hubei and Wuhan four collaborations, lead

In Hubei:

University of Traditional Chinese Medicine

Tongji

Concord

Wu Da

(see separate article)

4. Organize the combination of Chinese and Western forces, four collaborations, and lead

Hubei· Wuhan—Hubei University of Traditional Chinese Medicine

Shanghai - Fudan University

Tianjin - Nankai University

Shanghai - Shanghai University of Traditional Chinese Medicine

(see separate article)

5. Division of labor, each with a focus on achieving goals and achievements, achievements

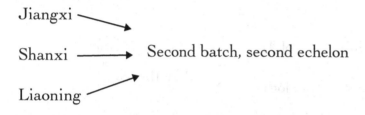

Jiangxi

Shanxi ⟶ Second batch, second echelon

Liaoning

(see separate article)

6. The task

1). To overcome the general attack of cancer

2). To establish a global demonstration of prevention and treatment hospitals (the combination of Chinese and Western medicine at the molecular level, prevention and treatment)

3). The preparation for "The Science City of conquering Cancer"

4). To establish multidisciplinary research institute

5). The preparation for Environmental Protection and Cancer Research Institute

6). To establish a cancer animal experiment center (all above are provincial)

(see separate article)

7. Hope: Establish the first "Science City for conquering cancer and launching the General Attack of Cancer Attack" in Hubei and Wuhan, and establish the world's first "Science City to overcome cancer and to launch the general attack of cancer."

Why is it set up in the university town of Huangjiahu?

Because it depends on Hubei University of Traditional Chinese Medicine (Chinese medicine, Chinese and Western medicine combined)

Wu Da ⟶
              Modern medicine
Huake University ↗

invite:

8. Chairman of the General Design and Academic Committee of Science City: Professor Xu Ze (Chinese Medicine)

Secretary General: Professor Zou Shengquan (Tongji)

Chief Dean: Professor Hong Guangxiang (Concord)

(see separate article)

invite:

9. "Conquering Cancer Science City" Chinese and Western Medicine combined with academic leaders: Academician Wu Xianzhong (Tianjin)

Academician Tang Wei (Shanghai)

Professor Xu Ze (Wuhan)

(see separate article)

Prevention cancer and anti-cancer

Conquer cancer and launch a general attack

(four)

"New Moon Plan or Cancer Moon Shot" (US) and "Dawning C Plan" (China)

- Moving forward together, heading for the science hall to overcome cancer

Situation analysis (2)

Scientific research plan

Original innovation

Secret level: Class A (A)

"New Moon Plan Cancer Moon Shot" (US) and "Dawning C Plan" (China)

- Moving forward together, heading for the science hall to overcome cancer

Situation analysis (2)

1. Race with the "Cancer moon shot", **why is it not to be led by the Oncology, Cancer Center or Provincial Cancer Hospital of some famous university affiliated hospitals in China or our province? They have superior equipment conditions and superb medical technology, but are led by the University of Chinese Medicine?**

Because the current status of modern medicine in the oncology and cancer centers of the affiliated institutions of higher education institutions in China and our province is:

- Life sciences, molecular biology, genetic engineering, and protein science groups are all studied and advanced from the United States, and they have no innovative patent inventions;

- Targeted therapeutic drugs and monoclonal antibody drugs are imported from the United States, and they have no innovative patents or inventions;

- Cancer diagnosis and treatment equipment and precision instruments are imported from the United States. They have studied and studied from the United States, and they have almost no innovation patents or inventions.

- New surgery for tumors or innovative new surgical techniques, from the United States to further study and study, without their own innovative patents, inventions;

- Minimally invasive technology and minimally invasive equipment, all imported from the United States, from the United States for further study and study, they have no innovative patents, inventions.

In short, modern medicine is sourced from Europe and the United States. In the past 100 years, American modern medicine has developed and advanced, and has developed into precision oncology medicine. Our oncology lacks innovative medicine, medicine and technology in our own oncology, innovative academics, theories, innovative patents and inventions.

<u>We must be self-reliant, independent innovation, original innovation, and breakthrough medical and scientific achievements. Only then can we have our own medical, pharmaceutical, and scientific achievements, and we can have our own medicine, medicine, and scientific and technological achievements to compete with others and race with others.</u>

Innovation is not only technology, product innovation, but also basic theoretical innovation, and theoretical innovation is the biggest achievement. Scientific development is based on the innovation of basic theory, which is the biggest invention.

2.   Why is it led by the University of Chinese Medicine?

It is because:

(1)   **We should give full play to China's advantages in areas where China has advantages. In the field of cancer research, traditional Chinese medicine is an advantage of China. We should play this advantage in cancer research and explore and develop effective Chinese herbal medicines for cancer prevention and anti-cancer.** In-depth research should be carried out to analyze and purify the active ingredients; to carry out research on the immunological pharmacology of traditional Chinese medicine; to carry out research on molecular level and gene level, so that the modernization of Chinese herbal medicines is in line with international standards.

(2)   **The combination of Chinese and Western medicine is the characteristics and advantages of Chinese medicine**. It comes from Chinese medicine, higher than Chinese medicine. It comes from Western medicine, higher than Western medicine, and is a combination of Chinese medicine and Western medicine. 1+1=2, 2>1, which makes the treatment of cancer combined with Chinese and Western medicine more perfect and reasonable, and improves the curative effect. Because traditional cancer therapy (surgery, radiotherapy, chemotherapy) reduces the body's immune function, and immune-regulated anti-cancer drugs increase the body's immune function, and become a comprehensive treatment, post-operative

+ immunity, radiotherapy + Chinese medicine immunity (immunotherapy) Chemotherapy + Chinese medicine immunization (immunotherapy) will inevitably improve its efficacy.

1). Why is Chinese herbal medicine the advantage of China in cancer research?

It is because treatment must be directed to the cause, pathogenesis, pathophysiology.

The following multidisciplinary and cancer-related relationships should be sought for treatment methods and drugs:

a, cancer and immunity have a positive relationship, should look for immunomodulatory drugs;

b, some cancers have a positive relationship with the virus, should look for antiviral drugs;

c, some cancers have a positive relationship with endocrine hormones, should look for drugs that regulate endocrine hormones;

d, some cancers are related to fungi, and anti-fungal drugs should be sought;

e, Some cancers are associated with chronic inflammation and should be searched for drugs that are resistant to chronic inflammation.

These immune regulation, adjustment of endocrine hormones, anti-virus, etc., are rare in modern medicine and western medicine. However, China's Fuzheng Guben and Tonifying Chinese herbal medicines are rich in resources, and have immune regulation, hormone adjustment, and anti-virus. Good function, and has a long history and clinical application experience and works. In recent years, some researchers and graduate students have carried out some experimental analysis and research on the molecular level of Chinese herbal medicines. It should be said that in the study of cancer, the richness of Chinese herbal medicine resources is an advantage.

2). Why is Chinese herbal medicine the advantage of China in the field of cancer research?

Our experiment has the following experimental basis and accumulated data of our own clinical verification.

It is because our laboratory has screened out 48 Chinese herbal medicines that have a good anti-tumor rate.

Existing anticancer drugs not only kill cancer cells but also normal cells, and have large adverse reactions. We have tried new cancer drugs in cancer-bearing mice to find new drugs that inhibit cancer cells without affecting normal cells. We spent a full three years on the anti-tumor screening experiments of cancer-bearing animals in 200 kinds of Chinese herbal medicines used in traditional anti-cancer prescriptions and anti-cancer agents reported in various places. As a result, 48 strains were screened for better tumor inhibition.

Looking for Chinese herbal medicine, screening anti-cancer, anti-metastatic new drugs:

The purpose is to screen out new anti-cancer, anti-metastatic, anti-recurring and intelligent anti-cancer drugs with no drug resistance, no toxic side effects, high selectivity and long-term oral administration.

To this end, we conducted an experimental study in the laboratory for screening anticancer and anti-metastatic drugs from traditional Chinese medicine for three years:

a. Using the method of in vitro culture of cancer cells, screening experiments on the inhibition rate of Chinese herbal medicine.

b. Manufacture of animal models of cancer-bearing animals, and conduct experimental studies on the rate of cancer suppression in cancer-bearing animals by Chinese herbal medicines.

Experimental results:

Among the 200 Chinese herbal medicines screened by animal experiments in our laboratory, 48 strains were selected to have certain or even excellent inhibitory effects on cancer cell proliferation, and the tumor inhibition rate was 75-90%. However, there are also some commonly used traditional Chinese medicines that are generally considered to have anti-cancer effects. After screening for animal tumors in vitro and in vivo, there is no anti-cancer effect. In this group, 152 kinds of anti-cancer effects were eliminated by animal experiment screening.

The 48 kinds of traditional Chinese medicines with good tumor inhibition rate were selected by this experiment, and then the anti-tumor experiments were carried out in vivo by optimizing the combination. Finally, the XU ZE China preparation with immunomodulation and anti-cancer Chinese medicine with Chinese characteristics was developed (XZ —C1-10).

XZ-C1 can significantly inhibit cancer cells, but does not affect normal cells; XZ-C4 can promote thymic hyperplasia and increase immunity; XZ-C8 can protect the marrow from hematopoiesis and protect bone marrow hematopoietic function.

3). Why is Chinese herbal medicine the advantage of China in cancer research?

Because our laboratory finds from the Chinese herbal medicine to promote thymic hyperplasia, prevent thymus atrophy, and improve immune control and regulation of traditional Chinese medicine.

We conducted a full 4 years of oncology research work in the laboratory. Our laboratory experimental results showed that the thymus of the cancer-bearing mice showed progressive atrophy, the volume was reduced, the cell proliferation was blocked, and the mature cells were reduced. By the end of the tumor, the thymus is extremely atrophied and the texture becomes hard.

From the above experimental studies, it is found that thymus atrophy and low immune function may be one of the pathogenic factors and pathogenesis of tumors, so it is necessary to try to prevent thymus atrophy, promote thymocyte proliferation, and increase immunity. The immune function of the body, especially cellular immunity, the function of T lymphocytes, and the immune regulation function of the thymus should be explored at the molecular level, and methods for immune regulation and effective drug research should be sought.

Where should I find new ways to regulate immune therapy?

In order to prevent thymus atrophy, promote thymocyte proliferation, and increase immunity, we look for both Chinese medicine and western medicine. The existing medicines of western medicine can improve immunity and promote the proliferation of thymus. So we changed to look for Chinese herbal medicine.

Why do you look for drugs that promote thymic hyperplasia, prevent thymus atrophy, and boost immunity from traditional Chinese medicine?

Because Chinese medicine's tonic drugs generally contain the role of regulating immunity. Chinese medicine has Chinese medicine and polysaccharide Chinese medicine.

a. tonic Chinese medicine, have the role of regulating the body's immune function. When the animal is at a low level of immune activity (such as dethymus, aging animals, or chemotherapy drugs cyclophosphamide inhibition and tumor animals), the tonic drugs improve the body's immunity is more significant.

b. Anti-cancer immunity of traditional Chinese medicine polysaccharides is progressing rapidly. A large number of immunopharmacological studies have been carried out at the molecular level. Polysaccharides can improve the body's immune surveillance system, including natural killer cells (NK), macrophages (MΦ), and killer T cells. (CTL), T cells, LAK cells, tumor infiltrating lymphocytes (TIL), interleukin (IL) and other cytokines are active to kill tumor cells.

Both Chinese medicine and western medicine have their own strengths, and each has its own shortness. Compared with western medicine immunopharmacology, traditional Chinese medicine immunopharmacology has its own characteristics and advantages, and each has its own shortcomings. The advantage of traditional Chinese medicine immunology is that a large number of Chinese medicines have the effect of regulating the body's immune function. Traditional Chinese medicine is rich in source and is an effective medicine for long-term clinical treatment. After extraction, it may obtain active ingredients and obvious pharmacological effects (including immunomodulatory effects). The research process saves people time and has high efficiency.

3. Why is the race proposed by our Experimental Surgery Research Institute of Hubei University of Traditional Chinese Medicine?

(1) For 28 years, we have achieved scientific research results and technological innovation series of cancer research:

Can participate in competitions, participate in learning, and inspire us to move forward

The goal of the competition is:

1), to prolong the survival time of cancer patients (long live), good quality of life, and fewer complications.

2), reduce the incidence of cancer, improve the cure rate and reduce the mortality rate.

(2) In the past 28 years, we have obtained research and research achievements in anti-cancer and anti-cancer metastasis, and scientific and technological innovation series:

A. New findings in experimental research, new theory, new theory

a. "thymus atrophy, low immune function is one of the causes and pathogenesis of cancer"

- propose a new concept of cancer treatment principles

b. "Theoretical Basis and Experimental Basis of XZ-C Immunomodulation Therapy"

—— Proposed the theoretical basis and experimental basis of cancer immune regulation therapy

B. Propose new concepts and new initiatives for cancer treatment

a. "Cancer treatment should change the concept, establish a comprehensive treatment concept"

- propose a new concept of cancer treatment principles

b. "A new model for the combination of multidisciplinary treatment of cancer"

- Proposing a new concept of the cancer treatment combination model

C. cancer metastasis research and theoretical innovation

a. "There are three main manifestations of cancer in the human body"

—— Proposed theoretical innovation of cancer metastasis treatment

b. "Two points and one line" in the whole process of cancer development

—— Proposed theoretical innovation of cancer metastasis treatment

c. "Three Steps of Anticancer Metastasis Treatment"

—— Proposing theoretical innovation of new concept of cancer metastasis treatment

—— Incorporate the "eight steps" of cancer cell transfer into "three stages" and try to break through

d. "Develop the third field of anti-cancer metastasis treatment"

—— Proposed the theoretical innovation of cancer metastasis treatment, found and proposed the third field of human anti-cancer metastasis treatment

—— **The circulatory system has a large number of immune surveillance cells, and the "main battlefield" of cancer cells on the way to annihilation is in the blood circulation.**

D. exclusive research and development products: XZ-C immune regulation anti-cancer Chinese medicine product series

a. "Overview of XZ-C Immunoregulation of Anticancer Traditional Chinese Medicine"

—— Using the method of in vitro culture of cancer cells to conduct screening experiments on the inhibition rate of Chinese herbal medicine

—— Manufacturing a cancer animal model and conducting an experimental study on the cancer suppression rate of Chinese herbal medicines in cancer-bearing animals

b. "Experimental study and clinical efficacy of XZ-C immunomodulation anticancer traditional Chinese medicine in the treatment of malignant tumors"

—— Animal experimental research and clinical application

—— XZ-C immunomodulation Chinese medicine is the result of the modernization of traditional Chinese medicine

c. "XZ-C immunomodulation anticancer Chinese medicine treatment of cancer cases list and some typical cases"

E. It is to Propose cancer treatment reform and innovation

a, "Cancer Treatment Reform and Innovation Research"

—— Adhere to the road of scientific research and innovation of anti-cancer transfer with Chinese characteristics

—— 1-8 of cancer treatment reform and innovation research

b, "Walked out of a new road to overcome cancer"

—— The theoretical system of XZ-C immunomodulation therapy has been initially formed, and it is undergoing clinical application and observation verification.

—— There are exclusive research and development products, XZ-C immunomodulation anti-cancer Chinese medicine series, there have been a large number of clinically validated cases

—— In the past 20 years, a new road to overcome cancer has been preliminarily

Now is the fourth stage of our research work, which is being carried out and carried out, research work, step by step, positioning the research target or "target" to reduce the incidence of cancer, improve the cure rate and prolong the survival period.

At present, the tumor hospital or oncology hospital model is fully focused on treatment. For the patients in the middle and late stage, the curative effect is poor, the human and financial resources are exhausted, and the incidence rate is not reduced, and the more patients are treated. The status quo is: the road that has passed in a century is to rectify the light, or to cure it. For many years we have only been working on cancer treatment. However, work on cancer prevention has been done very little and almost nothing has been done. As a result, the incidence of cancer continues to rise.

In short, anti-cancer has not been taken seriously, and prevention has not been taken seriously. The prevention of the old-fashioned talks is mainly based on failure to pay attention.

How to do? How to reduce the incidence of cancer? How to improve the cure rate of cancer? How to reduce cancer mortality? How to prolong the survival period? How to improve the quality of life?

It should be launched to overcome conquer and to launch the general attack of cancer, prevention and treatment are equally important.

The goal of conquering cancer should be:

reduce morbidity, increase cure rate, reduce mortality, prolong survival, improve quality of life, and reduce complications.

At present, global hospitals and hospitals in China are doing their best to treat, re-treatment and light defense.

At present, global hospitals and hospitals in China are all devoted to treatment, attach to treatment and light prevention, or only treatment without prevention.

XZ-C believes that this mode of hospitalization or cancer treatment is unlikely to overcome cancer and it is impossible to reduce the incidence. Global hospitals and hospitals in China must carry out an overall strategic reform of cancer treatment, focusing on treatment and focusing on prevention and treatment.

Therefore, we propose to launch a general attack plan and design to overcome cancer. XZ-C (Xu Ze-China) proposed to launch a general attack, that is, the three stages of anti-cancer, cancer control and cancer treatment were carried out in full swing.

Application report for "Necessity and Feasibility Report for Overcoming cancer and launching the General Attack of Cancer Attack"

Application report for "XZ-C Scientific Research Plan for Overcoming the General Attack of Cancer Attack"

In short, as mentioned above, China's modern medicine relies on imported medicine for cancer treatment, and its own inventions, patents, and intellectual property rights are small.

So how do you race? What to take to the game?

As mentioned above, in the field of cancer treatment, Chinese herbal medicine is China's advantage. In the past 28 years, the experimental research of our Experimental Surgery Research Institute and the clinical specialization of oncology clinics have confirmed the clinical trials in a large number of cases. It is confirmed that in the treatment of cancer, Chinese herbal medicine is China. The advantages can go international and benefit patients. Many cancer patients have significantly prolonged their survival.

Therefore, our country's advantages are:

1. Traditional Chinese medicine, anti-cancer traditional Chinese medicine, immune regulation traditional Chinese medicine, blood stasis anti-cancer suppository Chinese medicine

2. Combination of Chinese and Western medicine, combined with innovation 1+1=2

2>1

The advantages of the United States are:

Modern medicine, advanced diagnosis and treatment technology, targeted drugs

It should give full play to China's advantages, we should increase efforts to develop and explore the advantages of Chinese herbal medicine

Therefore, I think: it should be the game, and it should race

Chinese and Western medicines have their own strengths and shortcomings. The two should complement each other and combine advantages. One runs inside the ring, one runs outside the circle, one kills cancer cells, one focuses on boosting immunity, immune regulation, and advances together and going to the science hall to conquer cancer.

Running with the "New Moon Plan" is not a challenge or a challenge, but to motivate yourself to achieve the "Dawning C-type plan" and move forward together to reach the scientific hall of cancer.

Prevention cancer and anti-cancer

Conquer cancer and launch a general attack

(Fives)

"New Moon Plan or Cancer Moon Shot" (USA) and "Dawning C-type Plan" (China)

- Moving forward together, heading for the science hall to overcome cancer

Situation analysis (3)

Scientific research plan

Original innovation

Secret level: Class A

"New Moon Plan or Cancer Moon Shot" (USA) and "Dawning C-type Plan" (China)

- Moving forward together, heading for the science hall to overcome cancer

Situation analysis (3)

Conquering cancer, where is the road? - Where to go? How to go?

The analysis of the existing roads, what is the prospect? What is the future?

First

To analyze the situation of cancer occurrence and development in the past century.

I am a geriatric medical worker who has been in clinical practice for 60 years. What I have seen in Wuhan for 65 years is that I feel deeply that the incidence of cancer is rising. When we moved from Shanghai to Wuhan in 1951, when we moved to Shanghai from Shanghai, we were looking for a lung cancer patient to train our students. It was hard to find a cancer patient even if a phone call to the hospital was made one week earlier. In the past, there were no cancer departments in all hospitals, only tuberculosis. Today (65 years later) is a common disease, frequently-occurring disease, each hospital has an oncology department, and some large hospitals have cancer centers, the more patients are treated and the more the patients come.

Should it be analyzed, why?

Should be analyzed, what should I do? Where is the way out?

I am deeply aware that cancer should not only pay attention to treatment, but also pay attention to prevention, in order to stop at the source. The way out for cancer treatment is "three early" (early detection, early diagnosis, early treatment), and the way to fight cancer is prevention.

It should analyze, what should Wuhan do? How can we reduce the incidence? Improve the cure rate?

How can I "three early"? It is necessary to establish a full-range prevention cancer +cancer control + treatment hospital, change the hospital mode, and change the treatment mode.

How can I prevent it? A science city to overcome cancer should be established

We will establish the first "Science City for Cancer Prevention" in Hubei and Wuhan, which is the world's first science city to overcome cancer

Second

To analyze the current prospects of the three traditional treatments? What is the future?

Can you rely on three major treatments to conquer cancer and even overcome cancer?

Traditional cancer therapy (surgery, chemotherapy, radiotherapy) has been there for nearly a century, and it should review, reflect, summarize the lessons of success and failure.

The traditional concept holds that cancer is the continuous division and proliferation of cancer cells, and its therapeutic goal must be to kill cancer cells.

After more than half a century, how is the treatment outcome? The more patients are treated, the higher the mortality rate. Therefore, the above three major treatment methods must be further studied and improved. The problems and shortcomings of surgery, radiotherapy and chemotherapy should be analyzed and reviewed separately. **One**

One

The evaluation of chemotherapy

The comment on the problems and drawbacks of systemic intravenous chemotherapy for solid tumors

The current status of cancer chemotherapy, mainly systemic intravenous chemotherapy, the route of administration of this systemic intravenous chemotherapy is:

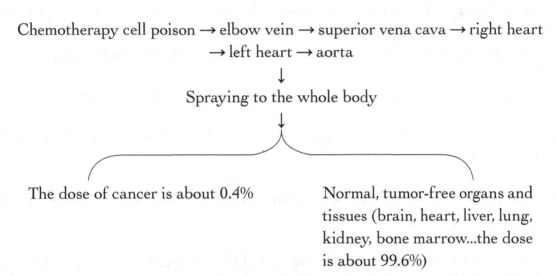

Chemotherapy cell poison → elbow vein → superior vena cava → right heart → left heart → aorta

↓

Spraying to the whole body

↓

The dose of cancer is about 0.4%   Normal, tumor-free organs and tissues (brain, heart, liver, lung, kidney, bone marrow...the dose is about 99.6%)

However, about the route of administration of systemic intravenous chemotherapy for such solid tumors, although it has been used in the world for decades, we should consider and analyze whether it is reasonable or not ? Is it scientific? Does it harm the patient? Does it cause toxic side effects?

It should be analyzed and commented:

Comment or /and Review 1: Evaluation of the route of administration of systemic intravenous chemotherapy for solid tumors

This route of administration, instead of targeted drug delivery, uses a heart pump to administer chemotherapeutic cell poisons to the whole body with blood, so that the cytotoxic drugs are distributed throughout the body and distributed throughout the body, so that the organs of the body are normal (brain, heart, liver, The lungs, kidneys, and bone marrow all obtained chemotherapy cell toxic drugs, which were damaged by them and caused toxic side effects. It is very unreasonable ad very unscientific, the result is:

1). Cancer lesion has very few drugs, only about 0.4%, and the curative effect is very small (because the cancerous area accounts for a small proportion of the total body surface area)

2). 99.6% of the cytotoxic drugs were killed to normal proliferating cells, causing toxic side effects of brain, heart, liver, lung, kidney, bone marrow, gastrointestinal system, hematopoietic system, immune system and endocrine system.

3). At present, no drug susceptibility test has been conducted in the hospital for chemotherapy. If the drug is resistant, the chemotherapy is all about killing normal tissue cells! It is especially inhibit bone marrow hematopoietic cells and immune cells! No effect on cancerous foci! (It's a white chemotherapy!)

4). So for every chemotherapy, does it kill cancer cells? It is not known.

How much has it killed? It is not known. It can only say that a chemotherapy job has been done.

Therefore, this route of administration is unreasonable, unscientific, and easily leads to iatrogenic side effects.

How to do? The route of administration should be changed into the target organ tissue intravascular chemotherapy, the drug is directly delivered to the "target organ", so the dose or drug amount is small, the curative effect is certain and positive and there is no toxic side reaction, which is beneficial or conducive to the patient.

Comment or/and Review 2: Evaluation of the dose of systemic intravenous chemotherapy for solid tumors

This is to extend the experience and methods of leukemia treatment to the treatment of solid tumors. The guiding ideology is to administer the whole body surface area. This is not sensible and unreasonable.

why?

Because leukemia cells are distributed in the systemic circulatory system, the "target" of treatment is also present in the systemic circulatory system, so systemic intravenous chemotherapy is reasonable, sensible, and consistent with targeted therapy.

However, solid tumors are limited to only one organ, and the "target" of treatment should be an organ with cancer, and targeted administration should be targeted by intravascular administration of the target organ. It is not wise and unreasonable to use the leukemia treatment experience to calculate the total body surface area.

However, solid tumors are now systemic intravenous chemotherapy. Calculating the dose according to the body surface area, in order to achieve the purpose of shrinking the cancerous foci, it is necessary to increase the amount of chemotherapy cells, which will lead to more toxic side effects and complications, and damage the patient. .

How to do?

The route of administration should be changed into the intravascular chemotherapy route of the target organ, the drug volume is small, the curative effect is certain, and there is no toxic side effect.

Comment 3: Analysis and evaluation of evaluation criteria for systemic intravenous chemotherapy of solid tumors

1). Why is the efficacy evaluation standard determined as relief?

At present, the clinical use of chemotherapy drugs can make the tumor shrink, but the effect is usually temporary, and can not significantly prolong the life of the patient. Therefore, the standard of efficacy evaluation is called "alleviation." - Generally calculated by day, week or month, if complete remission is only the tumor completely disappears, lasting for more than 4 weeks, that is to say, there may be recurrence and progression after 4 weeks.

2). Why can it only be alleviated?

a. The patient's chemotherapy to effectively kill cancer cells only 3-5 days of intravenous infusion, there is the role of killing cancer cells, then there is no killing of cancer cells, it is only a short time to kill (3-5 Days), cannot be done once and for all, after 3-5 days, the cancer cells continue to divide and proliferate, so it can only relieve short-term, can not be cured.

b. Chemotherapy cell poisons can only kill mature and mature cancer cells, and can not kill stem cells that have not yet matured. This chemotherapy kills mature and mature cancer cells. After some time, those stem cells that have not yet matured mature gradually mature. However, it continues to undergo sexual division and proliferation. It is divided into two, and the second is divided into four clones. This is a geometrical increase in value, so that the cancerous lesions are "wild fire, the spring breeze is born again", recurrence, metastasis, and progression.

Therefore, chemotherapy can not be cured, only relieved. Can only cure the symptoms, can not cure the disease, can not rely on chemotherapy to overcome cancer.

Comment 4: What is the adjuvant chemotherapy for abdominal solid tumors that failed to prevent recurrence and metastasis?

After abdominal solid tumor surgery, why failed to prevent recurrence and metastasis? Because of systemic intravenous chemotherapy cytotoxic drugs, it is not easy to reach the portal vein by the superior vena cava. The vena cava system is generally incompatible with the portal system. This route of administration is unreasonable and unscientific.

Where are the cancer cells of solid tumors of the abdomen (gastric cancer, colorectal cancer, liver cancer, biliary tract cancer, pancreatic cancer, abdominal cavity, etc.)? Mainly in the portal system, but the current global and Chinese hospitals for abdominal solid tumor postoperative adjuvant chemotherapy from the elbow vein → superior vena cava → right heart → double lung → left heart → aorta → spray to the whole body organs. However, it is not possible to enter the portal system directly. It is because the vena cava system is generally incompatible with the portal system.

Therefore, abdominal malignant tumors (stomach, intestine, liver, gallbladder, pancreas, abdominal cavity and other cancers), adjuvant chemotherapy for abdominal tumors from the venous vein → vena cava is unreasonable, unscientific, does not conform to anatomy Physiology and pathology, which does not meet the actual path of cancer cell metastasis, because this route of administration cannot directly enter the portal vein system in which cancer cells exist.

In the past half century, thousands of cancer patients all over the world and all over China have suffered from the extensive killing of normal cells by chemotherapy cell poisons. Clinicians should seriously think about, analyze, reflect, and evaluate this.

How to do?

The route of administration should be changed to the intravascular chemotherapy route of the target organ, so that the drug can be directly introduced into the portal vein. The above solid tumor should not be administered by the elbow vein, but should be changed to the intravascular administration of the target organ, so that the drug can be targeted to the target organ cancer, which will greatly reduce the dose and improve the curative effect. Turning or eliminating the side effects of chemotherapy, so that millions of cancer patients are protected from the pain and risk of adverse reactions to chemotherapy, and benefit patients. Reducing or eliminating the side effects of chemotherapy, it will greatly reduce the medical expenses, and will save more medical expenses for the country and patients, which will help solve the problem of difficult medical treatment and expensive medical treatment. This reform will benefit millions of cancer patients.

Comment 5: There are some important misunderstandings and drawbacks in current chemotherapy

a, chemotherapy inhibits immune function, inhibits bone marrow hematopoietic function, and reduces overall immune function. When the cancer is inhibited, the thymus is inhibited, and chemotherapy inhibits the bone marrow. It is like "adding frost", which damages the entire central immune organ and promotes further decline in immune surveillance. It may lead to chemotherapy and metastasis.

b. chemotherapy target kill cancer cells, is a one-sided treatment, neglecting the body's own anti-tumor ability, neglecting the host anti-cancer system anti-cancer system (NK cells, K cells, macrophages, LAK cells), anti-cancer cells Factor system (IFN, IL2, TNF, LT and other factors), anti-cancer gene system (Rb gene, P53 gene), neglecting the role of anti-cancer institutions and their influencing factors in the human body, ignoring the inherent factors of the body's own anti-cancer Not activated, mobilized, but only blindly killing cancer cells, this one-sided treatment concept is very unreasonable, which does not meet the biological characteristics and biological behavior of cancer cells.

Two

The evaluation of radiotherapy

Comment 1:

Radiation therapy can kill a large number of normal tissue cells while killing cancer cells, causing patients to suffer from radiotherapy complications, and the quality of life is degraded. The toxicity and damage of radiotherapy are generally persistent and irreversible. Therefore, we must pay attention to the prevention and treatment of complications of tumor radiotherapy.

Comment 2:

The most important problem in cancer treatment is how to resist metastasis. If the problem of cancer metastasis cannot be solved, cancer treatment cannot be advanced.

Radiotherapy is a local treatment, and cancer metastasis is a systemic problem. This is a major contradiction. How to play its role in anti-metastasis treatment must be seriously considered and studied in depth.

Three

The evaluations of surgical treatment

Comment 1:

Surgical operation is an effective and effective method for the treatment of malignant tumors. Even if cancer treatment is developed into multidisciplinary comprehensive treatment, surgery is still one of the most important and commonly used methods for the treatment of malignant tumors. It is an important part of multidisciplinary treatment.

Comment 2:

Surgical treatment is the main treatment for solid tumors, but the design of "radical surgery" needs further research and improvement to reduce postoperative recurrence and metastasis. Attention should be paid to intraoperative "tumor-free technology" to reduce or prevent the fallout, planting and metastasis of cancer cells during surgery. Should pay attention to the operation of light, stable, accurate, to reduce the intraoperative promotion of cancer cell metastasis and reduce the spread of cancer cells from the tumor vein. To prevent postoperative recurrence and metastasis, it must be started from the surgery. It must pay attention to the technology of no tumor, to prevent the transfer of the incision and drainage.

Comment 3:

Surgical treatment of solid tumors, after centuries of century history evaluation, remains the most important and reliable, the main treatment that can be relied

upon, is the main scientific technology and main treatment method to overcome cancer in the future.

In short:

As mentioned above, there are problems and drawbacks in radiotherapy and chemotherapy. It is difficult to overcome cancer, and it is necessary to find another way to overcome cancer.

Recognizing the problems and drawbacks of radiotherapy and chemotherapy, it is difficult to overcome the situation of cancer. We have taken a different approach and proposed: to overcome cancer, launch a general attack, and build a science city to overcome cancer.

Third

To analyze the next research prospects and the prospective assessment of cancer treatment.

—— *Molecular targeted drugs attract people's attention*

—— *The prospect of immunomodulatory drugs is gratifying*

—— *Immunotherapy opens a new era of cancer treatment*

—— *Biological therapy and combination of Chinese and Western medicine are two effective ways to fight cancer metastasis*

------ *Applying vaccine therapy is human hope*

—— *The way out for cancer treatment is "three early"*

—— *The way out to fight cancer is prevention*

1. Molecular targeted drug therapy attracts attention

The Philadelphia chromosome opened the door to targeted therapy. In 1960, researchers in Philadelphia, USA, found a chromosomal abnormality in patients with chronic myeloid leukemia (CML). A few years later, the researchers found that this was the result of the long arm translocation of chromosomes 9 and 22. Since this chromosomal abnormality was first discovered in Philadelphia (Phiadelphia), it was named the Philadelphia (Ph) chromosome. This chromosome has also become a target for CML targeted therapy marketed 40 years later. In 2001, the first drug that was proven to be resistant to Philadelphia molecular chromosome defects - imatinib.

The target drug trastuzumab, which targets human epidermal growth factor receptor 2 (HER2), is then used to treat HER2-positive breast cancer.

Bevacizumab, which targets VEGF, and cetuximab, which targets EGFR, treat colorectal cancer.

Gefitinib and erlotinib targeting EGFR are used for the treatment of non-small cell lung cancer.

Molecular targeting drugs are cell stabilizers, and most patients cannot achieve complete remission (CR) or partial remission (PR), but rather stable disease and improved quality of life. In addition to gefitinib, erlotinib, imatinib, more need to be combined with chemotherapy drugs.

Molecularly targeted drugs represent a new class of anticancer drugs, and Gleevec is a classic example of controlling cancer by inhibiting abnormal molecules that cause cancer without damaging other normal nuclear tissues. More and more molecularly targeted drugs have been used in cancer treatment. For example, rituximab (Trastuzumab) for treating breast of Rituximab for treating B cell lymphoma, Gifitinib for treating lung cancer, Erlotinib, and the like. Targeted therapy brings anti-tumor hope.

2.   The prospect of immunomodulatory drugs is gratifying

Regardless of the complexity of the mechanisms behind cancer, immune suppression is the key to cancer progression. By removing immunosuppressive factors and restoring the recognition of cancer cells by immune system cells, it is effective against cancer.

More and more research evidence shows that by regulating the body's immune system, it is possible to achieve cancer control. Treating tumors by activating the body's anti-tumor immune system is an area that is currently exciting for researchers. The next major breakthrough in cancer is likely to stem from this.

In order to explore the etiology, pathogenesis and pathophysiology of cancer, our laboratory has carried out a series of animal experiments in the laboratory for 4 years, and obtained new findings from the experimental results. New inspirations: thymus atrophy, low immune function is cancer One of the causes and pathogenesis, Xu Ze (Zu Ze) proposed at the International Oncology Society in 2013: the cause of cancer, one of the pathogenesis, Therefore, Xu Ze (Zu Ze) proposed at the International Society of Oncology in 2013: one of the causes of cancer, one of which may be thymus atrophy, low immune function, decreased immune surveillance and immune escape.

Therefore, the treatment principle must be to prevent progressive atrophy of the thymus, promote thymic hyperplasia, protect bone marrow hematopoietic function, improve immune surveillance, and provide experimental basis and theoretical basis for cancer immune regulation treatment.

Through the above four years to explore the basic experimental research on the mechanism of recurrence and metastasis, after 3 years from the natural medicine Chinese herbal medicine internal laboratory through the cancer-bearing animal experiment screening, 48 kinds of Chinese medicines were screened out to have a better tumor inhibition rate, and then The cancer-bearing animals were screened to form XZ-C1-10 anti-cancer immune regulation Chinese medicine.

After 20 years of clinical application of more than 12,000 patients with advanced cancer in the oncology clinic, the clinical observation and verification confirmed that the principle of immune regulation and treatment of "chest lifting" is reasonable and the curative effect is satisfactory. The application of immunomodulatory Chinese medicine has achieved good results, improved the quality of life, and significantly prolonged the survival period.

3.   ASCO Announces Major Progress in Clinical Oncology in 2015

Immunotherapy opens a new era of cancer treatment

On February 4, 2016, the American Society of Clinical Oncology (ASCO) announced the "2016 Annual Report: ASCO Clinical Oncology Progress" at Capitol Hill, Washington, DC. The report details the global clinical oncology in 2015. The research is summarized and at the same time, the future research direction is forecasted. ASCO rated the 2015 progress as "tumor immunotherapy."

ASCO President Julie M. Vose believes that the most important development in 2015 is the discovery of immunotherapy. She wrote in the foreword: "We are no longer determined by tumor type and staging as we have in the past. Treatment, in the era of precision medicine, we select or exclude treatment based on each patient and tumor genetic data. No other major advances, like immunology can be translated into clinical practice, so ASCO decided that the biggest progress in 2015 is immunotherapy."

The chairman of the committee, Professor Don Dizon, also believes that the annual research results are increasing, but from the perspective of being able to benefit patients, the most important development this year should be immunotherapy.

Prevention cancer and anti-cancer

Conquer cancer and launch a general attack

(six)

"New Moon Plan or Cancer Moon Shot" (USA) and "Dawning C Plan" (China)

- Moving forward together, heading for the science hall to overcome cancer

Situation analysis (4)

"New Moon Plan or Cancer Moon Shot" (USA) and "Dawning C Plan" (China)

- Moving forward together, heading for the science hall to overcome cancer

Situation analysis (4)

1.   **The goal of conquering cancer:**

To reduce the incidence of cancer, improve the cure rate, and prolong the survival period.

To Reach:

1/3 can be prevented

1/3 can be cured

1/3 can be treated to relieve pain, is a chronic disease

Survival with tumor, prolong survival

2.   **The road to overcome cancer**

The ways:

(1) Conquer cancer and launch a general attack

What is the total attack?

That is, prevention cancer + cancer control + cancer treatment, and at the same time,

(2) Prepare a science city to overcome cancer:

1). Innovative Molecular Oncology Medical College

-    and modern high-tech experimental talents

2). Innovative molecular tumors for prevention and treatment of Chinese and Western hospitals

3). Innovative Molecular Oncology Research Institute

4). innovative molecular tumor nano preparations pharmaceutical factory

5). Innovative Cancer Research Institute

6). Cancer Animal Experimental Center

(The following are provincial key disciplines)

3. **How to prevent it? Specific measures, feasible solutions (not empty talk), pragmatic**

4. **How to control? Specific measures, feasible solutions (not empty talk), pragmatic**

5. How to cure? Specific measures, feasible solutions (not empty talk), pragmatic

6. How to do it? Avoid empty talk, work hard, start off

7. How to get started?

1). First, it is to build the hospital with the preventing and controlling and treating cancer → establish various disciplines → establish each group

(Department)   (Study Group)

2). First, run a medical and education and research (section, group) at one-stop or at a dragon with emphasis, basic, clinical, three basic, three strict, theory, technology, experience

Cultivate all-round talents:

Have knowledge or learn, experience, technology, and theory, change the current status quo, have parts or points, and have the entire things

3). first run a graduate school, have talent training methods, ways;

a. first run the graduate tutor class, training classes, train talents and seeds, train and guide talents, put forward learning, how to overcome cancer and launch the general attack content of cancer, discussion

b. Talent seed plan: recruiting talents, experts, seeds, and learned experts and professors as seeds

Cultivating talent is seeding:

Recruit graduate students (Master degree, Ph.D degree) to cultivate seeds, work while learning, 100, all stay as new seeds, so generations of training, requires results, achievements, contribution (not only papers), that is, three years and five years later, the talents are very good and the results are numerous.

8.   How to carry out prevention cancer and anti-cancer work in Wuhan?

(1) To set up Department of prevention cancer at the top second level hospitals

Each of the top three hospitals is responsible for three community cancer prevention efforts.

Each of the top three hospitals' cancer prevention section or prevention departments needs to develop responsibilities and scope.

Not only to take vaccination, but to go deep into the community to carry out preventioncancer work

(2) The city' top second lever and three level hospitals have formulated the scope of prevention cancer and anti-cancer duties, and the division of labor is responsible for the work.

1). The top three hospitals in each province of the province are responsible for the prevention, control and treatment of the two regions.

The top three hospitals in each province are responsible for group medical treatment in two regions, consultation, solution, treatment, training, advanced training, grading diagnosis and treatment, and resolving the quality and level of technical problems.

2). The quality, level, talents and technology of the top three hospitals in the province must meet the quality level of the top three hospitals. It must be true, and it is necessary to solve the personnel training and technical level of the lower-level hospitals.

3). Establish a consultation system, brainstorm ideas, improve medical standards, solve difficult problems, and conduct inter-disciplinary consultations and inter-disciplinary consultations.

4). Tongji, Xiehe, People, Central South, and subordinate hospitals must solve the referral and consultation of the subordinate hospitals and solve the difficult problems.

5). Tongji Health System Trains the province's cancer prevention department, general practitioners, senior and intermediate health and epidemic prevention pre-scientific talents

6). Each community has prevention cancer, anti-cancer, carry out prevention cancer, supervision, mission group, responsibilities, tasks, division of labor

7). Provincial and Municipal Health Planning Commissions set up prevention cancer and cancer control offices, organize missions, guidance, and supervision

9.   How to carry out prevent cancer and cancer control work in the community?

It is to have the demonstration areas for cancer prevention, control and treatment in several communities.

It is to esstablish a system of prevention, control and governance, "China mode".

(1) Through the standardization of the "three early" information early warning system

The history of the following patients in the community is checked on schedule

1), history of blood in the stool, history of hemorrhoids, that is, it is to have colonoscopy

2), patients with a history of hematuria, that is, it needs to have cystoscopy

3), lumps, sarcoidosis, that should be percussion + surgery

4), hepatitis B, cirrhosis, half a year or once a year check

(2) Standardized community prevention cancer training

(3) Community registration, timely assessment

(4) Focus on "three early", precancerous lesions

It will greatly reduce the funds. This is used for three early examinations, different cancers, for prevention, early diagnosis, early treatment.

Chapter 21

Pathfinding and Footprint

(The scientific research footprint)

(To overcome cancer, where is the road?

- Where is the road? Where to go for ? How to go?)

Pathfinding and Footprint

(The scientific research footprint)

1. Causes

(1) Why do I study cancer?

(2) It was found from the results of follow-up

2. To find the way

(1) Why does it to find a way to conquer cancer, where is the direction of the road? Where is the road? Where is it to go?

(2) How to find a path? - it should follow the scientific research route.

(3) How to find this way? – it should be based on clinical actual problems and the experimental research findings

3. Footprint (scientific research footprint)

Pathfinding and Footprint

(The scientific research footprint)

1. Causes

(1) Why do I study cancer? I am a clinical surgeon, why do you study cancer? This is due to or caused by the result of the petition to a group of cancer patients after surgery.

In 1985, I conducted the petition for more than 3,000 patients who had undergone radical resection of thoracic surgery or general surgery operation for various cancer-related diseases (sending a letter from the operating room registration list). It was found that most patients relapsed and metastasized 2 to 3 years after surgery. This made me realize that although the operation is successful, the long-term efficacy is not satisfactory. Postoperative recurrence and metastasis are the key factors affecting the long-term efficacy of the operation. It also reminds us that prevention and treatment of postoperative recurrence and metastasis is the key to prolonging postoperative survival. **Therefore, clinical basic research must be carried out. Without breakthroughs in basic research, clinical efficacy is difficult to improve,** so we established the Institute of Experimental Surgery and conducted a series of experimental studies and clinical acceptance work.

(2) From the results of follow-up, it was found that:

1), the postoperative recurrence and metastasis are the key factors affecting the long-term efficacy of surgery;

2), it is to suggest or to prompt that clinicians must pay attention to and study the prevention and treatment of postoperative recurrence and metastasis in order to improve the long-term effect of surgery

2. Find the way

(1) Why is the pathfinding? How to find this way? Conquering cancer, where is the road? ——

- Where is the road? Where to go? How to go?

For more than a hundred years, many people with lofty ideals and scientific research elites are looking for it.

(2) How to find a path?

1). The research we conduct is based on the following research routes:

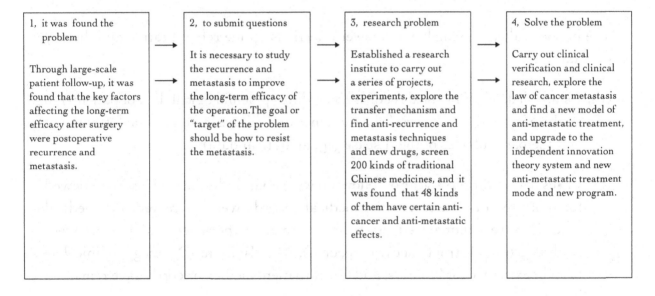

1, it was found the problem	2, to submit questions	3, research problem	4, Solve the problem
Through large-scale patient follow-up, it was found that the key factors affecting the long-term efficacy after surgery were postoperative recurrence and metastasis.	It is necessary to study the recurrence and metastasis to improve the long-term efficacy of the operation.The goal or "target" of the problem should be how to resist the metastasis.	Established a research institute to carry out a series of projects, experiments, explore the transfer mechanism and find anti-recurrence and metastasis techniques and new drugs, screen 200 kinds of traditional Chinese medicines, and it was found that 48 kinds of them have certain anti-cancer and anti-metastatic effects.	Carry out clinical verification and clinical research, explore the law of cancer metastasis and find a new model of anti-metastatic treatment, and upgrade to the independent innovation theory system and new anti-metastatic treatment mode and new program.

2). From clinical → experimental → clinical → re-experiment → re-clinical, return to the clinical to solve the problem.

3). Theory and practice are closely integrated. The chosen topics are all from the clinic. Looking for clinical focus and clinical breakthroughs, after experimental research and clinical verification, It is then applied to the clinic to solve clinical practical problems.

4). Take the road of combining Chinese and Western medicine → macroscopic combination → molecular level combination, using modern cancer cell molecular transfer mechanism and the latest theory of "eight steps" and "three stages" to find and screen anti-metastatic drugs from 200 ancient Chinese medicines. It protects immune organs, activates cytokines and immune factors, modernizes ancient Chinese medicines, and integrates with the international community, enabling modern medicine to combine with ancient Chinese herbal medicines at the molecular level and BRM level.

5). It was to establish Institute of Experimental Surgery, and to conduct a series of animal experiments and clinical basic research on cancer. Without a breakthrough in basic research, clinical efficacy is difficult to improve.

6). It was to establish a sputum tumor specialist clinic:

(a), it was to establish an outpatient medical record database, retain outpatient medical records, follow-up throughout the course, and long-term follow-up for many years.

The phone is always available to answer questions, guide rehabilitation and dietary precautions;

(b), Establish detailed medical records (including epidemiological data of patients) to analyze in depth the successful experience and failure lessons of each treatment and the particularity of the disease (eg, analytical data);

(c), Cases of 6 months to 1 year of follow-up were analyzed. The cases were reviewed for more than 3 years, and the medical records were extracted, the medical records were summarized, and the treatment experience and lessons were analyzed (eg, abstract medical records). The Twilight Oncology Clinic has been in existence for 21 years, and the outpatient medical records have remained intact.

7). A series of experimental studies were carried out by establishing animal models of various cancers through the laboratory of the Institute of Experimental Surgery;

To explore the etiology, pathogenesis, recurrence and metastasis mechanism of cancer, and carry out experimental research on effective measures to control cancer invasion, recurrence and metastasis. Through experimental research, we have obtained a series of experimental research findings.

(3) How to find this road? It should be based on clinical actual problems and experimental research findings:

The road we have been looking for for more than 20 years has come step by step:

1). The findings of follow-up results:

Postoperative recurrence and metastasis are the key factors affecting the long-term efficacy of surgery.

o   A——We must look for ways to prevent and treat cancer after recurrence and metastasis (method, medicine, technology, basic theory)

2). Discover the results of animal experiments:

As the cancer progresses, the thymus is progressively atrophy, and the host thymus is acutely progressively atrophied after inoculation of cancer cells, cell proliferation is blocked, and the volume is significantly reduced, thus revealing:

o   B - must find ways to prevent thymus atrophy, promote thymic hyperplasia, and boost immunity (method, medicine, technology, basic theory)

3). The findings of animal experiment research results:

The experimental results confirmed that the first immunosuppression, and then easy to have the occurrence and development of cancer, if no immune function decline, it is not easy to vaccinate successfully. The experimental results suggest that improving and maintaining good immune function, maintaining a good central immune organ thymus is one of the important measures to prevent cancer. Another experimental result in our lab suggests:

Metastasis is associated with immunity, low immune function, or the use of immunosuppressive agents to promote tumor metastasis. Thus the revelation:

o   C - must find the way to immune reconstruction of cancer patients

(method, medicine, technology, basic theory)

4). Through our proposed new concept of cancer metastasis treatment, the enlightenment of new theory:

The key to cancer treatment is anti-metastasis, how to eliminate cancer cells on the way to transfer

o   D – it must find the way to eliminate cancer cells on the way to transfer

(method, medicine, technology, basic theory)

Through the above research results:

We basically found the way to take the immune regulation method, and gradually established XZ-C immunomodulation therapy to treat cancer.

In the past 28 years, we have embarked the new path of conquering cancer of immune regulation and control with traditional Chinese medicine, regulating and controlling immune activity, preventing thymus atrophy, promoting thymic hyperplasia, protecting bone marrow hematopoietic function, and improving immune surveillance and western and Chinese medicine combines at the molecular level.

3. Footprint

(The scientific research footprint)

(1) Anti-cancer, anti-cancer metastasis research, scientific research achievements, scientific and technological innovation series

The following arguments in the XZ-C (XU ZE-China) series are the first to be presented internationally, all of which are original papers.

1). **"Thymus atrophy, low immune function is one of the causes and pathogenesis of cancer"**

-   New findings on experimental research on the etiology and pathogenesis of cancer

-   See the monograph "New Concepts and New Methods for Cancer Treatment" P.13

2). Theoretical basis and experimental basis of "XZ-C immunomodulation treatment" with protection of Thymus and increase of immune fucntion ——Proposed the theoretical basis and experimental basis of cancer immune regulation therapy

—— Because of the new enlightenment discovered by the above experimental research, the treatment principle must be to prevent progressive atrophy of the thymus, promote thymic hyperplasia, protect bone marrow hematopoietic function, improve immune surveillance, and control immune escape of malignant cells.

- See the monograph "New Concepts and New Methods of Cancer Treatment" P.17

3). "Cancer treatment should change the concept and establish a comprehensive treatment concept"

- propose a new concept of cancer treatment principles

—— The target or target of cancer treatment must establish a comprehensive treatment concept for both tumor and host

—— It should overcome or avoid the one-sided treatment concept of simply killing cancer cells

- See the monograph "New Concepts and New Methods for Cancer Treatment" P.28

4). "New Combination of Multidisciplinary Treatment of Cancer"

- Proposing a new concept of the cancer treatment combination model

- The new model for multidisciplinary treatment is:

Long-term treatment mainly: surgery + biological treatment + immunotherapy + Chinese medicine, Chinese and Western combined treatment

Short-course treatment is supplemented: radiotherapy, chemotherapy, not long-range, not excessive

- See the monograph "New Concepts and New Methods of Cancer Treatment" P33

5). "Analysis, evaluation and questioning of systemic intravenous chemotherapy for solid tumors and four evaluations"

—— Analysis of the problems and drawbacks of systemic intravenous chemotherapy for solid cancer

—— Question and evaluation of systemic intravenous chemotherapy for solid tumors, calculation of drug volume, evaluation of efficacy

- See the monograph "New Concepts and New Methods for Cancer Treatment" P.57

6). "Initiatives for the treatment of abdominal solid tumor systemic venous chemotherapy should be reformed as target organ intravascular chemotherapy, reform initiatives for traditional cancer chemotherapy"

—— Because systemic intravenous chemotherapy cytotoxic drugs cannot directly reach the portal system by the superior vena cava administration, the vena cava system and the portal system are generally not connected, and it is difficult to reach the portal vein by the superior vena cava.

—— Where are the cancer cells of abdominal solid tumors (stomach, colorectal, liver, gallbladder, pancreas, spleen, abdominal cavity, etc.)? Mainly they are in the portal system, postoperative adjuvant chemotherapy from the venous vein to the vena cava is unreasonable, does not meet the anatomy, physiological pathology, because it can not directly enter the portal system

- Therefore, the route of administration should be changed to the endovascular treatment of target organs.

- See the monograph "New Concepts and New Methods of Cancer Treatment" P.63

7). "There are three main forms of cancer in the human body"

—— Proposing theoretical innovation of new concept of cancer metastasis treatment

—— This third manifestation is proposed to be a group of cancer cells on the way to metastasis. The treatment target of cancer should be directed to the above three forms of existence, especially for cancer cells on the way to metastasis.

- See the monograph "New Concepts and New Methods for Cancer Treatment" P.38

8). "Two Points and One Line" in the Whole Process of Cancer Development

—— Proposed theoretical innovation of cancer metastasis treatment

- One of the purposes of cancer treatment is to prevent metastasis

The whole process of cancer metastasis development can be summarized as "two points and one line"

—— Traditional cancer treatment only pays attention to "two points" and ignores "first line".

The new concept believes that both "two points" should be emphasized, and that "one line" should be cut off.

- See the monograph "New Concepts and New Methods for Cancer Treatment" P.43

9). "Three Steps of Anticancer Metastasis Treatment"

—— Proposed theoretical innovation of cancer metastasis treatment

—— Incorporate the "eight steps" of cancer cell transfer into "three stages" and try to break each transfer step.

- See the monograph "New Concepts and New Methods of Cancer Treatment" P.47

10). "Developing the Third Field of Anti-Cancer Metastasis"

—— Proposed the theoretical innovation of the new concept of cancer metastasis treatment, and found and proposed the third field of human anti-cancer metastasis

—— The circulatory system has a large number of immune surveillance cells, and **the "main battlefield" of cancer cells on the way to annihilation is in the blood circulation.**

Proposed to conquer cancer and to launch the general attack of cancer, this is unprecedented work

11). For the first time in the world:

"XZ-C Scientific Research Plan for Overcoming cancer and launching the General Attack of Cancer"

—— The overall strategic reform and development of cancer treatment in China

- Avoid empty talk, work hard, start to act or to walk

No matter how far the road to conquer cancer is, you should always take a walk.

—— Proposed to overcome the general attack of cancer, this is unprecedented work

12).For the first time in the world:

"Necessity and Feasibility Report on Overcoming cancer and launching the General Attack of Cancer"

—— The overall strategic reform of cancer treatment in China will shift focusing on treatment into prevention and treatment at the same attention and level.

—— XZ-C proposes the general idea and design of conquering cancer

------ What is the total attack on cancer and the goal of the total attack?

—— XU ZE proposes ideas, strategies, plans, blueprints to overcome cancer and launch a general attack

13). For the first time in the world:

"Preparing to build the hospital of cancer prevention and treatment during the whole process of cancer occurrence and development"

(Global Demonstration Cancer Prevention and Treatment Hospital)

—— The current problems in the hospital hospital hospital model

—— The road of how to overcome cancer lies in researching the establishment of hospitals with cancer prevention and treatment during the whole process of cancer occurrence and development, and reforming the current mode of hospitalization with heavy treatment and light prevention

—— XU ZE's strategic thinking, planning sketch, prevention and treatment of cancer during the whole process of cancer occurrence and development

14). For the first time in the world:

"To build a general plan to overcome cancer and the basic design of the Science City"

1)).Equivalent to designing an overall framework for Chinese characteristics to overcome cancer design

2)). How to form the basic idea and design to conquer cancer and launch the general attack of cancer

3)). How to overcome cancer?

The Cancer Animal Experimental Center must be established.

Innovative Molecular Oncology Medical School must be established.

Cancer and Multidisciplinary Research Institute must be established.

4)). How to overcome cancer?

It is necessary to "prepare a medical, teaching, research, and science base to conquer cancer and launch the general attack of cancer - Science City"

(2) Publishing a monograph on cancer research

Professor Xu Ze continued to study after he retired. Science is on the go, continue to achieve the following series of scientific research results.

In 1996, I was 63 years old and I was retired. After I retired, I have been living in a small building for 20 years. I have been working alone and fighting alone. I have continued a series of experimental studies and clinical verification observations. I have achieved the following series of scientific research results. The following monographs have been published.

Three monographs, Chinese version, domestic issue

Four monographs, English edition, Washington publication, international distribution

These seven monographs are the results of four different levels of research, four hardships, hard climbs, four different scientific research stages, and four different levels of mountain results.

1). 67-year-old flower year published the first monograph "New understanding and new model of cancer treatment" Hubei Science and Technology Press, Xu Ze, January 2001.

2). The 73-year-old ancient rare year published the second monograph "New Concepts and New Methods for Cancer Metastasis Treatment", published by Beijing People's Military Medical Press, Xu Ze, January 2006. In April 2007, the People's Republic of China Publishing Office issued the "Three One Hundred" original book certificate.

3). The 78-year-old ancient rare year published the third monograph "New Concepts and New Methods for Cancer Treatment", published by Beijing People's Military Medical Press, Xu Ze, Xu Jie/, October 2011. Later, the American medical doctor Dr. Bin Wu and others translated into English, and the English version was published in Washington, DC on March 26, 2013.

4). The 80-year-old is published in the third edition of the English edition, "New Concept and New Way Of Treatment of Cancer", published in Washington, March 2013, in English, internationally

5). 82-year-old published the fifth monograph "On Innovation of Treatment of Cancer" - "On Cancer Treatment Innovation", published in Washington, December 2015, full English, globally distributed

6). At the age of 83, he published the sixth monograph "New Concept and New Way of Treatment of Cancer Metastais"

- "New Concepts and New Methods for Cancer Metastasis Treatment"

In August 2016, Washington published a full English version, globally distributed.

7). At the age of 83, he published the seventh monograph "The Road To Over Come Cancer" --- the road to Conquer cancer, published in Washington, December 2016, full English, globally distributed

(3). Some of the Pictures for the Contribution as the following:

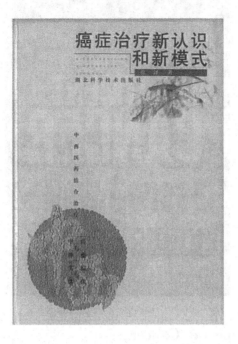

The First Monograph was published in January, 2001 by Beijing Publication Inc at the age of 67

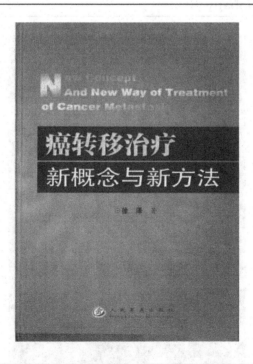

The second Monograph was published in January 2006 by Beijing Publication Inc at the age of 73

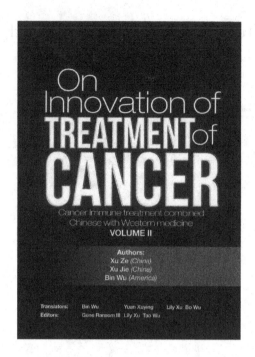

On Innovation of Treatment of Cancer

It was published in December 2015 by Authorhouse Publication Inc in English version, Distributed Globally

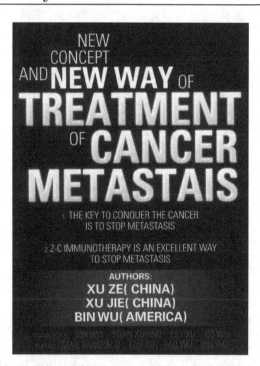

<New concept and new way of treatment of cancer metastasis> was published in Augest by Authorhouse in English version and distributed globally

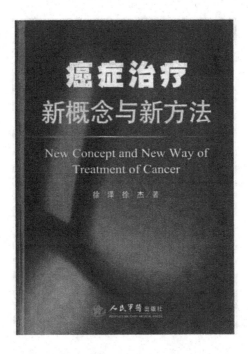

The third monograph was published in October 2011 by Beijing publication Inc at the age of 78

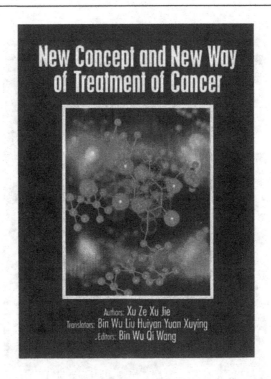

The English version for the third monograph was published in March 2013 by Authorhouse Publication Inc at the age of 80 and distributed globally

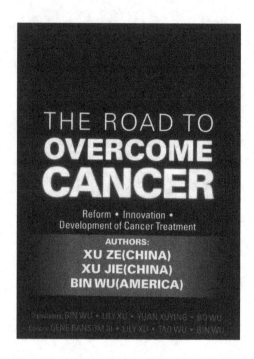

The road to overcome cancer was published in English version
by Authorhouse Publication Inc and distributed globally

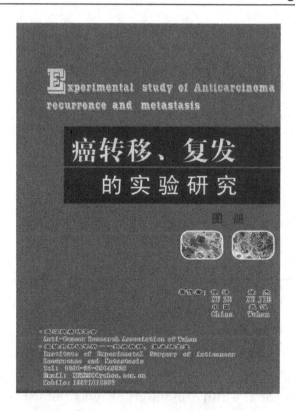

In 2009 this gift was given to the Huston cancer research institution when visiting
USA, which included the scientific results and the color pictures of the experiments

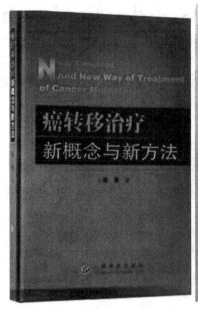
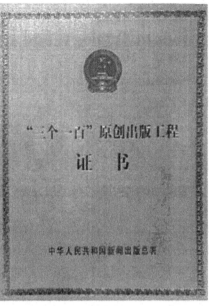

This is the "the three one-hundred" award certificate of <New concept and new way of treatment cancer mestastasis> (the book is in the life side and the certificate is in the right side

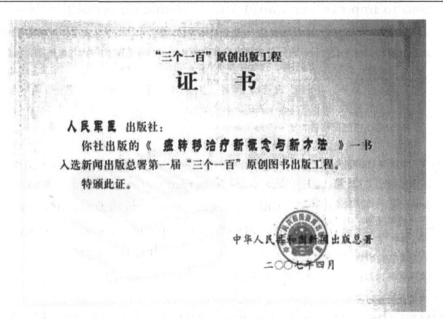

This is the another certificate for the three one-hundred award in Chinese version

(4) Report cancer research papers at the American Society of International Oncology, and research papers go international

1). Received an invitation from the American Association for Cancer Research AACR to Xu Ze.

In September 2013, he reported "XZ-C immunomodulation anticancer therapy" at the International Cancer Society in Washington, USA. It has aroused widespread attention and high attention from the international oncology community.

2). From October 27 to 30, 2013, he attended the 12th International Conference on Cancer Research of the American Association for Cancer Research (AACR) in Washington, DC, which attracted great attention from the oncology community.

3). On February 14, 2014, Dr. Bin Wu gave a lecture on "The thymus atrophy and immunocompromised cancer is one of the causes and mechanisms of cancer" in the academic lecture hall of the Library Building in US. The report, as well as the "protection of the thymus and increase of immune function" (protecting the thymus to improve immunity), the academic report of the theoretical basis and experimental basis for the treatment principle of "protecting the marrow to produce blood" (protecting bone marrow hematopoietic stem cells) was warmly welcomed and highly valued by the participants.

4). World-class oncology immunoscientists such as Stanford University School of Medicine, University of California, San Francisco, Harvard Medical School, etc. fully affirmed Professor Xu Ze's research results, and agreed that the immune system can enhance the anti-recurrence and metastasis of cancer patients themselves. It is agreed that immune regulation and control can enhance the anti-recurrence and metastasis immunity of cancer patients, and can fully improve the quality of life of patients with advanced cancer. It is the most effective anti-cancer pathway after surgery, radiotherapy and chemotherapy.

(5) Visiting the Stirling Cancer Institute in Houston, USA

In order to strengthen the exchanges and cooperation of international scientific and technological organizations, on December 10, 2009, we were invited to visit the Stirling Cancer Institute in the United States, and were warmly welcomed and warmly welcomed by the fellows of the Institute. The 86-year-old professor and a number of professors, researchers, nude animal model laboratories, and anti-cancer drug analysis laboratories participated in the discussion and exchanges, and reported the latest scientific research results with slides.

We presented the color map of the Institute of Cancer Metastasis and Recurrence in our institute to the Institute of Oncology, USA. This paper introduces the experimental research on the tumor-free technique in radical surgery and the experimental study on the removal of thymus to produce cancer-bearing animal models. And the exclusive development of Z-C immune regulation of anti-cancer, anti-metastasis Chinese medicine series Z-C1-10 related information. And presented the monograph "New Concepts and New Methods for Cancer Metastasis Treatment" published by me.

The three hundred original books that won the book award in China were warmly welcomed and appreciated by the researchers.

(6)   Basic planning and design of XZ-C launching general attack

Professor Xu Ze (XU ZE) proposed the overall design of the Science City to overcome cancer and launch the general attack of cancer.

Dawning or Shuguang scientific research spirit

Hard work and striving and struggle:

20 years of cold window, hard work

Review and reflection:

Follow-up, summarizing successful treatment experience (typical cases in the second monograph); rethinking the lessons of treatment failure (the first monograph failed to prevent recurrence and failed to prevent metastasis).

Open-up and Innovation

Screened out a series preparations or medications including 48 kinds of XZ-C immunomodulation Chinese medicine with the better cancer inhibition rates from 200 kinds of Chinese herbal medicine in the animal inhibition experiment and realized the rise to theoretical knowledge, new concepts and new models.

Facing Future medicine or Future-oriented medicine

Recognizing the shortcomings and problems of traditional therapy in the 20th century, and recognizing the direction of the 21st century.

Insight and Look forward:

Suggest:

- Establish an innovative molecular oncology hospital – to train senior oncology researchers for the country.

- Establish innovative molecular cancer, occurrence and development of the whole process of prevention and treatment of hospitals (in combination with Western medicine at the molecular level) - to benefit more cancer patients and serve more cancer patients.

- Establishing an Innovative Molecular Oncology Institute – researching cells to begin malignant transformation – to CT can be found for a significant period of time to reach the three-early target, "target" metastasis, cancer lesions, and precancerous conditions.

- Establish an innovative molecular oncology drug factory – stepping out of a new path to overcome cancer with Chinese characteristics.

- Establish an environmental protection and cancer prevention research institute and carry out anti-cancer system engineering

(7) The theoretical system of XZ-C immunomodulation and cancer treatment has been formed.

In the book "New Concepts and New Methods of Cancer Treatment", Professor Xu Ze published a series of research papers on basic and clinical research results, which was published in the form of a new book, with 20 years of self-reliance and hard work. .

This book has initially formed the theoretical system of XZ-C immune regulation and treatment of cancer, and the clinical basis and experimental basis for cancer treatment are undergoing clinical application observation and verification.

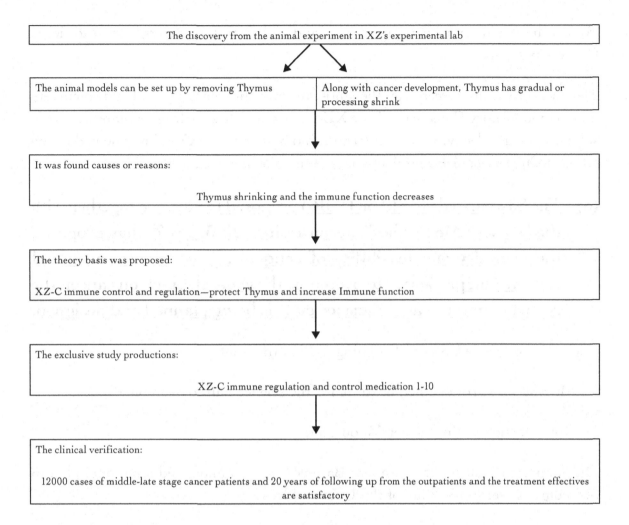

The discovery from the animal experiment in XZ's experimental lab

The animal models can be set up by removing Thymus

Along with cancer development, Thymus has gradual or processing shrink

It was found causes or reasons:

Thymus shrinking and the immune function decreases

The theory basis was proposed:

XZ-C immune control and regulation—protect Thymus and increase Immune function

The exclusive study productions:

XZ-C immune regulation and control medication 1-10

The clinical verification:

12000 cases of middle-late stage cancer patients and 20 years of following up from the outpatients and the treatment effectives are satisfactory

The theory system of XZ-C immunological regulation and treatment of cancer (XZ-C)(XU ZE-China)(China-Xu Ze)

Exclusive research and development products: XZ-C immune regulation anti-cancer Chinese medicine series products

(introduction)

The self-developed XZ-C (Xu Ze China) immune regulation anti-cancer series of traditional Chinese medicine preparations, from experimental research to clinical verification, applied to clinical practice on the basis of the success of animal experiments, after more than 12,000 clinical cases in 20 years, it has the Significant effect. Clinical application can improve symptoms, good spirits, good appetite, significantly improve the quality of life, significantly prolong the survival period, independent innovation, independent intellectual property rights.

To search for and screen new anti-cancer and anti-metastatic drugs from traditional Chinese medicine:

The purpose is to screen out the anti-cancer, anti-metastatic and anti-recurrent immunomodulatory Chinese medicine XZ-C1-10 which has no drug resistance, no toxic side effects, high selectivity and long-term oral administration. (XZ-C immunomodulation series of Chinese medicine products, see the first volume, the eighth volume)

(8) The 83-year-old year (April 2016) proposed to advance together with the "Cancer Moon Shot", because since 2013, Xu Ze has proposed the necessity and feasibility of conquering the general attack of cancer. And proposed "to overcome the general attack on cancer, the report to build a cancer science city" is being planned and designed.

"New Moon Plan" (US) and Dawning C Plan (middle)

- Moving forward together, heading for the science hall to overcome cancer

1). "Introduction to the Cancer Moon Shot"

On January 12, 2016, US President Barack Obama announced a national plan to overcome cancer in his State of the Union address:

Plan Name: "New Moon Plan"

Goal: Conquer cancer

Nature: National plan to overcome cancer

Announcer: President Obama

The person in charge of the plan: Vice President Biden

Announced: January 12, 2016

The specific plan of the plan: unknown

2). Dawning or Shuguang C-type plan introduction

a. Before January 12, 2016, the progress of the XZ-C Scientific Research Plan for Overcoming the General Attack of Cancer Attack was put forward.

334

b. Before January 12, 2016, we have carried out research results in the field of cancer research, technology innovation series

c. Shuguang C-type plan (developed in July 2015)

I. "Overcome the general attack of cancer"

II. "Preparation of the whole process of prevention and treatment of hospitals"

III. "Preparing to build a cancer science city"

IV. "Forming a Multidisciplinary Research Group"

V. "Vaccine is the hope of mankind"

VI. "The prospect of immunomodulatory drugs is gratifying"

3). The situation analysis

a. Analyze their respective technological advantages

b. Analyze the current status quo

c. Analyze the next research prospects

d. Outline of the realization of scientific and technological innovation in the "Dawning C-type plan"

e. How to implement this unprecedented event in human history?

f. expected results

(9) Conducting anti-cancer metastasis research is an urgent need

1). Conducting anti-cancer and anti-cancer metastasis research is an urgent need for the development of oncology. "Oncology" is one of the most backward disciplines in medical science. Its "name" is not yet unified. Some people write it as "tumor" and "Cancer, cancer, malignant tumor, new organism. Because a disease name is defined, its cause and pathogenesis must be clarified. Because the etiology, pathogenesis, and pathophysiology of oncology are not well understood, the oncology discipline is still a scientific virgin for scientific research, and it needs a lot of basic scientific research.

2). Anti-cancer metastasis and recurrence, basic research must be carried out on animal models of cancer-bearing animals. Currently, many large hospitals have not established laboratories and cannot carry out basic research on cancer. It is necessary to establish various cancer metastasis animal models in nude mice to study cancer cell metastasis. The law and mechanism (the author's laboratory uses pure Kunming mice to make cancer-bearing animal models about 10,000 times), because without the breakthrough of basic research, the clinical efficacy is difficult to improve.

3). Research on anti-cancer and anti-cancer metastasis focuses on the study of unknown knowledge. Researchers should look ahead and face the science of the future. Science is an infinite frontier. Researchers must surpass the old knowledge and constantly update with a developmental perspective. Constantly surpassing, constantly developing and moving forward.

(10).How to innovate in science and technology? How to leave a scientific research footprint?

An old cement road, with hundreds of people walking every day, will not leave footprints, only a new cement road, every step will leave eternal footprints, so scientific research must have innovative thinking, must be innovative Results.

In the past 30 years (1985-), our research history and cancer research work have achieved scientific and technological innovation series of scientific research achievements in animal experiments, clinical basic research and clinical verification work. Only the results catalogue (scientific research footprint) is listed here, and each scientific research result is Belonging to original innovation or independent innovation, it is every eternal scientific research footprint.

(11) In his 85-year-old year, he published the medical monograph "Agglutination Wisdom, Conquering Cancer - Benefiting Mankind". XZ-C proposed: How to overcome cancer? How can I prevent cancer? I see how to treat cancer.

Professor Xu Ze proposed:

The scheme diagram of the engineering planning for how to overcome cancer

This medical monograph is a practical, applied, research-oriented, implementation of how to overcome the outline of cancer. This set of scientific research programs, scientific research design, scientific research planning, and blueprints can be used by countries, provinces, and states to implement the vision of cancer and benefit humanity.

The main project of this implementation outline is:

a. Overcoming cancer and launching the general attack of cancer

b. Prevention and control and treatment of cancer at the same attention and move together and at the same level and at the same time

c. Create a scientific research base for multidisciplinary and cancer-related research – the Science City

The two-wing project is:

A wing - how to prevent cancer? To reduce the incidence of cancer

B wing - how to treat cancer? To improve cancer cure rate

The goals or aims:

A: Reduce the incidence of cancer

B: Improve cancer cure rate, prolong patient survival and improve quality of life

Chapter 22

Guide Reading

How to overcome cancer? How to prevent cancer? How to treat cancer? How to conquer cancer and launch the general attack of cancer?

Professor Xu Ze (XZ-C) summed up the collection, agglutinated wisdom, and proposed 1-8 of "walking out of the new road to overcome cancer" for clinical application and reference.

XZ-C's scientific thinking, scientific research design, academic thought, scientific dedication and summary of conquering cancer and launching the general attack are summarized and collected as the following monographs. The following is a guide to the "Monographs":

1. **Walk out of a new road to overcome cancer - 1 (a)**

(Volume I)
"Conquering cancer and launching the general attack of cancer" – cancer prevention and cancer control and cancer treatment at the same attention

   [Introduction]

The focus is:

- What is the "conquering cancer and launching the general attack on cancer"?

- Why is it proposed to conquer cancer and to launch the general attack of cancer?

- How to implement the "conquering cancer and launching the general attack on cancer"?

- XZ-C proposes to the vision, design, planning, and blueprint for conquering cancer and launching the general attack on cancer

- XZ-C proposes to conquer cancer and to launch the general attack of cancer, this is unprecedented work

- How to overcome cancer? How can I treat cancer? by I see

How can I prevent cancer? by I see

- XZ-C proposed the XZ-C Scientific Research Plan to overcome cancer and launch the general attack on cancer.

- Presented the "Necessity and Feasibility Report for Overcoming cancer and launching the General Attack of Cancer"

- Put forward the "the establishment of the hospital with Cancer Prevention and treatment during the whole cancer occurrence and development and Prevention process"

(Global Demonstration Cancer Prevention and Treatment Hospital)

• XZ-C proposed:

Why is it to put forward the "conquering cancer and launch a general attack of cancer" and the need for launching the general attack".

1. Because the goal of conquering cancer is:

(1),reduce the incidence of cancer

To improve cancer cure rate, significantly prolong patient survival, improve quality of life, and reduce cancer mortality

(2),

It is up to or to reach to:

1/3 can prevent

1/3 can be cured

1/3 can extend life through treatment

- How can it be to reduce the incidence of cancer?

It should be prevention-oriented, control-oriented, prevention-oriented

But the road we have traveled for decades is to focus on or to rectify the heavy treatment with light prevention of cancer, or just have treatment cancer without preventing it.

Therefore, **the incidence of cancer is increasing, and the more patients are treated and the more new patients show up.**

- How to do?

It should be prevention-oriented, control-oriented, and implement the principle of prevention

Only by paying attention to preventing cancer can reduce the incidence of cancer.

Therefore**, cancer prevention should be the most important.**

- Professor Xu Ze (XU ZE) proposed to launch the general attack, which is actually the prevention, control, and treatment at the same attention.

To refer to the prevention of cancer as an important part, in fact, it is to **implement the "prevention-based" health work policy. Our medical predecessors, the world's medical sages, put forward the "cancer prevention and anti-cancer" and the cancer prevention is priority. This policy is very correct, but unfortunately our medical juniors have not paid attention to it.**

For a century, cancer prevention has not paid attention to it, which has led to such a high incidence of cancer today. The more patients are treated, the more new cases of cancer

In China there are about 4.292 million (1.4 billion people in China) in 2015.

11922 people had new cancer, and 8 people were diagnosed with cancer every minute. Such amazing data should be a major event for the people's livelihood.

- XZ-C proposes to overcome cancer and launch the general attack of cancer— cancer prevention, cancer control, and cancer treatment at the same attention. The goal is to reduce the incidence of cancer, improve the cure rate of cancer, and significantly prolong the survival of cancer patients.

- **To change the mode of running a hospital:**

To reform the current mode of hospitalization that is to have heavy treatment with light prevention or only have treatment without prevention.

- **To change the treatment model:**

To reform the current treatment mode with a focus on the middle and late stages of treatment.

- **To Shift treatment alone without preventing into preventing and controlling, and treating at the same time and the same attention**

- **The way out to cure cancer is "three early", early cancer treatment is good, and it can be cured.**

- **It is necessary to establish a hospital for prevention, control and treatment according to the occurrence and development of cancer.**

- **The overall strategic reform of cancer treatment in China should change only focusing on treatment into prevention and treatment at the same time and attention.**

- XZ-C proposed the general attack design, blueprint and implementation rules and plans·

- **Conquering cancer and launching a general attack is an unprecedented event in human history. It is at the forefront of science and can revitalize China and benefit mankind.**

- How to implement this plan to overcome cancer, Professor Xu Ze (XZ-C) elaborated the planning, blueprint for the general design, master plan, specific plan, talents of the team.

The general design, blueprint and preparation work for the Science City to overcome cancer and launch the general attack of cancer was put forward.

The chief designer and subject operator of the "Science City for conquering cancer and launching the total Attack of Cancer and the Creation of a Science City for conquering Cancer" is the XZ-C Professor Xu Ze, who has published a series of research articles on cancer prevention and cancer treatment.

2. Walked out of the new road to overcome cancer - 2 (two)

> (Volume II) (Part I)
>
> "Walked out of a new way of immune regulation and control with the combination of Chinese and Western medicine for cancer treatment"

- How to overcome cancer? How to treat cancer?

(Part I)

[Introduction]

The key points are:

• How did we find the new way of cancer treatment with immune regulation and control?

In the past 30 years, we have made research work in the field of cancer research, and we have achieved a series of scientific research achievements, scientific and technological innovation series. The road we are looking for conquering cancer was walking out as the following step by step:

(1). New findings from the follow-up results:

Looking for the road of the research to prevent recurrence and postoperative recurrence

(2). **The New findings from experimental results of animal models: looking for ways to prevent thymic atrophy, promote thymic hyperplasia, enhance the path of increasing immunity, and find a way to rebuild immune**

It is to put forward the new concept of "immunity control and regulation with protection of Thymus and increase of immune function for cancer treatment"

(3). The key to studying cancer treatment is anti-metastasis:

looking for ways to eliminate cancer cells on the way to metastasis, and put forward the "two points and one line theory", not only paying attention to two points, but also cutting off one line, which is the new concept of fcancer treatment.

- Why should we take the new path of immune control and regulation for treatment of cancer?

It is because Western medicine or drugs are few which can increase immune function, Chinese medicine has a large number of prescriptions to enhance immunity, especially polysaccharides and tonics have the effect of regulating immune activity.

- How did our laboratory conduct an experimental study on screening anticancer and anti-metastatic drugs from traditional Chinese medicine?

(1) Screening experimental study on cancer suppression rate of Chinese herbal medicine by using in vitro culture method of cancer cells

(2) Experimental study on making the cancer-bearing animal models and conducting the cancer inhabitation rate of Chinese herbal medicine in cancer-bearing animals

- Experimental research •Chinese medicine immunopharmacology and at the molecular level the research of the combination of Chinese and Western medicine

- **Walking out of the new way of cancer treatment with XZ-C immune control and regulation, of the combination of Western and Chinese medicine at the molecular level.**

- **Stepped out of a new way of using Chinese medicine immune regulation and control, regulating immune activity, preventing thymus atrophy, promoting thymic hyperplasia, protecting bone marrow hematopoietic function, improving immune surveillance, and combining Western medicine at the molecular level to overcome cancer.**

- **Has formed the theoretical system of XZ-C immune regulation and treatment of cancer, the theoretical basis and experimental basis of immunotherapy**

- **We have embarked on a new road of XZ-C immune regulation, molecular level Chinese and Western medicine combined with cancer treatment - "Chinese anti-cancer" new road**

- XZ-C immunomodulation anticancer Chinese medicine is the result of the modernization of traditional Chinese medicine

> (Volume II)
>
> Part II
>
> Walked out of the new road of cancer treatment with immune regulation and control of combination of western and Chinese medicine

- How to overcome cancer? How to treat cancer?

(Part II)

[Introduction]

The key points are:

- New findings in experimental research on the etiology, pathogenesis, and pathophysiology of cancer

Thymus atrophy and immune dysfunction may be one of the causes and pathogenesis of cancer, and explore ways to curb tumor progression, progressive atrophy of thymus and immune reconstruction

- Theoretical basis and experimental basis for cancer treatment

Animal experiment enlightenment:

The theoretical basis and experimental basis of XZ-C immunomodulatory therapy and "chest lifting" should protect, regulate and activate the anti-cancer immune system in human body.

- Principles of cancer treatment – should change the concept and establish a comprehensive treatment concept

- Cancer treatment model – a new combination of cancer multidisciplinary treatment

- Principles of cancer metastasis treatment

The key to cancer research is anti-metastasis

The basic principle of cancer treatment is anti-metastasis

- "It is an empty talk to not study cancer metastasis and improve efficacy"

- Innovation must challenge traditional ideas and reforms can develop

- Analysis, evaluation and evaluation of systemic intravenous chemotherapy for solid tumors:

Evaluation of the route of administration of systemic intravenous chemotherapy for solid tumors

The current route of administration of systemic intravenous chemotherapy for solid tumors is:

chemotherapy cell poison → elbow vein → superior vena cava → right heart

→ double lung → left heart → aorta → spray to the whole body

{
Normal normal tumor-free organs, tissue (brain, liver, lung, kidney, bone marrow...) obtained about 99.6% of a dose.

The dose of cancer is about 0.4%
}

This route of administration is not a targeted drug delivery, but a blood pump is injected into the body through a heart pump, so that the cytotoxic drugs are distributed systemically, so that all organs of the body have obtained cytotoxic drugs, which is unreasonable and unscientific, the result is:

(1) The cancer has few drugs, only about 0.4%, and the curative effect is very small (because the cancerous area accounts for a small proportion of the total body surface area)

345

(2) 99.6% of the cytotoxic drugs kill normalized proliferating cells, causing toxic side effects of brain, heart, liver, lung, kidney, gastrointestinal system, hematopoietic system, immune system and endocrine system. These toxic side effects are caused by unreasonable treatment design and route of administration and should be avoided.

(3) At present, all hospitals have not tested for drug susceptibility. If the drug is resistant, the chemotherapy will kill normal tissue cells! Especially inhibit bone marrow hematopoietic cells and immune cells! It has no effect on cancerous foci.

(4) So every chemotherapy, kill cancer cells? do not know. How much has it killed? I don't know, I can only say that I have done a chemotherapy job.

Therefore, this route of administration is unreasonable and easily leads to iatrogenic side effects. How to do? The route of administration should be changed to the intravascular chemotherapy route of the target organ, and the drug can be directly delivered to the "target" organ, so that the drug amount is small, the curative effect is affirmative, and there is no toxic side reaction, which is beneficial to the patient.

- **When cancer patients receive chemotherapy, the immune organs such as thymus, bone marrow, and lymph nodes are damaged, which reduces the overall immune function. The thymus has been inhibited during cancer, and chemotherapy inhibits the bone marrow, which is like "adding frost", so that the entire central immune organ is affected. Damage is not effectively protected. Therefore, XZ-C recommends: after chemotherapy, you should add immunoregulatory Chinese medicine to protect the bone marrow hematopoietic function, increase immunity or can be called chemotherapy + immunity, immunotherapy.**

3.   **Walked out of a new road to overcome cancer - 3 (three)**

(Volume III)
"Research on Immunoregulation of Anticancer Traditional Chinese Medicine" - Experimental Research and Clinical Application Verification

-   How to overcome cancer? How to treat cancer?

[Introduction]

The focus is:

- Experimental research + clinical application + case + list

- **XZ-C immunomodulation anticancer Chinese medicine is a kind of Chinese herbal medicine that has a good tumor inhibition rate from more than 200 traditional Chinese medicines in China. After compounding the compound, the anti-tumor effect of the compound cancer+mouse in vivo was greater than the single-spot inhibition rate, and XZ-C1 had a significant anti-tumor effect, and did not kill normal cells. For mouse sarcoma S180, the tumor inhibition rate is as high as 98.9%, which has the effect of strengthening the body and improving the immune function of the human body.**

- **Self-developed XZ-C (XU ZE-China) (Xu Ze - China) immunomodulatory anti-cancer series of traditional Chinese medicine preparations, from experimental research to clinical verification, applied to clinical practice on the basis of successful animal experiments, after 24 years More than 12,000 cases of clinical validation, significant efficacy, independent innovation, independent intellectual property rights.**

- Exclusively developed products: XZ-C1-10 immune regulation anti-cancer Chinese medicine series product introduction.

- XZ-C1-10 immunoregulation of traditional Chinese medicine for anti-cancer, metastasis, recurrence, clinical application

- Typical case series

- Case list

- Pharmacodynamic studies of XZ-C from our laboratory have shown that it has a high tumor inhibition rate for Ehrlich ascites, S100 and H22 hepatoma.

- No acute toxic side effects by mouse acute toxicity test. In the long-term clinical oral administration (after 2-6-8-10 years), no obvious side effects were observed.

- Patients with advanced cancer are mostly debilitating, fatigue, fatigue, loss of appetite, and taking XZ-C immunomodulation Chinese medicine for 4-8-12-16 weeks, can significantly improve appetite, sleep, relieve pain, and gradually restore physical strength, can significantly extend the survival period.

- XZ-C proposes: Cancer treatment must take a new path of immune regulation and treatment. In the research of cancer, traditional Chinese medicine is the advantage of China. The research that exerts this advantage should be a strategic vision with international significance.

- At present, world scientists agree that tumor formation is summarized into three processes:

In the first step, carcinogenic factors act on the body and interfere with cell metabolism;

The second step is to disrupt the genetic information in the nucleus and cause cancer of the cell;

The third step is that the cancer cells escape the body's immune alert defense system. The body's immunity is an internal cause. The external cause is caused by internal factors. The cancer cells must escape the body's alarm system and break through the body's immune defense. Tumor. Therefore, finding ways to improve the body's immunity is a key measure to prevent cancer and cure cancer.

Chinese herbal medicine is an extremely important advantage. There are many immune Chinese herbal preparations and rich sources of medicine. It should be used as an important anti-cancer and anti-cancer resource. It should be organized for research and development.

- Traditional Chinese medicine is the essence of Chinese culture. One of the essence of traditional medicine is Chinese medicine.

4.   Walked out of a new road to overcome cancer - 4 (four)

(Vol. IV)

"Clinical Application Theory Innovation of Cancer Prevention and Management Research in the 21st Century"

[Introduction]

The focus is:

• Our cancer research has reached the forefront of the world

In the past 30 years, we have made scientific research achievements in the field of cancer research. The following points in the "Scientific" series of scientific and technological innovations are presented for the first time in the world. They are all original papers, international firsts, international leaders, and have reached the world's leading position.

Its main contents are as follows:

The XZ-C was first proposed internationally:

(1) First proposed internationally: "Thymus atrophy, low immune function is one of the causes and pathogenesis of cancer"

-   New findings on experimental research on the etiology and pathogenesis of cancer

(2) For the first time in the world, the theoretical basis and experimental basis of "ZHU-C immune regulation treatment"

—— Proposed the theoretical basis and experimental basis of cancer immune regulation therapy

(3) The first international initiative: "Cancer treatment should change the concept and establish a comprehensive treatment concept"

(4) The first international initiative: "A new model for the combination of multidisciplinary treatment of cancer"

(5) For the first time in the world: "Analysis, evaluation and questioning and evaluation of systemic intravenous chemotherapy for solid tumors"

(6) For the first time in the world, the "Initiative of Intravascular Chemotherapy for Abdominal Solid Tumors for Intravascular Chemotherapy of Target Organs and Suggestions for Reform"

(7) For the first time in the world, "There are three main forms of cancer in the human body"

(8) For the first time in the world, the "two points and one line" theory of the whole process of cancer development

(9) For the first time in the world, the "Three Steps of Anticancer Metastasis Treatment"

(10) For the first time in the world, "Developing the Third Field of Anti-Cancer Metastasis"

(11) For the first time in the world, the "XZ-C Scientific Research Plan for Overcoming the General Attack of Cancer"

How to overcome cancer? XZ-C proposes to overcome the general attack of cancer, this is unprecedented work.

(12) For the first time in the world: "Necessity and Feasibility of Overcoming the General Attack of Cancer Attack"

(13) For the first time in the world, it is proposed to "build a cancer prevention and development hospital for prevention and treatment"

(14) For the first time in the world, the "General Plan for Overcoming Cancer and the Basic Design of Science City"

(15) For the first time in the world, "To overcome the general attack of cancer, to prevent and control"

—— Changed the current hospitalization mode of re-treatment and light defense

(16) For the first time in the world, the "Scientific City for Scientific Bases to Acquire Cancer"

- established an overall framework for the fight against cancer

(17) For the first time in the world, "Getting out of a new road to overcome cancer"

—— Prevent postoperative recurrence and metastasis

(18) For the first time in the world, how to overcome cancer? XZ-C proposes "Dawning C-type plan No. 1-6"

(19) International initiative: independently developed XZ-C immunomodulation anticancer traditional Chinese medicine series products

(20) For the first time in the world:

How to overcome cancer?

XZ-C proposes:

Cancer is a disaster for all mankind. It is necessary for the people of the world to work together.

"Cancer moon Shot" (US) and "Dawning C-type plan" (middle)

- Going forward together, heading for the science hall to overcome cancer, why do you say that you can move forward together? What are you together? Analysis of the respective advantages of China and the United States, complementary advantages

(21) Over the past 100 years, the history of cancer has been proposed

----- Two US presidents have successively proposed a national plan to "catch cancer"

—— A Chinese physician XZ-C proposed the general design, plan, specific plan, blueprint for conquering cancer, and published five monographs (English version, global release), and wrote a book.

(22) For the first time in the world, how to overcome cancer? XZ-C proposes two wheels, A wheel, B wheel

(23) For the first time in the world, how to overcome cancer? XZ-C proposes need A wheel, A runway

B wheel, B runway

(24) For the first time in the world, how to overcome cancer? XZ-C proposes to target three targets A, B and C

(25) XZ-C proposes that several treatments of traditional Chinese medicine can be applied to the treatment of tumors.

(26) For the first time in the world, XZ-C proposes:

To overcome cancer, we must create the Environmental Protection and Cancer Research Institute and carry out cancer prevention system engineering. This is the first time in the world to conduct cancer prevention research, find cancer-causing factors, detect the source of carcinogens or carcinogenic factors, and try to stop these carcinogenic factors damaging on the human body.

Cancer prevention research should conduct the cancer prevention research:

Air pollution, the relationship with cancer, the relationship between water pollution and cancer, the relationship between soil pollution and cancer, the relationship of chemical, physical, biological factors and cancer, the relationship of diet, lifestyle, clothing, food, housing, travel, house decoration, etc. To research, testing, monitoring these sources of pollution and trying to stop at the source.

(27) XZ-C proposes that research ethics should be advocated, medicine is benevolence, and ethics is the first

(28) XZ-C proposes how to carry out the general attack on cancer in Hubei

(29) After the introduction of comprehensive skills - how to implement, how to achieve this comprehensive design, plan, planning, blueprint for cancer, in short, the above items, if it is implementation and achievement, it should be able to overcome cancer.

1)) The goal of conquering cancer:

It is to reduce the incidence of cancer, improve the cure rate of cancer, reduce the cancer mortality, significantly prolong the survival of cancer patients, and improve the quality of life of patients.

2)) To reach:

1/3 can be prevented, 1/3 can be cured, and 1/3 can be prolonged by treatment.

(30) Internationally It was proposed for the first time:

XZ-C proposed Dawning cancer prevention program A, B, D for scientific anti-pollution, pollution control, scientific cancer prevention, anti-cancer

How to overcome cancer? How can I prevent cancer?

How can I treat cancer?

XZ-C put forward the above 30 internationally initiated innovative academic arguments, all of which are clinical application theory innovations, which can be used in clinical practice to promote the new progress of 21st century oncology medicine.

Stepping out of a new road to conquer cancer (6) (Volume VI)

> **Created to overcome cancer multidisciplinary and the Science City of Cancer related Research Science Base**
>
> --------------**Promoting new advances in 21st century oncology medicine**

[Introduction]

- Established an overall framework for the fight against cancer, which is the only way to overcome cancer

—— Proposed the overall design, plan, plan, blueprint and implementation rules of Science City

- Equivalent to designing an overall framework for Chinese characteristics to overcome cancer

- The following is the implementation of XZ-C's outline of how to overcome cancer:

The main project to implement the outline of how to overcome cancer is:

The structural work:

To overcome cancer and to launch the general attack of cancer, focusing on prevention, control, and governance

To create a scientific research base for multidisciplinary and cancer-related research - Science City

Two-wing project:

A wing - how to overcome cancer? How to prevent cancer? - to reduce the incidence of cancer

B wing - how to overcome cancer? How to treat cancer? - to improve cancer cure rate

The aims:

A: Reduce the incidence of cancer

B: Improve cancer cure rate, prolong patient survival, and improve patient quality of life

If it is to implement and realize the overall design of cancer, planning blueprints, it is possible to overcome cancer.

How to implement, how to achieve this general guideline to overcome cancer, programs, plans, blueprints, should be set up to "conquer the general attack of the cancer attack team."

Invite famous experts, professors, academic leaders or leading scientists to support scientists, entrepreneurs, leaders, and volunteers who have overcome the general attack on cancer, and invite them to work together to make an unprecedented event in human history, "to overcome the general attack of cancer," and "create A science city that conquers cancer, for the benefit of mankind.

The Preparation for setting up the following:

"The first science city in the country to overcome cancer research base"

"The world's first science city to conquer cancer research base"

Chapter 23

Guide the Action

How is it to implement this scientific plan to overcome cancer and to launch the cancer attack and to build a scientific city to conquer cancer, which was it proposed by XZ-C?

How to implement it ? how to proceed it ? How to achieve it ? The following is a brief description:

(1) The goal of conquering cancer:

Reduce the incidence of cancer, improve the cure rate of cancer, and prolong the survival of cancer patients

To achieve:

1/3 can prevent

1/3 can be cured

1/3 can be treated to relieve pain, is a chronic disease and survival with tumor, prolong survival

The criteria for assessing the efficacy of cancer patients should be:

1). live a long time, prolonged survival

2). good quality of life

3). no complications, or less complications

(2) The road to conquer cancer

The route or the way:

1). To conquer cancer and launch a general attack

What is the total attack?

That is, cancer prevention + cancer control + cancer treatment at the same time and simultaneously

2). to build a science city of conquering cancer:

a, how to overcome cancer?

It must start the "Innovative Molecular Oncology Medical School" and graduate school and modern high-tech experimental talents

b, how to overcome cancer?

It must establish the "innovative molecular tumor prevention and treatment of Chinese and Western combined hospitals"

c, How to overcome cancer?

It must start the Institute of Innovative Molecular Oncology and the Multidisciplinary and Cancer Research Group

d, how to overcome cancer?

It must establish "Innovative Molecular Tumor Nano-Preparation Pharmaceutical Factory"

e, How to overcome cancer?

It must establish the "Innovative Environmental Protection and Cancer Research Institute" and carry out anti-cancer system engineering

f, how to overcome cancer?

It must establish the Cancer Animal Experimental Center

This is the only way to overcome cancer.

(3) How to prevent? How to control? How to cure?

All of these specific measures, feasibility plans, plans, blueprints are formulated.

(See the establishment of the C-station of the Cancer Working Group) preliminary planning and design of the test area (I) (II) (III) (IV)

(4) How to get started?

1). First, to build the hospital with prevention and control and treatment → to establish various disciplines (sections) → establish each group (study group)

2). First, to set up the whole team or the whole dragon with medical, teaching, research (section, group) and prevention, control, treatment, at one-stop; prevention and treatment at the same attention with the basic and the clinical parts; there are "three early", there are precancerous lesions.

3). First, it is to run a graduate school, talent training methods, ways;

The key to overcome cancer is to cultivate multi-disciplinary talents. It is cultivated through experimental research and clinical practice.

a. Firstly, the postgraduate tutor class, seminars, and training of talents, how to overcome the general attack content of cancer, discuss, divide the work, and conduct special and special research.

b. Talent training plan:

The graduate School recruits 100 graduate students (PhD, Master degree), who work while studying; after graduation, all stay in Science City, so it is to train them from generation to generation, and it is to require the results, achievements, contribution, patents (not only papers); after three years or/and five years, there will be rich in talent and scientific research results or there will be huge talented people and scientific research results.

• To Conquer cancer and launch a general attack, prevent cancer + control cancer + treat cancer at the same attention, this policy is the right way to overcome cancer.

- To create a scientific base of overcoming cancer and launching the general attack of cancer-----the Science City is the only way or the necessity method for how to set up agglutination wisdom and how to conquer cancer, this policy is the right way to overcome cancer.

How is it to implement these?

- It is necessary to establish a test area for the cancer working group (station) to explore the experience in prevention, control and treatment.

- This set of plans, programs, and general designs to overcome cancer can be applied to a country, a province, and a city.

- Because cancer is a disaster for the people of the world, the people of all countries, people of all countries, and the people of all provinces and cities must fight for it.

It is condensing wisdom, conquering cancer, and launching a general attack for the benefit of mankind.

Conquering the general attack of cancer is an unprecedented event in human history and the frontier of science.

- Emphasis on cancer prevention, cancer control, and cancer treatment. The way out for cancer treatment is "three early".

- Emphasis on the prevention of cancer, the establishment of the Cancer Prevention, Cancer Control, and Cancer Research Institutes. It is because 90% of cancers are related to the environment, we must prevent cancer from the environment and small environment, and prevent cancer from air, water, and soil. From clothing, food, housing, and anti-cancer, from changing lifestyle habits, changing life hobbies to prevent cancer.

(5) XZ-C proposes that in order to overcome the general attack of cancer, it must establish the Cancer Research Institute and the anti-cancer system project.

In the search for the cause and condition of cancer, the most prominent thing is that more than 90% of cancers are caused by environmental factors.

How is it to implement the creation of this cancer research institute?

Professor Xu Ze XZ-C proposed the general design of cancer prevention and proposed prevention cancer system engineering:

To study how to reduce or prevent these carcinogens

Because cancer patients cover the whole world, the pollution of industrial and agricultural wastewater, waste residue and waste gas also covers the whole world, therefore, it is necessary to globally attack the cancer attack.

Professor Xu Ze suggested:

1). All countries, provinces and states should establish prevention cancer research institutes (or institutions), carry out prevention cancer system projects, and carry out prevention cancer work for their own country, province and city.

2). Countries establish cancer prevention regulations and carry out comprehensively (some should be legislated)

3). I will use this project to recommend the World Health Organization to hold a prevention cancer campaign, with the goal of reducing the incidence of cancer. Conquering cancer is a frontier of science and a worldwide problem. Cancer is a human disaster, covering the whole world. People all over the world are eager to hope that one day they can overcome cancer and benefit mankind.

4). Professor Xu Ze suggested or proposed:

It is to advocate scientific research ethics, medical is benevolence, ethics first

The Scientific Research ethics:

Products should have ethical standards

The Standard:

It should be based on the standard of not damaging human health

Pay attention to cancer prevention regulations

The Basic ethics:

All products and people are harmless and do not harm people's health, especially for children.

(To be beautiful, living environment and living environment)

5). The health administrative department shall protect or guide life and protect health, and shall master, lead, support, and guide cancer prevention measures, cancer prevention projects, cancer prevention tests, and cancer prevention monitoring.

Cancer is a disaster for all mankind. It must fight globally. The people of the whole world must work together. Human beings should not sit still. Doctors should not do nothing. The health administrative department should not do nothing and should lead and lead the cancer prevention research series, be moving forward together, work together, and to take complementary advantages, to lead and to guide to overcome cancer and launch a general attack.

(6) Prof. XZ-C put forward the followings:

Professor Xu Ze XZ-C proposed:

Scientific ethics should be advocated, medicine is benevolence, and the ethics is the first.

The Research ethics:

Products should have ethical standards

Standard:

should be based on the standard of not damaging human health

Basic ethics:

All products and people are harmless and do not harm people's health, especially for children.

(To be beautiful, living environment and living environment)

The health administrative department shall guard, protect, and protect health. It shall lead, lead, support, and guide anti-cancer measures, anti-cancer projects, anti-cancer tests, and anti-cancer monitoring.

Cancer is a disaster for all mankind. It must fight globally. The people of the world must work together. Human beings should not sit still. Physicians should not do nothing. The health administrative department should not do nothing. It should guide and lead the series of prevention cancer research projects, and move further together and work together and have complementary and have the leadership and become guidance to overcome cancer and launch a general attack.

(7). The Post review - how to implement, how to achieve this overall design, program, planning, blueprint for cancer

"Condensing wisdom and conquering cancer - for the benefit of mankind" This is a more complete, more systematic, more comprehensive design, more specific planning how to overcome cancer medical monographs.

The book is divided into two parts:

1). How to overcome cancer? How can I prevent cancer?

2). How to overcome cancer? I see how to cure cancer.

A.   This book discusses how to prevent cancer, specific plans, plans, and blueprints in four tenths. How to overcome cancer? How can I prevent cancer? It is to put or position the research goal or "target" on how to reduce the incidence of cancer.

The current status quo is:

more and more cancer patients, the incidence rate continues to rise, the mortality rate remains high. The road that has passed in a century is to attention the heavy treatment with light prevention, or to only have treatment without prevention. In the cancer prevention work, it has done very little prevention or almost nothing has been done on the prevention cancer, and the prevention cancer has not been taken seriously, and prevention has not been taken seriously, so the incidence of cancer is rising.

How to prevent cancer? Where is the goal or "target" of cancer prevention? There must be specific cancer prevention targets, clear goals, and operability.

Professor Xu Ze proposed how to prevent cancer by I see (1), (2), (3), and (4) which proposed that it should analyze what is the cause or the factor to increase the incidence of cancer. The more patients are treated and the more the new patient shows up; the incidence rate is rising, and 90% of them are related to the environment. Research and discussion should be conducted on environmental carcinogenic factors (external environment and internal environment).

The cause of cancer is related to the external environment and the carcinogenic factors of the internal environment.

If we have a deeper understanding of the cause of cancer, then in the future we can ask: how to prevent cancer-causing factors, how to monitor which carcinogenic factors, which will eliminate which carcinogenic factors, so that we are away from cancer and prevent cancer.

Therefore, Professor Xu Ze proposed that:

It should prevent cancer from the big environment, small environment and should prevent cancer from clothing, food, shelter, and walking.

B. This book discusses how to treat cancer with 6/10 pages. It was positioning the research goal or "target" on how to improve the cure rate of cancer, prolong the survival of cancer patients, improve the quality of life, and propose how to treat cancer by I see.

The road of that we walk on for cancer treatment is the new way of combination Chinese medicine and western medicine at the molecular level. It is the new way for our laboratory to find immunomodulatory methods and drugs based on the new findings on the animal experiments. After years of animal screening and clinical validation, finally, we are looking for this new way of cancer treatment with immune regulation and control including XZ-C1-10 immunomodulating anti-cancer Chinese medicine series.

- From our laboratory experiments results, it was found that the host's thymus was acutely progressively atrophied after being inoculated with cancer cells, and the volume was significantly reduced.

- From the above experimental results, thymus atrophy, immune function is low, may be one of the etiology and pathogenesis of the tumor occurrence, therefore, its treatment principles must try to prevent thymus atrophy, promote thymocyte proliferation, increase immunity.

- In order to prevent thymus atrophy, promote thymocyte proliferation, and increase immunity, we look for both Chinese medicine and western medicine. The existing medicines of western medicine which can improve immunity and promote the proliferation of thymocytes are just few. So we went to the Chinese medicine to find because Chinese medicine has a general immunomodulatory effect.

- After 7 years of laboratory research, we have screened out XZ-C1-10 from the natural medicine to control the anti-cancer, anti-metastatic Chinese medicine, which can have Thymus function enhancement and increase immune function, and protect the marrow to produce blood. The clinical validation work was carried out on the basis of the success of the animal experiment. After 20 years of clinical application of more than 12,000 oncology clinics, good results have been achieved.

- After the experimental research and the anti-cancer research of Chinese medicine immunopharmacology with the combination of Chinese and Western medicine, it walked out of the new way of conquering cancer with XZ-C immune regulation and control, regulate immune activities, prevent thymic atrophy, promote thymocyte proliferation, protect bone marrow hematopoietic function, improve immune surveillance at the molecular level of the combination of Chinese and Western medicine.

C. **This medical monograph is practical, applied, research-oriented, and the outline of the implementation of how to overcome cancer. This scientific research program, scientific research design, scientific research plan, and blueprint can be used by countries, provinces and states to implement the concept of conquering cancer for the benefit of mankind.**

The main project of this medical monograph implementation outline is:

The main project	**Overcoming** the general attack of cancer, prevention + control + governance
Two-wing project:	**A scientific** research base for multidisciplinary and cancer-related research - Science City

A wing - how to prevent cancer - to reduce the incidence of cancer

B wing - how to treat cancer - to improve cancer cure rate

Aims:

A: Reduce the incidence of cancer

B: Improve cancer cure rate, prolong patient survival and improve quality of life

If the overall design and the planning blueprint of conquering cancer is implemented and achieved, it is possible to overcome cancer.

D. The work for the next step is that how to implement and how to achieve this overall design, scheme, plan, and blueprint for conquering cancer.

It should set up a team to tackle the cancer and launch the general attack.

To overcome cancer and to launch the general attack on cancer, talent is the key, and the first team should set up a research team.

The conditions or criteria for the Research team, academic committee :

Really academic, academic achievements and academic results in cancer research, basic research or clinical work, and there are monographs, editors, special issues, international papers; there is practical clinical experience; there is experimental research results, which it is to be the "overcome cancer" as the research direction of the academic and the research.

The leaders Leading and organizing cancer and the scientists, entrepreneurs, leaders, and volunteers who are supporting cancer prevention research, supporting cancer treatment research, supporting who have overcome cancer must have both ability and moral/political integrity, medicine is benevolence, and ethics is the first.

To overcome cancer and to launch the general attack of cancer, talent is the key. First, the organization should organize a research team and issue an invitation to form:

1. The Wuhan Anti-Cancer Research Society has tackled the research team for the general attack on cancer, which was established on December 6, 2017.

2. Invite domestic fellows to participate in the research team to overcome cancer and to launch the general attack of cancer

3. Inviting international fellows to participate in the research team to overcome cancer and to launch the general attack of cancer

Invitation from the chief designer of the "Science City to Conquer cancer and to launch the General Attack and Create a Multidisciplinary and Cancer-Related Research Base - Science City"

Invite famous experts, professors, academic leaders or leading scientists and scientists, entrepreneurs, leaders and volunteers who support of conquering cancer and launching the general attack on cancer.

Drafting

Within the province: Invitation to the team

Domestic: Invitation to the team

International: Invitation to the team

Professor Dr. Xu Ze
- Chief designer — "Overcoming the general attack on cancer and creating a scientific research base for cancer research - Science City"
- Project Leader of "Overcoming the General Attack of Cancer"

Postscript

Xu Ze, Xu Jie, Bin Wu

Where do these 8 medical monographs come from? Some of the first drafts came from the original record of "Think of it in the morning" and then compiled into a manuscript. I sent it to the street to copy the typing room and put it into a book. From the years of the flower, to the age of the ancient, to the year of the shackles, sent to the street copying typing room to type hundreds of times. Sometimes my wife and I went to the typing room to print the manuscript. She is the first reader and supporter of my "Monograph".

After I retired at the age of 63, I continued to research, self-reliance, self-financing, and the journey of Science was non-stop. Still struggling, arduously climbing, four different scientific research stages of one scientific research footprint, four different levels of mountain results. A mountain is better than a mountain scientific research landscape. It is to be Perseverance and be persistence. Since 1980, I have insisted on memorizing scientific research diaries, scientific research records, the accumulation of these scientific research original materials and the record of scientific thinking, and some have also been selected as the material of this series of "monographs".

I read five years of private school in my childhood (at the time of the early 1930s, there was only one elementary school in a county, and the villages were mostly private). I loved the ancient books and poems. In addition to medical research, you can enjoy yourself.

A. In this poem, Dr. Xu Ze express that Dawn is precious time for him to have all of these scientific ideas and all of these great monograph done in Chinese poem version.

晨起想到
二00六年春

万籁无声寂
鸡鸣报晓时
曙光潜入内
轻唤已黎明
一夜酣甜睡
醒来脑清新
灵思一闪现

靶点豁然明
迅起披衣坐
挥毫录万千
医籍添新贵
斯哉为黎民

B. In this poem, Dr. Xu Ze express his spirits of hard working and persistence for scientific research and human health no matter the age. Keep persistence of hard work. Don't give up

自　咏
二00六年春
年逾古稀犹自奋
赛因征途不停蹄
躲进小楼研机理
灵思一现靶点明
老骥伏枥志未已
为控转移究歧黄
十裁卓然成夙志
晚霞迷人似晟曦

(8)　How to carry out "to overcome cancer and to launch the general attack of cancer" in Hubei and Wuhan?

It should be to propose:

1). Conducted an academic report on "Proposal to Overcome cancer and to launch the General Attack of Cancer"

2). Set up a team of "conquering cancer and launching the general attack"

3). To formulate the tasks and achievements of each team member, not to name but to seek truth, to strive to achieve results, it must be truly practical, and it must have both ability and moral/political integrity, the medicine is benevolence, the ethics first.

The contribution of each team member, the tasks and indicators of each member, the tasks and indicators of the team must clearly define the goals and objectives, and strive for innovation.

1. Can cancer be overcome?

It should be able to overcome cancer. It is because 90% of cancer is caused by the environment.

It is that the environmental factors lead to genetic mutations that lead to chromosomal deletions and abnormalities.

The environmental factors are possible or can be managed to do research, find ways to solve them.

"Condensing wisdom, conquering cancer - for the benefit of mankind" is a medical monographs with the comprehensive design, specifically planning of how to overcome cancer, is the outline of the implementation of how to overcome cancer. This set of scientific research plans, scientific research programs, and blue maps are available everywhere as the Reference application.

2. Do cancers need to be overcome?

It must be and urgently overcome because the incidence rate is rising and the mortality rate is high. The number of cancer deaths worldwide is 8.18 million. About 8550 people in China are diagnosed with cancer every day, and 6 people are confirmed to be cancer every minute. Therefore, research to overcome the scientific research work of cancer attack, can not walk slowly, should run forward, save the wounded. Because people all over the world are eager to hope that one day they will be able to overcome cancer and stay away from cancer for the benefit of mankind.

3. How should cancer be gotten rid of it?

(1). It should conquer cancer and launch the general attack of cancer, and put the attention on prevention + control + treatment of cancer at the same level and at the same attention and the same time.

(Change the current mode of hospitalization for heavy treatment with light prevention, and change the current treatment mode that focuses on the middle and late stages of treatment)

(2). It should be implemented and realized in accordance with the report and the proposal book on "Conquering cancer and launching the general attack on cancer"

The next step is how to implement, how to achieve this overall design, program, plan, blueprint for conquering cancer.

The steps, plans, programs, and general design of conquering cancer and launching the general attack of how to achieve have been completed, and have been published globally.

Why publish English books worldwide? It is because cancer patients cover the whole world, the pollution of industrial and agricultural wastewater, waste residue and waste gas also covers the whole world. Therefore, it is necessary to globally conquer cancer and to lauch the general attack to cancer.

(3). The above-mentioned plan, planning, general design, and blueprint for conquering cancer and launching the general attack of cancer can be applied to a country, a province, a state, and a market reference application to conquer cancer and even conquer cancer.

4. How is it to implement the creation and building of this cancer prevention research?

XZ-C proposed the cancer prevention general design and cancer prevention system engineering

Professor Xu Ze suggested:

(1) All countries, provinces and states should establish anti-cancer research institutes (or institutions) to carry out cancer prevention system projects and carry out cancer prevention work for their own country, province, state and city. (It is because there are a large number of cancer patients in various countries, provinces and cities)

(2) Countries should establish cancer prevention regulations and control and carry out comprehensive development (some should be legislated)

(3) I will use this project to recommend the World Health Organization to hold an cancer preventioncampaign, with the goal of reducing the incidence of cancer.

Conquering cancer is at the forefront of science and a worldwide problem. Cancer is a human disaster. The whole world and the people all over the world are eager to hope that one day they can overcome cancer and benefit mankind.

(4) Research ethics should be advocated, medicine is benevolence, and ethics is the first

The Research ethics:

Products, achievements, and patents should all have ethical standards.

The Standard:

The bottom line should be based on standards that do not harm human health. In particular, it must not contain carcinogens.

The Basic ethics:

All products, achievements, patents, goods and people are harmless and do not harm people's health, especially for children. Do not contain carcinogens.

(5) **XZ-C proposes scientific ethics, and should recommend to WHO that all products, achievements, and patents should be the bottom line of moral standards that do not harm human health, especially the carcinogens. E.g:**

1). Women's cosmetics, hair dyes, children's toys... should be tested without carcinogens, without damaging human health

2). The house decoration, materials ... should be tested without carcinogens

3). Food additives, preservatives, food processing packaging ... should be tested without carcinogens

4). Leather products, cloth dyes ... should be tested, no carcinogens

5). The feed of collectively fed pigs is not allowed to contain hormones, auxins, vegetarian meat, growth-promoting hormones... all should be tested without carcinogens.

6). Group feed chicken, duck feed must not contain hormones, auxin ... should be tested without carcinogens

(6) **The health administrative department shall protect and protect health, and shall lead, master, support, and guide cancer prevention measures, cancer prevention projects, cancer prevention tests, and cancer prevention monitoring.**

(7) XZ-C proposes to establish the "Cancer Prevention Research Institute" and carry out cancer prevention system engineering:

- The way in which so many carcinogens or carcinogenic factors should be studied

- These sources of pollutants should be studied and managed to stop at the source.

- These carcinogenic mechanisms should be studied, their carcinogenic effects, and environmental factors leading to genetic mutations.

- It is necessary to study the "two-type society" resource-saving and environment-friendly community to prevent cancer (to achieve a beautiful green environment and living environment with beautiful flowers and birds).

Professor Xu Ze proposed how to overcome cancer? how to prevent cancer? By I see:

Situation analysis: (1) - how to prevent cancer, cancer incidence is rising

Situation analysis: (2) - Cancer incidence is related to the environment

1. Why does the increase in cancer incidence have a relationship with the environment?

2. The cause of cancer is related to the external environment and the carcinogenic factors of the internal environment.

3. If we have a deeper understanding of the causes of cancer, then we can come up with more valuable suggestions in the future: how to prevent cancer-causing factors, how to monitor which carcinogenic factors, and which cancer-causing factors to clear, so that we can stay away from cancer, prevent cancer.

Situation analysis: (3) - Prevention should be based on improving the carcinogenic factors of external factors (external environment) and internal factors (internal environment).

Professor Xu Ze proposed:

The establishment of an innovative cancer prevention research institute and an innovative cancer prevention system project. This is an unprecedented work and must be practiced in person to seek health and welfare for human beings.

XZ-C proposed the general design of cancer and cancer prevention system engineering.

Situation analysis: (4) – it should set up the Environmental and Cancer Research Group

Monitor environmental pollution-causing factors and data, develop cancer prevention, cancer control measures, and research and development interventions.

a, from clothing, food, shelter, anti-cancer

b, from the big environment of life to prevent cancer

c, from the small living environment to prevent cancer

d, from life behavior, life hobbies, living habits to prevent cancer

Under the guidance of Xi Jinping's characteristic socialism under the new era, he is struggling to open up a new phase of scientific research in the new era and overcome the scientific research work of cancer. We will strive to follow the path of independent innovation with Chinese characteristics and adhere to the road of independent innovation of Chinese and Western medicine combined with "Chinese-style anti-cancer".

Innovation--------We have accumulated 30 years of anti-cancer basic and clinical research on anti-cancer metastasis and came out the road of a "Chinese-style anti-cancer", the combination of Chinese and Western medicine with immune regulation and control of the treatment of cancer. We have accumulated more than 12,000 clinical application experiences in 20 years, which can be pushed to the whole country, can go to the world, can connect with the "A Belt and A Road",

make Chinese medicine go to the world, and make "Chinese-style anti-cancer" and Chinese and Western medicine combined with immune regulation and treatment. Cancer not only develops and enriches the content of immunology and cancer treatment, but also brings China's medical modernization into line with international standards and is at the forefront of the world.

Chapter 24

Annex

1. Three "one hundred"

2. The Academician letters

3. Introduction to the Institute of Experimental Surgery in Hubei University of Traditional Chinese Medicine

4. The science and technology research topics

5. The cooperation letter of intent

6. Major progress in cancer research in the past 100 years

   Postscript (with the pictures)

Attachment 1

The Award Certificate of The National Book Award which was won the "Three One Hundred" Original Book (Chinese version with English translation)

The English version as the following:

"Three hundred" original publishing project

Certificate

People's Military Medical Press:

The book "**New Concepts and New Methods of Cancer Metastasis Treatment**" published by your agency was selected into the first "Three One Hundred" original book publishing project of the General Administration of Press and Publication.

Specially issued this certificate.

Press and Publication Administration
of the People's Republic of China
April 2007

The Chinese verision as the following:

"三个一百"原创出版工程

证　书

人民军医 出版社:

你社出版的《癌转移治疗新概念与新方法》一书入选新闻出版总署第一届"三个一百"原创图书出版工程。特颁此证。

中华人民共和国新闻出版总署

二〇〇七年四月

Create an environmental protection and cancer prevention research institute and carry out cancer prevention system engineering

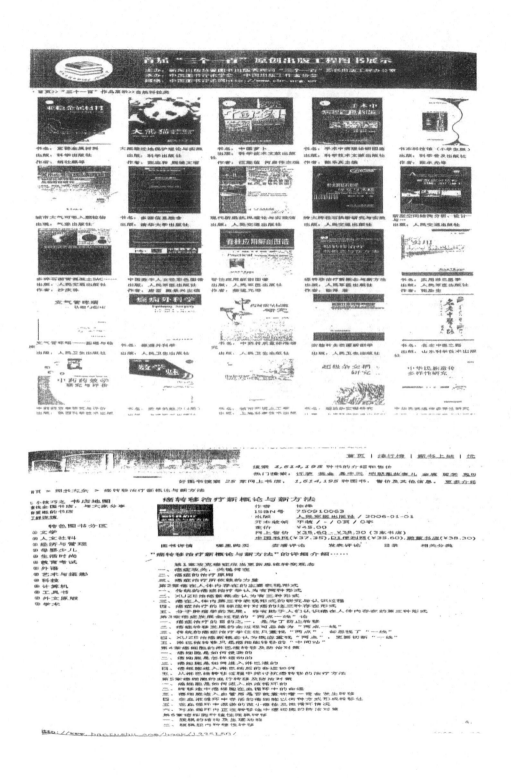

377

癌转移治疗新概念与新方法 - Google 搜索   http://www.google.cn/search?rlz=1B3GGGL_zh-CNCN246

网页 图片 地图 资讯 视频 博客 更多▾

Google

癌转移治疗新概念与新方法   Google 搜索 | 高级搜索 | 使用偏好

所有网页 中文网页 简体中文网页 中国的网页

网页 集体中文 和 简体中文网页中，约有 683,000 项符合癌转移治疗新概念与新方法的查询结果，以下是第 1-10 项 （搜索用时 0.28 秒）

癌转移治疗新概念与新方法
癌转移治疗新概念与新方法在搜狐网上书店销售，读者在搜狐搜狗网页可了解到癌转移治疗新概念与新方法作者、价格、内容介绍等信息。欢迎购买癌转移治疗新概念与新 ...
www.bxb.cn/books/23/219708.html - 13k - 网页快照 - 类似网页

癌转移治疗新概念与新方法-希望书店
网上销售癌转移治疗新概念与新方法,作者:徐泽,出版社:人民军医出版社,出版日期:2006-1-1,定价:￥45元,书店价:￥42.8元,全国125省上门，提供货到付款服务。
www.hopebook.net/yw/product/184365.htm - 19k - 网页快照 - 类似网页

癌转移治疗新概念与新方法(精)/徐泽-图书-卓越亚马逊
癌转移治疗新概念与新方法(精). 市场价：￥45.00. 本站价：￥35.50 折扣：78折 节省：9.70元.
VIP 价：￥34.30 SVIP价：￥33.60. 信用产品任何价格均免费图运：...
www.amazon.cn/mn/detailApp?ref=DT_RV&uid=000-0000000-0000000&prodid=zjbk270585 - 55k - 网页快照 - 类似网页

癌转移治疗新概念与新方法-当当图书
癌转移治疗新概念与新方法 » 推荐给朋友 · 查看更大图片. 作者：徐泽著, 出版社：人民军医出版社. 出版时间：2006-1-1; 字数：354000; 版次：1; 页数：229 ...
product.dangdang.com/product.aspx?product_id=2128276 - 50k - 网页快照 - 类似网页

癌转移治疗新概念与新方法- 原价：￥45.00 现价：￥35.50
购买《癌转移治疗新概念与新方法》图书的图片及详细介绍，该书属于医学专业书籍分类下的肿瘤学书籍。读书频道：￥45.00 现价：￥35.50 如其您想购买癌转移治疗新概念 ...
www.39world.com/buybooks/0320422T20064226d.html - 21k - 网页快照 - 类似网页

癌转移治疗新概念与新方法-购书网
关于癌转移治疗新概念与新方法的简介,本书是一部癌症转移治疗的专著,其30章,作者将自己50年来肿瘤外科临床治疗经验和10多年的实验室研究成果进行认真地分析 ...
www.61goushu.com/10192895.html - 26k - 网页快照 - 类似网页

癌转移治疗新概念与新方法-协讯-全国打折全国送货
图书《癌转移治疗新概念与新方法》提供网上书店观看方订价! 系统订购 | 首页 | 购物车 | 购物指南 | 我的帐户 | 繁体系 | 简繁/简体 ...
www.boukyen.cn/book/Alzhuanyizhiliaoxingainianyuxinfangfa.html - 37k - 网页快照 - 类似网页

【图书简介】- 癌转移治疗新概念与新方法|图书信息|购买|阅读-异悦图书馆
作为《癌转移治疗新概念与新方法》图书的图片及详细介绍,该书属于医学肿瘤转移概念一、癌症成为、关键词包含二、癌症的治疗原则三、癌症治疗所做新的力量第2章癌症人体内容 ...
bc.ykle.net/302/1120692/ - 23k - 网页快照 - 类似网页

癌转移治疗新概念与新方法 肿瘤学 医学书店 专业书店 四川省专试书店 ...
作者将自己50年来肿瘤外科临床治疗经验和50多年的实验室研究成果进行认真整理、归纳总结，形成了其有自己特色的癌转移新认识、新概念和思路抗转移治疗新技术。新 ...
www.77manhai.com/goods.php?id=56240 - 43k - 网页快照 - 类似网页

癌转移治疗新概念与新方法-时代网
癌转移治疗新概念与新方法,徐泽著,人民军医出版社,肿瘤学;医学卫生;图书,85折优惠;定价45;快递货上门，货到付款。
www.vev1.com/852815.html - 33k - 网页快照 - 类似网页

1 2 3 4 5 6 7 8 9 10   下一页

新！ www.G.cn —— 最短域名上谷歌，立刻试试看！

.5.

赞助商链接

5分钟 获得 你想要的答案
无须等问答，自助分类检索；
保证你的问题第一时间被解答！
WenDa.TianYa.cn

在此展示您的广告

Annex 3

Brief Introduction of Experimental Surgery Research Institute of Hubei College of Traditional Chinese Medicine

The Attachment 3
(Two version of English and Chinese)

The Chinese version as the following:

湖北中医学院实验外科研究所
情 况 简 介

实验外科在发展医学科学方面极其重要，它是打开医学禁区的一把钥匙，许多疾病的发现及防治方法都是经过无数次动物实验研究，取得了稳定性成果才应用于临床、促进医学事业的发展，提高医疗质量开展新的防治方法。结合我院医学科研实际情况的需要，湖北中医学院实验外科研究所于1991年3月成立。

一、实验外科研究所的基础建设和发展情况

（一）实验室的创办与发展

本研究所的前身为实验外科研究室，更前身为肝腹水实验室1980年5月，在省血研会召开的晚期血吸虫病外科治疗座谈会上，裘法祖教授将"晚期血吸虫病顽固腹水外科治疗"的研究究任务分配给我院外科。起初我们与长虹工厂合作试制了腹腔——静脉转流装置，但由于没有动物实验室，没有经费，实验面临困境、研究面临搁浅。

80年7月3日，我们向医院领导作了汇报，第3天医院就批准成立"外科肝腹水科研小组"，并上报省卫生厅，省科委，第4天学院领导也听取了汇报。各级领导部门对研究工作给予了高度的重视和大力支持，省科委正式批准"这一科研项目，至此，组织形式，经费来源，人事安排均有了保障，实验外科实验室始宣告成立。

实验室的创办还得到了省财政厅、省血防办的有力支持，同时我们还荣幸地得到了我国著名外科专家裘法祖教授的亲切关怀与热情指导，加上本室同志们因陋就简，艰苦创业，为实验外科研究所的成立，打下了坚实的基础。实验外科实验室于1980年组建，十年来在徐泽教授主持下进行了肝硬化顽固性腹水外科治疗的实验研究及发病机制的实验研究，用实验外科方法探讨肺日本血吸虫病的病理、病理生理、发病机理的实验研究，日本血吸虫病肝硬变门脉高压发病机理的实验研究，肝纤维化微观定量测定的实验研究及肝细胞移植于脾形成第二肝脏治疗肝衰的实验研究等国家和省科研课题。

1987年开始转为实验肿瘤研究，进行癌细胞移植，实验肿瘤动物模型，探索其发病机制，转移机理和规律，免疫机能变化，进而探讨防癌有效的中草药，对抗癌抑癌的中草药进行严格的科学的反复筛选研究，现正在进行八项中草药防癌抗癌的实验研究，已取得一定的成效和进展。

实验外科实验室已参加了全国癌肿研究协作组，并牵头在全省部分地区组织了癌肿的研究协作组，在本院牵头组织了多学科对消化系肿瘤研究协作组，为了发展防癌抗癌事业，致力于深入研究发掘防治癌肿的中草药。

（二）实验室已完成的和正在进行的科研课题。

1.已完成了中国医科院科学基金、国家自然科学基金中央血办、省科委、省卫生厅、省

379

血研会等课题15项。并继续开展正在进行的新课题研究有8项。

2.1987年起，转为实验肿瘤研究：开展癌细胞移植和对受体微血管建立，微循环建立规律的观察寻找抑制癌转移的方法；中草药抗癌转移的作用；中晚期消化道抗癌转移的实验；中草药抗癌作用对NKC和免疫调节影响的实验等。实验研究旨在将现代科学与传统中医中药相结合，从伟大的祖国医药宝库中发掘防癌抗癌的有效方法和制剂。

（三）已取得的科研成果：

1.完成的课题成果

（1）、Z～CI型腹腔——静脉转流装置治疗肝硬变顽固性腹水的实验研究及临床应用。1982年在湖北省科委主持下召开鉴定会，为国内先进水平，获湖北省科技成果二等奖。成果论文发表于《中华外科杂志及同济医科大学英德文版学报；先后有10个国家医科院或大学医院来函索取资料。成果在10多个省市医院推广应用。

（2）、"用实验外科方法对日本血吸虫病的病理、病理生理、发病机理的实验研究"，国家自然科学基金课题、1986年在湖北省卫生厅主持下召开鉴定会，为国际水平。获湖北省科技成果二等奖，省卫生科技成果一等奖。

2.科研论文及学术交流情况：

（1）、十年来有80篇（45万字）科研论文在全国性或省级医学杂志发表或在国际、全国或省级学术会议上报告交流。

（2）5次出席国际学术会议，报告本所科研学术论文：

①1933年中日两国寄生虫病学术讨论会；

②1985年第四届世界微循环卫星会议；

③1988年国际肝病学术会；

④北京国际癌症讨论会；

⑤1990年澳大利亚国际肝病研究会学术年会。

本室5次国际学术会议交流论文均被收入其英文资料汇编中。

3.人材培养：

培养了4名硕士研究生及1名博士研究生毕业、现有2名硕士研究生在读。

4.资料积累和管理工作：

创立了拟临床动物实验资料记录法，建立了完整的资料体系。本室资料的管理体系及完整性受到有关方面的关注和重视，《健康报》曾两次派员专程来访报道，省卫生厅科教处曾在本室召开了医学科研资料积累与管理的现场会。

（四）、实验室现有设备条件：

现在实验外科有一栋二层楼房的实验室，楼上有动物无菌手术室、器械间、洗手间，楼下有病理室、生化免疫室、癌细胞生物学细胞工程室、微循环室、动物术后观察室及动物室及储藏室，设备有病理切片机、生物显微镜、系列型微镜、照相显微镜、微循环显微机、血压血流计、精密分析天平、深低温冰箱、心电图机、恒温箱、干燥箱、高速离心机、腹水转流机，有生化免疫、细胞移植的各项化验仪器设备及全套手术器械基本设备，受体病理切片基本设备，微循环检测设备，细胞工程基本设备。十年来已形成了一套实验外科动物手术室、实验室、动物病群、术后饲养观察的管理、工作常规程序。本所现有条件及仪器设备可

380

供现有所承担课题任务的完成（现有国家自然科学基金、省科委、省卫生厅、省血防办、省教委课题）

二、实验外科研究所的宗旨、研究目标和任务

（一）、宗旨：

实验外科在医学科学的发展中，有着极其重要的地位和作用。本所宗旨即以充分运用现代科学技术，以现代科学实验方法为手段，开展挖掘祖国医药学宝库，致力于癌肿防治事业，深入研究发掘防癌抗癌中草药，着眼于三早（早期发现、早期诊断、早期治疗）开展中西医结合，防治癌肿的工作，为攻克癌肿，造福于人类而做出贡献。

（二）、研究目标和任务：

实验外科研究所主要是对癌肿的攻关，其次是对肝硬化腹水，血吸虫肝病、肺病等实验研究，重点是用实验外科方法，对癌肿进行实验癌肿的基础研究和临床癌肿病人的防治研究，发掘防癌抗癌的中草药的动物实验研究及应用中西医结合，中医中药防癌治癌的临床研究，本所实验肿瘤研究室，采用癌细胞生物工程技术及基因工程技术，开发肿瘤的生物治疗肿瘤的免疫治疗的基础研究与临床实践，发展和推动防癌抗癌事业。

此外本所还发展抗癌防癌的保健咨询，癌症患者的心理咨询，肿瘤防治教学及研究生的培养等任务。以及建立我省一些癌症高发地区的普查网。

（三）、组织机构

实验外科研究所设：

顾问指导：裘法祖（同济医大名誉校长、国际著名外科教授）

名誉所长：夏穗生（同济医大器官移植研究所所长、国际著名外科教授）

所　　长：徐　泽（外科教授）

副所长：王抗生（外科教授）

　　　　胡军谱（外科副教授）

下　　设：

1.实验医学动物实验研究室

2.临床肿瘤外科研究室

3.实验肿瘤研究室

以徐泽教授为首的湖北中医学院实验外科研究所在实验肿瘤研究方面已经取得了相当的成就；研制成功Z—CⅠ型腹腔——静脉转流装置（pVS），治疗肝炎后肝硬变顽固性腹水及晚期日本血吸虫病肝硬变顽固性腹水，经十年来大量临床病例应用疗效显著；采用癌细胞生物工程技术，探索癌肿新的生物治疗及免疫治疗方法的实验研究，发现了免疫治疗新方法的可喜苗头；对48项传统抗癌中草药进行了严格的科学的反复重复的癌动物模型的实验筛选，淘汰去无稳定效果的，筛选出确有疗效的武汉中草药抗癌1～6号胶囊。正在实验及临床验证。本研究所今后将以攻克癌肿为研究方向，以现代医学科学实验方法为手段，深入发掘祖国医药学宝库，研究防癌抗癌的中草药及开发肿瘤的生物免疫治疗，造福人类。

The English Version of the above as the following:

Brief Introduction of Experimental Surgery Research Institute of Hubei College of Traditional Chinese Medicine

Experimental surgery is important in the development of medical science. It is a key to opening the medical exclusion zone. The discovery and prevention methods of many diseases have been carried out through numerous animal experiments, and the results of stability have been applied to the clinic, promote the development of medical undertakings, and improve the quality of medical treatment to develop new prevention methods. Combined with the actual needs of medical research in our hospital, the Institute of Experimental Surgery of Hubei College of Traditional Chinese Medicine was established in March 1991.

First

Infrastructure and development of the Institute of Experimental Surgery

(One)

The establishment and development of the laboratory

The predecessor of this institute is the laboratory of experimental surgery. The previous predecessor was the Liver Ascites Laboratory in May 1980. At the Symposium on Surgical Treatment of Advanced Schistosomiasis held by the Provincial Blood Research Institute, Prof. Qi Fazu assigned the research task of "Surgical treatment of advanced schistosomiasis in stubborn ascites" to our hospital. At first, we cooperated with Changhong Factory to try out the abdominal cavity-venous bypass device. However, due to the lack of animal laboratories and no funds, the experiment was faced with difficulties and the research was stranded.

On July 3, 1980, we reported to the hospital leadership. On the third day, the hospital approved the establishment of the "Surgical Liver Ascites Research Group". And reported to the Provincial Health Department, the Provincial Science and

Technology Commission, the fourth day of the academic commander also heard the report. The leading departments at all levels gave high attention and strong support to the research work. The Provincial Science and Technology Commission officially approved the scientific research project. At this point, the organizational form, funding sources, and personnel arrangements were guaranteed, and the experimental surgery laboratory began to be established.

The founding of the laboratory has also received strong support from the Provincial Department of Finance and the Provincial Department of Blood Prevention. At the same time, we are also honored to receive the cordial care and enthusiasm of our famous surgeon, **Prof. Qi Fazu**, and the comrades in this room are simple and hard-working. It laid a solid foundation for the establishment of the Institute of Experimental Surgery. The experimental surgery laboratory was established in 1980. In the past ten years, under the auspices of Professor Xu Ze, the experimental research and pathogenesis of cirrhosis refractory ascites have been carried out. The experimental surgical method explores the pathology and pathophysiology of pulmonary schistosomiasis. Experimental study on pathogenesis, experimental study on the pathogenesis of hepatic cirrhosis and portal hypertension in schistosomiasis, experimental study on microscopic quantitative determination of liver fibrosis, and experimental study on hepatocyte transplantation in the spleen and formation of second liver in the treatment of liver failure And provincial research projects.

In 1987, beginning to turn into experimental tumor research, transplant cancer cells, experimental tumor animal models, explore its pathogenesis, transfer mechanism and regularity, immune function changes. Furthermore, it is necessary to conduct a rigorous scientific and repeated screening study on prevention cancer effective Chinese herbal medicines and Chinese herbal medicines against cancer and inhibiting cancer. Eight experimental studies on prevention cancer and anti-cancer of Chinese herbal medicines are underway, and some achievements and progress have been made.

The experimental surgical experiment has participated in the National Cancer Research Collaborative Group and led a research collaboration group that organized cancer in some parts of the province. It led a multidisciplinary research group on the digestive system of swollen oil in order to develop prevention. I am interested in anti-cancer career and are committed to in-depth research and discovery of Chinese herbal medicine for preventing and treating cancer.

(Two)

The research courses of that the laboratory has completed and ongoing

1. Completed 15 projects including the Science Foundation of the Chinese Academy of Medical Sciences, the Central Co-organizer of the National Natural Science Foundation, the Provincial Science and Technology Commission, the Provincial Health Department, and the Provincial Association and continue to carry out 8 new research projects.

2. Since 1987, it has been converted to experimental tumor research:

Carry out cancer cell transplantation and establishment of microvessels in the recipient, and establish a regular observation of microcirculation to find a way to inhibit cancer metastasis.

(Three)

Scientific research achievements that have been obtained:

1. Completed project results

(1) Z-Cl type abdominal cavity-venous bypass device Jinchuan cirrhosis refractory ascites experimental study and clinical application. In 1982, under the auspices of the Northern Science and Technology Commission, the appraisal meeting was held, which was the domestic advanced level and won the second prize of Hubei Province Science and Technology Achievements. The results paper was published in the Journal of Chinese Journal of Surgery and Tongji Medical University. There are 10 national medical colleges or university hospitals to obtain information. The results are promoted and applied in more than 10 provincial and municipal hospitals.

(2) "Experimental research on the virulence or/and pathology, pathophysiology, and pathogenesis of schistosomiasis in Japan",

The National Natural Science Cluster Project was held in the Health Department of Hubei Province in 1980 to hold an appraisal meeting for the international level. He was awarded the second prize of Hubei Province Science and Technology Achievements and the first prize of provincial health science and technology achievements.

2. Research papers and academic exchanges:

(1). In the past ten years, 80 papers (450,000 words) have been published in national or provincial medical journals or reported at international, national or provincial academic conferences.

(2). 5 times attending international academic conferences and reporting academic papers on scientific research.

1). 1983 Sino-Japanese Parasitic Disease Symposium;

2). 1 985 Fourth World Microcirculation Satellite Conference;

3). 1988 International Association of Liver Diseases,

4). Beijing International Pain Symposium;

5). 1990 Australian International Liver Disease Research Association Academic Annual Meeting. The five international academic conference exchanges in this room were all included in the compilation of English materials.

3. Talent cultivation:

Four graduate students and one doctoral graduate have been trained, and two graduate students are currently enrolled.

4. Data accumulation and management work:

The establishment of the clinical animal experiment data recording method, the establishment of a complete Jia system, the knowledge system of the wooden room data and the integrity of the relevant aspects of attention and attention, "Health News" has sent personnel to visit the report twice. The Department of Science and Education of the Provincial Health Department once held a site meeting on the black and management of the school.

(Four)

The existing conditions of the laboratory:

Now experimentally bred a laboratory of a two-story building, with a sterile aseptic surgery animal room, a device room, a toilet, a pathology room downstairs, a biochemical immunization room, a cancer cell engineering room, a microcirculation room, and an animal. Postoperative observation, serial microscope, photographic microscope, microcirculation microscopy, blood pressure blood flow meter, precision analytical balance, deep bottom temperature refrigerator, electrocardiogram, thermostat, drying oven, high speed centrifuge, ascites transfer machine, There are various biochemical immunity, cell transplantation equipment and a complete set of basic equipment for surgical instruments, basic equipment for pathological sectioning, microcirculation testing equipment, and basic equipment for cell engineering. A set of experimental surgical animal rooms and experiments have been formed in the past ten years. Room, animal anesthesia, postoperative maintenance observation management, routine work procedures, the existing conditions and equipment of the Institute can be used to complete the task of the existing tasks (existing National Natural Science Foundation, Provincial Science and Technology Commission, Provincial Health Department, Provincial Association Defense Office, Provincial Education Commission)

Second

The purpose, research objectives and tasks of the Institute of Experimental Surgery

(1). The purpose:

Experimental surgery has an extremely important position and role in the development of medical science. The purpose of the Institute is to make full use of modern science and technology, to use modern scientific experimental methods as a means to carry out the excavation of the treasure house of the motherland, to devote to the prevention and treatment of tumors, and to study and discover the anti-pain and anti-drug Chinese herbal medicines. (early discovery, early diagnosis, early treatment) to carry out the work of the combination of Chinese and western medical treatment of cancer prevention and treatment, to overcome cancer and to contribute for benefit the human beings.

(2). Research objectives and tasks:

The Institute of Experimental Surgery is mainly for the research of tumor or cancer, followed by experimental research on cirrhosis ascites, schistosomiasis liver disease, lung disease, etc. The focus is the research of the prevention and treatment about the basic research on experimental cancer and of clinical painful patients with the experimental surgical methods, is the research for exploring Chinese herbal medicine for prevention cancer and anti-cancer and the application of the combination of Chinese and western medicine.

The Institute of Experimental Oncology uses cancer cell bioengineering technology and genetic engineering technology to develop basic research and clinical practice of tumor immunotherapy for biological treatment of tumors, and to develop and promote cancer prevention and cancer prevention.

In addition, the Institute also develops health consultations for prevention of cancer and anti-cancer, psychological counseling for patients with symptoms, cancer prevention and teaching, and training for graduate students. And establish a census wind in some high-incidence areas of our province.

(3) Organizations

Institute of Experimental Surgery:

Consultant Guidance: Qi Fazu (Honorary President of Tongji Medical University, Professor of Internationally Famous Surgery)

Honorary Director: Xia Suisheng (Director of the Institute of Transplantation of Tongji Medical and Miyajima, Professor of Internationally Famous Surgery)

Director: Xu Ze (Surgery Professor)

Deputy Director: Wang Kangsheng (Surgery Professor)

Hu Junpu [Associate Professor of Surgery)

Under:

1. Experimental Medical Animal Experimental Research Laboratory

2. Clinical Tumor Surgery Laboratory

3. Experimental tumor research laboratory

The Institute of Experimental Surgery of Hubei College of Traditional Chinese Medicine, led by Professor Xu Ze, has made considerable achievements in experimental tumor research; successfully studied zc I type abdominal cavity-venous bypass device (pV), treatment of 1H hard refractory ascites after hepatitis and cirrhotic refractory ascites in advanced schistosomiasis, after a decade of clinical use of a large number of clinical cases, the use of cancer cells Engineering technology, exploring the new biological treatment and immunotherapy methods, the more experimental research, found a new way of immunotherapy, and the screening of 48 traditional anti-cancer Chinese herbal medicines. The sputum has no stabilizing effect, and the Wuhan Chinese herbal medicine anti-cancer 1 to 6 capsules have been screened out. Experimental and clinical validation is underway. In the future, the Institute of Wood will focus on the research of cancer, and use modern medical science experimental methods as a means to explore the treasure house of the motherland, research on anti-cancer and anti-cancer Chinese herbal medicines, and develop biological and immunotherapy for swelling and pain for the benefit of mankind.

The introduction for the experimental and clinical research lab

The Chinese version:

我国山上实验外科实验室，坐落一栋两层楼房的动物实验室，由徐琼教授于1980年亲手创建，建立了本实验外科研究所，承担了国家科委、卫生部、中央血液、中国医学科学院、省科委、省卫生厅等15项科研课题，为湖北中医学院培养了110名硕士研究生、为国际医学院培养了两名博士研究生毕业，发表科研论文206篇，取得了多项科研成果，其中二项获湖北省科技成果二等奖，一项获湖北省卫生厅一等奖。"膜水"科研成果上了高等院校教科书外科学。十个国家索函索取资料，国内38家医院推广，"血瘀实病"成果资料已上交联合国文献小组存档，成为国际先进水平，

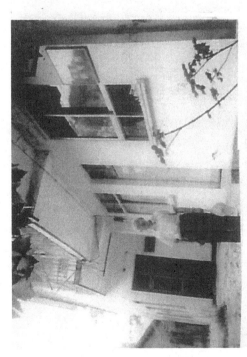
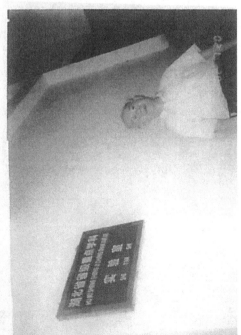

The English version:

There is a experimental surgery lab in the garden mountain, which is a two floor animal experimental lab, built by Dr. Xu Ze in 1980 and built the institution of the experimental surgery which carried out 15 scientific research projects and trained 10 Master degree students for Hubei traditional Chinese medicine university and 2 Ph.D degree students for Tongji University and published 206 scientific research papers and got many scientific research achievement, including two were awarded the second level prizes in Hubei scientific technology results, one was awarded the first prize in Hubei healthy department. The scientific results of "Ascites" was selected as the medical university text books. Ten country wrote letters for asking the information, in the country there are 38 hospital which used. The achievement of the "blood warm disease" have submitted to the eduation group to keep into record, all of which are the leading level.

Annex 4:

Topics in Science and Technology (English and Chinese version)

1. The Chinese version of the contract:

专题合同编号:

密级

专 题 类 别: A类

"八五" 国家科技攻关计划

专 题 合 同

专 题 名 称: 中医药治疗胃癌癌前期病变
的临床及实验研究

专 题 负 责 人: 徐 泽

专题合同起止年限: 1991年12月至1995年12月

课题编号、名称: 85—019—01 中医对恶性肿瘤的防治研究

项目编号、名称: 85—919 中医防治重大疾病的研究

国家科学技术委员会
一九九一年十一月十日

The Number of special topic contract:

The kind of this special topic : A type Secret

The plan of "eight-five" country scientific technology research

The contract of the special topics

The name of topic: The clinic and experimental research of that Chinese medications treat the precancerous lesion of stomach cancer

The charger of the special topics: Xu Ze

The starting and ending date of this contract: 12-1991 to 12-1995

The name and number of this project:

Prevention and treatment of research of tradition medication impact on Maligency 85-919-01

The number and name of this project:

85-819 The research of the prevention and treatment of the serious diseases.

The committee of country science and technology

11-10-1991,

THE CHINESE VERSION:

九、国家政关拨款偿还计划

偿还总金额 （万　元）	分　年　度　偿　还　金　额　（万　元）				
	年	年	年	年	年

十、专题参加人员表

	姓　名	性别	年龄	职　称	职　务	专　业	单　位	在本专题中的分工	在本专题中的劳务量(人年)
负责人	徐泽	男	58	教授	所长	普外	湖北中医学院	负责人	全年
						实验外科	实验外科研究所		
主要参加人员	胡军谱	男	50	副教授		实验外科	实验外科研究所		
	吕继渭	男	64	主任医师		中医	实验外科研究所		
	涂少川	男	68	主任药师		中药	实验外科研究所		
	朱思平	男	31	研究生		实验外科	实验外科研究所		
	邹少敏	男	26	研究生		实验外科	实验外科研究所		
	石月仙	女	48	主管护师		实验外科	实验外科研究所		
	张益麟	女	48	主管技师		免疫	实验外科研究所		
	李柳	男	48	主治医师		实验外科	实验外科研究所		
	赵立	男	32	医师		实验外科	实验外科研究所		
	王国荣	男	48	医师		病理	实验外科研究所		
	胡义平	男	25	医师		实验外科	实验外科研究所		
	吴晓阳	女	24	医师		实验外科	实验外科研究所		
	姜永宏	男	24	医师		实验外科	实验外科研究所		
	余津	女	37	技师		生化	实验外科研究所		

THE English version as the followings ;

Nine. The project of the country research funding with distribution, payment and return

Total funding	the reimbursement by year			
Ten thousand	Year	Year	Year	Year
Yan				

Ten. The table of the participants for the special topics

Name	Sex	Age	Profession	Responsibity	Specialty	Union	the function in project	The work load in Project
Xu Ze In Charge	Male	58	Professor	chief	general Surgery	Hubei tradition medicine school		

The Chinese version form:

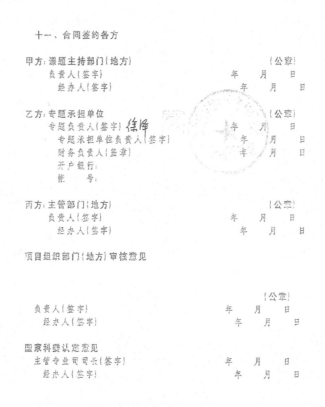

The eleven

The signature for each part of the contract

A : the project holding department

Manager

The executor

B: the union of doing this project

The responsibility and manager and the executor: Dr. Xu Ze

The Chinese version for this project as the following:

"八五" 期间重点科技攻关项目建议书

密级

一、项目名称:

进一步发掘防癌抗癌中草药对肝癌、胃癌和胃癌的癌前期病变的抗癌抗转移中西医结合防治的实验和临床研究

Ⅰ 研究中草药芦、灵、蟾、蒜、青汁……等抗癌作用和对自然杀伤细胞及免疫调节功能以及微量元素硒、钼等测定的实验研究

Ⅱ 研究中药逆转胃癌的癌前期病变,研制对肝癌、胃癌抗淋巴转移的新型系列防癌抗癌中药剂,中西医结合防治消化道癌的实验及临床研究

主管单位: 国家科委
承担单位: 湖北中医学院
起止日期: 1991年1月—1995年12月

The advocate of "eight-five" period important scientific and technology research topics

1. The name of the project

    The experiments and clinic research of further exploring the prevention cancer and anti-cancer function of the prevention and anti-cancer Chinese herbs for the anti-cancer and anti-metastasis on the liver cancer, stomach cancer and early stage or pre-cancerous lesions.

A. The research study of anti-cancer function and function on NK cell and immune regulation and control function from Chinese herb Lu, lin, chan, onion and green liquel etc and the measurement of Selenium and molybdenum.

B. The research of the Chinese medicine which can reverse the precancerous lesion of stomach cancer and the study of the new prevention cancer and anti-cancer Chinese herbsfor for resisting the lymphatic metastasis, and the experimental and clinical study of the combination of western and Chinese medicine to prevent and to treat the digestive track.

The main union: Country Scientific Associate

The executive union: Hubei Chinese medical university

The starting date: 1991, 04---1995, 02

The Chinese version as the following:

九、建议承担单位和协作单位: (应包括最终使用或最后的商品生产单位)

本项目承担单位: 湖　北　中　医　学　院
　　　　　　　　湖北中医学院实验外科研究所

项目课题负责人: 徐　泽教授

协　作　单　位: 同济医大核医学研究室协助作
　　　　　　　　NCA自然杀伤细胞测定

最后系列抗癌中药成药生产: 武汉健民制药厂

Nine. The suggestion of the charging union and the cooperation Union (including product unit for the final use and late final union)

THE Union of charging this project:

Hubei traditional Chinese medical university

The experimental surgery institution of Hubei traditional Chinese university

The executive person of this project Dr. Xu Ze

The cooperative union: the nuclear medicine department in Tongji medical university cooperation for assessment of NKC(nature killing cells)

The production of the final series of anti-cancer traditional Chinese medication is produced by Wuhan healthy people pharmacy factory

The Chinese version as the following:

十、专家意见（请有关专家评议）

研究癌肿转移以及为何防止转移是当前一个极重要的课题。通过实验研究寻找在临床上的防治方法是可行的。本课题的设计科学性强，有临床上的实用价值。该研究单位有一定的实验研究条件和一定的技术力量，可以承担此一课题研究。

Ten, the suggestion of the specialists and the professional(the invitation of the related specialists)

To study the cancer metastasis and the prevention of metastasis is the important projects currently. Through the experiment to explore the prevention method in the clinics it is feasible. This program designation has strong scientific and have the clinical practical volume. This institute has certain experimental research condition and certain technology ability, it can take charge of this program research.

Professor Qi fazu

Annex 5:

Shanghai Cooperation Letter of Intent

(The English and Chinese Verison)

It was to put forward the academic level, evaluation, recognition of the academic value of the book and the suggestion for promotion to the whole country.

The Chinese version as the followings:

合作意向书

1、徐教授倾其毕生精力以一颗伟大的慈爱心、责任心，从临床到科研，创造性的提出并建立癌症转移治疗理论体系，通过两本著作《癌症治疗新认识和新模式》、《癌转移治疗新概念与新方法》进行全面系统总结。并在临床的基础上，实现中药现代化，将其及时应用到癌症转移治疗中。这对当前乃至今后肿瘤治疗领域具有重要的现实的深远的意义与价值，不仅有理论上方向上的指导，而且有实践上的方法和措施！应该尽快地最大范围地在广大肿瘤患者、临床医疗界推广开来，以促动当今肿瘤治疗的革新。在当今市场化了的医疗界受利益因素影响，传统疗法要彻底革新可以说是举步为艰，一套新理论要推广开来并得到重视，不亚于一场"革命"，必须相当的付出和人力、物力、财力的投入、资源的整合，有思路有计划有步骤地开展自下而上的自民间到政府的宣传教育。这种付出和投入必须需要动员社会资源和力量的参与，企业是其中的一支重要依靠力量，尤其是多年来扎根在肿瘤事业上的企业，更是最好的力量。否则，倘若依靠徐老个人的不懈努力和坚持付出，即使能够在一定范围内一定阶段产生一定影响，却很难得到真正地全面推广，惠及广大的肿瘤人群。徐教授对于癌转移开辟性的理论著述，其推广过程应该探索一条非常之道，一条"科企结合，科企合作"的路子是值得研究和尝试的。只有这样，徐老的科技成果才能真正产生经济效益和社会效益，徐老造福广大肿瘤病友奉献社会和人类的的愿望才能由理想变为现实，徐老一辈子的心血才能在晚年开花结果，无憾终身。

2、上海德今，作为一家科技企业，10多年来，一直专心专注于肿瘤事业。十年来，我们与包括中国科学院、中国药科大学在内的全国十多个著名科研单位密切联系和深入合作，与包括上海肿瘤医院在内的全国二十多个临床医疗单位密切联系和深入合作，与包括北京抗癌乐园在内的全国三十多家抗癌民间组织密切联系和深入合作，接触和结交了国内数十名科研及临床专家、学者、康复明星，更是通过十多种抗癌产品的独立开发或经销推广，在国内近三十个省市建立市场推广网络和社会资源，与数万名肿瘤患者和家属产生往来关系。正是这样，我们对肿瘤的认识更加清楚，对肿瘤病人认识更加清楚，对当前行业的弊病和由此反映的社会阶段性矛盾认识更加清楚。我们也由此，更加坚定了要闯出一条"经济效益和社会效益并举"道路的决心，同时也让我们更加清楚地认识到，要从观念、方法和措施上找到适应当前社会和行业的解决之道。所以，一方面我们一直利用自己的资源对接有利于抗癌事业的理念及成果，另一方面又把视野放开不断搜寻更多更好的理念及科技成果，一旦找到以后，经过我们有思路有计划有步骤地推广，就能产生非常好的经济效益和社会效益，并与合作双方实现双赢。

——如果以上两方能够成功对接，那么我们一定要达到并能够达到这样的目的：让最新抗癌理念深入人心，让最新抗癌科技成果得到推广应用，让肿瘤病人康复得更好，让合作双方实现经济利益并由此推动社会效益。

为了更好的推广徐教授的癌转移治疗理论以及相关的的科技成果，

我们认为应该抓住问题的关键和重点，分近期和远期稳步实施。目前的重点首先应该是宣传和推介徐教授的癌症转移治疗的理论理念，以两部著作为重点，然后结合徐教授多年的临床成果或者可以向社会赛选产品应用到癌症转移治疗中。在此基础上，整合国内外最优质的资本和人才实现徐教授的"两条路线"（一是建立大型新型肿瘤医院配合徐教授的癌症治疗新理念；二是将临床成果按药物程序进行国家级申报应用）。

按照以上思路：

一、近阶段合作重点：

推广徐泽教授关于癌症治疗的最新理念。所谓一切皆成于势，而非力；革命工作，政治宣传先行。有大家对一种理论认可了，形成了新的观念，并因此带动一大片，形成气候，其他一切工作才能水到渠成，科技推广更是如此，必须理论科普先行。合作的最终落脚点或者说是依托，应该是解决问题的方法。兼顾合作双方的合作目的，以促进患者康复为出发点；合作的落脚点应该是：德今公司的主打产品胞逆康和徐泽教授的 Z—C 系列。这两者有一个共同点，都是科研界为肿瘤病人贡献的一份解决癌转移问题的科技成果，是爱和责任的产物。不同的是前者是一个把企业目标定位在抗癌事业并精心耕耘十载的有良知的企业把国内知名科研院所的科技成果产业化的结晶；后者是一位把毕生精力贡献给抗癌事业尤其是在癌转移研究方面有突出贡献的专家呕心沥血研制的科技成果。前者的局限性在于应用时间短，有待进一步临床实践，不断提升品质，同时与最新抗癌理念对接；优势在于已经建立一支专业的专职的产品推广团队，已经历经国内各大科研机构实验及部分临床验证，并经过一系列药理检验得到卫生部批号，已经在全国主要大中城市应用推广。后者的优势在于长达数年的临床应用观察，并不断进行基础研究，加之有着最新抗癌理论指导。局限在于只能在徐教授现在的门诊推广，受国家政策职能部门的管理影响，一方面没有专业专职的团队推广；另一方面又不能在各大医院药店这种传统正统渠道推广，这就很难在短时间内放大影响，不能很好的发挥应有的社会效应和经济效应，不能很好的支持徐教授的肿瘤治疗新理念以及持续的科学研究。这样长时间下去，对于肿瘤治疗、肿瘤人群乃至于整个社会留下无尽的遗憾！造成不可估量的损失！所以，我们觉得，两者的结合，资源共享，优势互补，应该可以创出一条打破传统，有益于肿瘤病人和社会的科技应用新路子来。

二、近阶段合作内容规划：

（一）、建立"癌症转移治疗上海科普基地"

建立科普基地是科普推广有效实施，并长效运行逐步达到宣传教育目的的重要渠道。而上海是国际大都市，利用上海的人才、信息、资源、国际国内影响力等诸多优势可以很好的做好科普工作。该基地工作要良好运作，包括五方面的机构平台或者说渠道支流。

400

1、设立"中国癌症转移治疗"专业网站

网站以徐泽教授对癌症研究的最新理论为基本依托，兼顾国际国内最新抗癌的研究及信息，制作成一个立足癌症尤其是癌转移理论研究和科技成果推广，面向国际面向未来的专业化高水准网站，并以中英文版向全球推介。

网站的内容设计由徐泽教授指导，网站的建设、维护、推广由上海德今公司聘请专门人才设立专门部门进行专项工作开展，并提供建设和维护推广费用。

2、创办内部刊物——《癌症转移治疗简讯》

该刊物面向徐泽教授已有的病人网络及德今公司全国各地的病人网络，以及双方的科研网络、医院网络和民间抗癌组织网络。以邮寄或现场发放的形式发行。该刊物编辑部设在上海，由德今公司安排专人负责编辑、制作，所发生的费用由德今公司独家承担。徐泽教授题写刊名，内容由徐泽教授指导。刊物的主办方定位：癌症转移治疗专家委员会、癌症转移治疗上海科普基地、湖北中医学院抗癌转移、复发研究室。该刊物暂定为每季一刊。

3、 成立癌症转移治疗专家委员会

该专家委员会是一个学术科普和治疗服务的团体。由徐泽教授任主任委员，组成成员为徐泽教授推荐的相关专家及德今公司现有网络选拔的部分专家组成。人数可以逐步增加。专家委员会负责对科普基地的宣传教育进行全程指导，包括撰写相关科普文章，开展科普讲座，进行癌转移诊疗服务等。专家委员会设在上海，相关运行费用由上海承担。

4、设立癌症转移治疗科普讲坛

该讲坛是开展科普宣传的一个重要途径，讲坛设在上海，相关运行费用由上海独家承担。讲坛包括以下三方面活动：

（1）针对广大癌症患者的科普讲座，可以每月进行一次，分主题进行。率先在上海试点。今后可以在全国大中城市巡回讲座。

（2）针对广大肿瘤临床界义务人员的培训交流。可以率先在德今公司各地资源系统里的医务人员进行培训交流。

（3）针对国际国内专家、学者的学术论坛。可以在国家权威机构的牵头下进行，邀请国际国内的专家参与，进行癌转移治疗的专题研讨。

5、创建上海肿瘤专科门诊

随着条件成熟，考虑在上海成立肿瘤专科门诊，整合各地的专家资源，配合徐教授的最新治癌理念以及其他成功的肿瘤门诊经验，直接对广大的肿瘤人群进行诊治。由于上海医疗是全国的窗口，可以辐射影响全国各地！

以上即为现阶段近期初步合作项目规划。请徐泽教授审阅，斧正，不足或不当之处，双方再进一步协商修订补充并在此基础上具体细化，直至操作实施。一旦达成共识后，我们双方签约约定。

上海德今生物科技有限公司

二零零七年七月十一日

The Cooperation Letter of Intent

1. Professor Xu devoted his life to a great compassion and responsibility, from clinical to scientific research, creatively proposed and established a system of cancer transfer therapy. Through two books, "New Understanding and New Model of Cancer Treatment", "New Concepts and New Methods for Cancer Metastasis Treatment", a comprehensive systematic summary, and on the basis of clinical, modernization of traditional Chinese medicine, timely application of cancer metastasis treatment. This has far-reaching significance and value for the current and future areas of cancer treatment. There are not only theoretical guidance, but also practical methods and measures! It should be promoted as soon as possible in the vast majority of cancer patients and clinical medical circles to promote the current cancer treatment innovation.

In today's market-oriented medical sector, influenced by the interests of the factors, the traditional innovation to be completely reformed can be said to be difficult, a set of new rationale must be paid for and the manpower, the theory should be promoted and paid attention to, no less than one The field "revolution", the input of material and financial resources, the integration of resources, and the idea of systematic and step-by-step development of the bottom-up propaganda and education from the people to the government. This kind of effort and investment must involve the participation of social resources and strength. The enterprise is one of the important relying forces, especially the enterprises that have been rooted in the cause of the tumor for many years, and it is the best force. Otherwise, if you rely on Xu Lao's unremitting efforts and perseverance, even if it can have a certain impact in a certain period of certain difficulties, it is difficult to get a truly comprehensive promotion, benefiting the majority of cancer patients. Professor Xu's theoretical writing on the development of cancer metastasis should explore a very special way in the promotion process. A path of "combination of science and technology, cooperation between science and technology" is worth studying. Only in this way can Xu Lao's scientific and technological achievements truly produce economic benefits and social benefits. Xu Lao's desire to contribute to the society and human beings of the majority of cancer patients can turn the white ideal into reality. Xu's life will be able to bear fruit in his later years. No regrets for life.

2. Shanghai Dejin, as a technology company, has been focusing on the cause of cancer for more than 10 years. In the past ten years, we have closely contacted and cooperated with more than ten famous scientific research units including the Chinese Academy of Sciences and China Pharmaceutical University, and have close contact and deep cooperation with more than 20 clinical medical units including Shanghai Cancer Hospital. Close contact and in-depth cooperation with more than 30 anti-cancer civil organizations including Beijing Cancer Park, and contacted and made dozens of domestic scientific and clinical experts, scholars, and rehabilitation stars, and more than 10 kinds of anti-cancer The independent development or distribution of products has established market promotion of private network resources in nearly 30 provinces and cities in China. It has a relationship with the family of tens of thousands of people who have a tumor, and it is precisely this way that our understanding of the tumor is more clear, and the patients who have swollen tumors are more aware of the current industry's ills and the private stage. Contradictions and understandings are even more clear, and we have thus become more determined to find a way to "both economic and social benefits", and at the same time let us know more clearly. It is necessary to find solutions to the current society and industry from the concepts, methods and measures. Therefore, on the one hand, we have been using our own resources to connect with the ideas and achievements that are conducive to the cause of cancer, and on the other hand, we have opened our eyes and constantly searched for more ideas and scientific achievements of Xia Duo, once found. After we have ideas, planned and step-by-step promotion, we can produce very good economic and social benefits, and achieve a win-win situation with both partners.

If the above two parties can successfully dock, then we must achieve and achieve this goal: let the latest anti-cancer concept be deeply rooted in the hearts of the people, let the latest anti-cancer scientific and technological achievements be promoted and applied, so that cancer patients can recover better, so that the partners can achieve Economic benefits and thus promote social benefits.

In order to better promote Professor Xu's theory of cancer metastasis treatment and related scientific and technological achievements, we believe that we should grasp the key and key points of the problem and implement it steadily in the near and long term. The current focus should be on promoting and promoting Professor Xu's theory of cancer metastasis treatment, focusing on two books, and then combining Professor Xu's many years of clinical results or using social selection products to apply to cancer metastasis.

Follow the above ideas:

First, the focus of cooperation in the near stage:

Promote Professor Xu Ze's latest concept on cancer treatment. Everything is in the power, not power; revolutionary work, political propaganda first. Some people have recognized a theory, formed a new concept, and thus led a large piece of film to form a climate. All other work can be achieved. Science and technology promotion is even more so. It must be preceded by theoretical science. The ultimate goal of cooperation is to rely on it. It should be the way to solve the problem. Taking into account the cooperation purposes of the two parties, to promote the recovery of the interests of the people as the starting point; the focus of cooperation should be: the main products of the company today, the company's products, the company's Z-Mao series. The two have one thing in common. They are scientific and technological achievements that solve the problem of cancer metastasis contributed by research patients with cancer. They are products of love and responsibility. The difference is that the former is a crystallization of the scientific achievements of well-known research institutes in China, which are targeted at the anti-cancer cause and carefully cultivated for ten years. The latter is a life-saving contribution to anti-cancer. The cause is especially the scientific and technological achievements of the loss-making efforts that have made outstanding contributions to cancer metastasis research. The limitation of the former lies in the short application time, further clinical practice, continuous improvement of quality, and docking with the latest anti-cancer concept. The advantage lies in the establishment of a professional full-time product promotion team, which has undergone experiments with major domestic research institutions. Part of the clinical verification, and a series of pharmacological tests to obtain the Ministry of Health batch number, has been promoted in major major cities in the country. The latter's strength lies in years of clinical application observations, and ongoing basic research, coupled with the latest anti-cancer theory guidance. The limitation lies in the promotion of Professor Xu's current outpatient clinic and the influence of the management of the national policy function department. On the one hand, there is no dedicated team to push the factory: on the other hand, it cannot be promoted in the traditional orthodox channels of major hospital pharmacies. It is difficult to amplify the influence in a short period of time, and it is not possible to play a proper social and economic effect: it does not support Professor Xu's new concept of cancer treatment and continuous scientific research. This long time goes on, leaving endless regrets for cancer treatment, cancer patients and even the whole society! Cause immeasurable loss! Therefore, we believe that the combination of the two, resource sharing, and complementary advantages should create a new way to break the tradition and benefit the scientific application of cancer patients and society.

Second, the recent phase of cooperation content planning:

(1) Establishing "Shanghai Science Popularization Base for Cancer Metastasis Treatment"

The establishment of a popular science base is an important channel for the popularization of science popularization and the long-term operation to be gradually transferred to the education of Lu. Shanghai is an international metropolis. It can do a good job in science and technology by leveraging the talents of Shanghai, the letter, the resources, the international and domestic influences, etc.: The work of the base should be well-functioned, including the five-factory platform. Or old channel tributaries.

First, the focus of cooperation in the near stage:

Promote Professor Xu Ze's latest concept on cancer treatment. Everything is in the power, not power; revolutionary work, political propaganda first. Everyone has a long-term understanding of a kind of coin, and has formed a new concept, and thus has driven a large piece of land to form a climate. All other work can be accomplished, and technology promotion is even more so. It must be preceded by theoretical science. The ultimate goal of cooperation or support is to be the solution to the problem. Taking into account the cooperation purposes of the two partners, to promote the rehabilitation of patients as the starting point; the focus of cooperation should be: the main products of the company today, the company's products, the company's z-c series. The two have one thing in common. They are the scientific and technological achievements that the research community contributes to cancer patients and solve the problem of cancer metastasis. They are the products of love and responsibility. The difference is that the former is a crystallization of the scientific achievements of well-known research institutes in China, which are targeted at the anti-cancer cause and carefully cultivated for ten years. The latter is a life-saving contribution to anti-cancer. The cause is especially the scientific and technological achievements made by the losers who have made outstanding contributions to the research on cancer metastasis. The limitation of the former lies in the short application time, further clinical practice, continuous improvement of quality, and docking with the latest anti-cancer concept. The advantage lies in the establishment of a professional full-time product promotion team, which has undergone experiments with major domestic research institutions. And part of the clinical verification, and after a series of pharmacological tests to obtain the Ministry of Health batch number, has been promoted in major major cities in the country. The latter's strength lies in years of clinical application observations, and ongoing basic research, coupled with the latest anti-cancer theory guidance. The limitation lies in the promotion of Professor Xu's current outpatient clinic, which is affected by the management of the national policy function department. On the one hand, there is no professional full-time team to push the factory; on the other hand, it cannot be promoted in the traditional orthodox channels of major hospital pharmacies. It is difficult to amplify the impact in a short period of time, and it is not possible to give full play to the social and economic effects it deserves: it does not support Professor Xu's new concept of cancer treatment and continuous scientific research. This long time goes on, leaving endless regrets for cancer treatment, cancer patients and even the whole society! Cause immeasurable loss! Therefore, we feel that the combination of the two, resource sharing, and complementary advantages should create a new way to break the tradition and benefit the cancer patients and society.

Second, the recent phase of cooperation content planning:

(1) Establishing the "Shanghai Science Popularization Base for Cancer Metastasis Treatment" The establishment of a science popularization base is an important channel for the popularization of science popularization and long-term operation to gradually reach the educational education. And Shanghai is an international metropolis. Liyue Shanghai's talents, information, resources, international and domestic influences, etc. can do a good job in science work. The base work should be well operated, including a 50,000-faced institutional platform or Said channel

1. Established the "China Cancer Metastasis Treatment" professional website

The website is based on Professor Xu Ze's latest theory of cancer research, taking into account the latest international anti-cancer research and information, and is making a high-quality professional website for the future of cancer, especially cancer transfer research and technology promotion. And promoted to the world in Chinese and English.

The content design of the website is guided by Professor Xu Ze. The construction, maintenance and promotion of the website are hired by Shanghai Dejin Company to set up special departments to carry out special work and provide construction and maintenance promotion expenses.

1. Establish a special website for recognizing cancer transfer treatment in China

The website is based on the latest theory of cancer research by Professor Takizawa, taking into account the latest research and information on cancer prevention at home and abroad, and making a theoretical and scientific research promotion based on cancer, especially cancer metastasis, and specializing in the international future. High-level website, and promoted to the world in Chinese and English.

The content design of the website is guided by Professor Xu Ze. The construction, maintenance and promotion of the website Shanghai Dejin Company hires specialized personnel to set up special departments to carry out special work and provide construction and maintenance promotion expenses.

2, the establishment of internal publications - "Cancer Metastasis Treatment"

The publication is aimed at Professor Xu Ze's existing patient network and the patient network across the country, as well as the research network, hospital network and civil anti-cancer organization network. Issued by mail or on-site distribution. The editorial department of the publication is located in Shanghai, and the company has arranged a special person to edit and produce it. The expenses incurred by the company are exclusively borne by Dejin Company. Professor Xu Ze inscribed the title, the content is guided by Professor Xu Ze. The organizer of the publication is the Expert Committee of the Cancer Metastasis Office, the Shanghai Science Popularization Base for Cancer Metastasis, and the Anti-cancer Metastasis and Recurrence Research Office of Hubei College of Traditional Chinese Medicine. The publication is tentatively scheduled for each quarter.

3. Establish a committee of cancer transfer therapy experts

The Expert Committee is a group of academic science and therapeutic services. Xu Zejiao was appointed as the chairman, and the members were composed of relevant experts recommended by Professor Xu Ze and some of the existing network selections of Dejin. The number of people can be gradually increased. The Expert Committee is responsible for the whole process of publicity and education of the popular science base, including writing relevant popular science articles, conducting science popular lectures, and conducting cancer transfer diagnosis and treatment services. The expert committee is located in Shanghai and the relevant operating costs are borne by Shanghai.

3. Establish a committee of cancer transfer therapy experts

The Expert Committee is a group of academic science and therapeutic services. Xu Zejiao was appointed as the chairman, and the members were composed of relevant experts recommended by Professor Xu Ze and some of the existing network selections of Dejin. The number of people can be gradually increased. The expert committee is responsible for the whole process of publicity and education of the science base, including writing relevant science articles, conducting science lectures, and conducting cancer transfer services. The expert committee is located in Shanghai and the relevant operating costs are borne by Shanghai.

4. Establish a science forum for cancer metastasis treatment

This forum is an important way to carry out popular science propaganda: the forum is located in Shanghai, and the relevant operating expenses are exclusively borne by Shanghai. . The forum includes the following three activities:

(1). A science lecture for a wide range of cancer patients can be conducted once a month, sub-theme. Take the lead in piloting in Shanghai. In the future, you can tour lectures in large and medium cities across the country.

(2). Advise the training and exchange of volunteers in the clinical field. You can take the lead in Shi Dejin's medical staff in the resource system of the company to carry out training and flow.

(3). Academic forums for international and domestic experts and scholars. It can be carried out under the leadership of national authorities, and invites international and domestic experts to participate in the seminar on cancer metastasis treatment.

4. Establish a science forum for cancer metastasis treatment

This forum is an important way to carry out popular science propaganda: the forum is located in Shanghai, and the relevant operating expenses are exclusively undertaken by Shanghai.

The forum includes the following three activities:

(1) Science lectures for a wide range of cancer patients can be conducted once a month, sub-theme. Take the lead in piloting in Shanghai. In the future, you can tour lectures in large and medium cities across the country.

(2) For the majority of tumors, the clinical obligation is less and the training of the staff is exchanged. You can take the lead in Shi Dejin's medical staff in the resource system of the company to carry out training and flow.

(3) Academic forums for international and domestic experts and scholars. It can be carried out under the leadership of national authorities, and invites international and domestic experts to participate in the seminar on cancer metastasis treatment.

5. Create a Shanghai Oncology Clinic

With the maturity of the conditions, consider setting up an oncology clinic in Shanghai, integrating the expert resources from all over the world, and cooperating with Professor Xu's concept of the most cancer treatment and Qi's successful oncology experience, directly to the majority of the fat, _ feet Hao Hao in the diagnosis ; Shanghai Medical is a national window that can radiate across the country!

The above is the preliminary plan for the initial cooperation of the recent bullying. Professor Xu Ze is murdered, Busy, insufficient or inappropriate, double-entry

One step of consultation and revision, and on this basis, specific refinement to the operation of the first two. Once the consensus is reached: our two parties signed the agreement.

Shanghai Dejin Biotechnology Co., Ltd.
2007, July 11

Annex 6

The Major Progress in Cancer Research in the Past 100 Years

A Great Progress in Study on Tumor over 100 Years

In Apr. 2007, American Association for Cancer Research (AACR) invited the famous tumor scholars all over the world to review the history of study on tumor, which is now briefly extracted as follows:

1907	It was discovered that the solar exposure was related to skin cancer and later it was proven by the animal model that sunlight and ultraviolet radiation could lead to skin cancer.
1908	The tumor was successfully transferred to another animal from one animal with cell-free concentrate. Fowl leukosis, lymphadenoma and sarcomata model was established and this discovery was later deemed as the evidence that the filterable taddecheese would lead to tumor.
1915	The first animal model of chemical-induced tumor was established. Repeated painting of tar could produce skin tumor on rabbit.
1916	It was discovered that the incidence of breast carcinoma on mice could be reduced after removal of the ovary, indicating ovarian hormone may lead to breast carcinoma.
1924	It was discovered by the study on metabolism that the tumor was manifested as anoxia metabolism.
1928	It was deemed that "gene mutation was the basic reason of producing the carcinoma".
1928	The cells of cervical carcinoma were observed through the exuviation smear of vagina. The method of detecting the <u>suspected</u> patient with cervical carcinoma with smear method was widely accepted by the people step by step and used as the effective detection and prevention method of the cancer until Pap smear method was applied in 1960.
1928	It was discovered that X-ray could lead to mutation. X–ray could lead to the gene mutation of common fruit fly, which was the theoretical basis of the carcinogen participation in tumorigensis.
1930	Benzopyrene, the first chemical carcinogen was separated form the coal tar and the carcinogenesis of these chemical constituents was made clear through the animal model experiment.
1932	The artificial hormone was injected to induce the breast carcinoma of mice.
1937	The leucocythemia of the mouse was transfected through transplantation of the single leukemic cell.
1938	It was discovered through study that chemical carcinogenesis process was divided into two different stages including excitation stage and promotion stage.

1939   The transplanted animal tumor could produce the blood vessel. The tumor transplanted on the ears of the rabbit could produce the vascular net, which was the early evidence of formation of the blood vessel, later the anti- angiogenesis became one target of the treatment of tumor.

1940   The heat control could reduce the incidence of tumor on the mice.

1941   The hormone dependence of prostatic carcinoma was proven. Physical castration therapy and estrogen chemical castration therapy could reduce tumor load of the metastatic prostatic carcinoma while the androgen injected could promote the metastasis.

1946   The nitrogen mustard was firstly used for tumor chemotherapy. It was observed that after contacting the nitrogen mustard, the soldiers in time of war could meet with reduction of white blood cells, enlightening the people on using the nitrogen mustard for tumor chemotherapy and the intravenously injected nitrogen mustard for treating the lymphadenoma and leukemia that could not be controlled by radiotherapy, in this way, the disease was remitted for several months. The nitrogen mustard was used for tumor treatment initially in 1949.

1948   The first chemotherapy on leukemia of children was successful. The artificial folic acid antagonist was applied to 16 children with leukemia among which 10 patients got a relieving course of 3 months.

1950   It was discovered by the study on epidemiology that smoking was related to pulmonary carcinoma.

1951   The virus spread the leucocythemia of mice. It was discovered by the study that the leucocythemia could be spread through virus from one mouse of one germ line to another mouse of another germ line and spread from one generation to the next generation vertically. Before this, it was deemed by the people that the tumor was a hereditary disease, which laid a foundation for the study on other tumor viruses and of the mice and other species in the future.

1951   Co-60 (^{60} Co) radiation equipment came out.

1951   The ultrasonic detection was firstly used for diagnosis of tumor.

1958   It was proven that the food additive prohibited by the food additive modification organ could induce the occurrence of carcinoma on human or animal.

1959   The leucocythemia induced by the food additive was related to the radioactive dose. It was proven that the radiation could induce the human carcinoma and the natural characteristics of the relation between radioactive dose and effect were also illuminated.

1963   Hodgkin lymphoma was treated with chemical method. In 1960, Hodgkin lymphoma was reported in the Sahara in Africa, which was featured in regional distribution. In those days, it was deemed that it was induced by the virus and the tumor induced by the virus was firstly successfully cured and later it was proven as Epstein virus.

1964   Luther L. Terry, an American surgeon proposed that the smoking was related to the pulmonary carcinoma.

1969   The tumor was successfully transplanted to the nude mice of different germ line.

1970   The multi-drug resistance of cell line was proposed. The multi-drug resistance of cell toxicant was the main reason of failure of chemotherapy.

1971   The growth of tumor depended on the regenerative blood vessel. Since the discovery of the tumor metastasis, it had been known that the tumor could not grow in the tissue without blood vessel. It was shown by the continuous experiments that the tumor growth factor could promote the generation of the new blood vessel and the growth of the tumor. Finally, these gene factors offered the basis for the molecular-targeted therapy of tumor.

1971   President Nixon presented an anti-cancer slogan in the address in UN.

1972   The paclitaxel, the extract from the natural vegetables could be used for chemotherapy.

1976   The virus oncogene existed in the related proto-oncogene in the normal cells. Through hybridzation technique (before DNA precedence ordering), it was discovered by the researcher that the virus oncogene existed in the chicken's cells, and so did in other families (such as mice and human kind) through study.

1977   Tamoxifen was approved for the clinical treatment of breast carcinoma.

1978   Nitrosamine in the tobacco leaf was proven as the cancerogenous substance in the cigarette. The nitrosamine derived from nicotia in the cigarette was discovered in the animal model that it was cancerogenous and soon later it was proven to be related to pulmonary carcinoma and oral carcinoma of human being.

1979   p53 gene was discovered, which was initially deemed as a kind of oncogene and finally proven as a kind of anti-oncogene by the subsequent study.

1979   Discovery of protein-tyrosine kinase (PTK) and illumination of the tyrosine phosphorylation process. One new kind of protein-tyrosine kinase (PTK) was discovered, which was related to gene products of T antigenic conversion protein and rous sarcoma virus in the polyoma virus. This discovery told us that the maladjustment of tyrosine phosphorylation process catalyzed by activated protein-tyrosine kinase could result in the malignant transformation of cells. In the following several years, the pathogenic protein-tyrosine kinase depressant was approved for clinical treatment.

1980   The degradation of peripheral collagen of the tumor impelled the metastasis of tumor. In the tumor metastasis process, it was necessary for the cancer cells to break through the epithelial layer and the true skin layer so as to invade the circulating system. It was proven by the study that tumor cells could excrete collagenase so as to degrade the peripheral collagen while the cell strains with relatively high excretion level of collagenase would be metastatic more easily.

1980   The prostate specific antigen (PSA) was discovered. Detection of PSA level in the body is the first kind of routine detection method to screen and prevent the carcinoma of prostate with tumor markers through assessing the risks of suffering the carcinoma of prostate.

1980   The importance of DNA methylation in the occurrence and development of carcinoma was revealed.

1982   The primary oncogene concept was launched. The conclusion that the oncogene in the normal cell genome could meet with variance and carcinomatosis was made through combination of the previous findings.

1982   The helicobacter pylori (Hp) was separated from the gastric ulcer of human. It was indicated by the findings over the past 10 years that the virus was cancerogenous, however, it was accepted by the people after several years that the infection of Hp would lead to the gastric ulcer while the continual Hp infection and inflammation would result in canceration.

1983   Papilloma viral infection of human was one of the pathogenic factors of cervical carcinoma. Type 16 and 18 papillomavirus of human separated from the biopsy specimen was proven to be related to the height of cervical carcinoma. This discovery would encourage the people to research, develop and use the corresponding bacterin to prevent the cervical carcinoma.

1983   American Academy of Science issued the report named "Diet, Nutrition and Carcinoma" and proposed American Association of Carcinoma to guide the healthy diet of the public so as to reduce the incidence of the carcinoma.

1990   National Institutes of Health and Department of Energy officially launched the human genome project.

1991   The specific variance of p53 gene in the hepatic carcinoma was related to the environmental carcinogen, namely aflatoxin.

1994   The carcinoma originated from the normal cells that could be transformed into cancer cells and it was shown by the survey that the stem cells in the normal tissue with clear source was most possible to develop into the cancer cells in the process of renovation.

2004   The bacterin for anti human papillomavirus (HPV) could prevent the cervical carcinoma. The type of the most common carcinogenic human papillomavirus that the bacterin can prevent mainly included HPV16 and HPV18, which could prevent 70% of the cervical carcinoma all over the world.

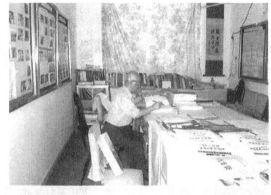

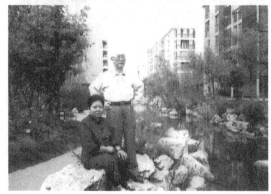

徐泽别名子久
医学教授
七旬之后
医研之余
吟以自娱

Postscript

Where did these 18 medical monographs come from? Some of the first drafts came from the original record of "Morning in the morning" and then compiled into a manuscript. I sent it to the street to copy the typing room and put it into a book. From the years of the flower, to the age of the ancient, to the year of the shackles, sent to the street copying typing room to type hundreds of times. Sometimes my wife and I went to the typing room to print the manuscript. She was the first reader and supporter of my "Monograph".

After I retired at the age of 63, I continued to research, self-reliance, self-financing, and the journey of Science was non-stop. Still struggling, arduously climbing, four different scientific research stages of one scientific research footprint, four different levels of mountain results. A mountain is better than a mountain scientific research landscape. It is to perseverance and persistence. Since 1980, I have insisted on memorizing scientific research diaries, scientific research records, the accumulation of these scientific research original materials and the record of scientific thinking, and some have also been selected as the material of this series of "monographs".

I read five years of private school in my childhood (at the time of the early 1930s, there was only one elementary school in a county, and the villages were mostly private). I loved the ancient books and poems. In addition to medical research, you can enjoy yourself.

斯　医　挥　迅　靶　灵　醒　一　轻　曙　鸡　万　　　二
哉　籍　毫　起　点　思　来　夜　唤　光　鸣　籁　　　〇
为　添　录　披　豁　一　脑　酣　已　潜　报　无　　　〇　晨
黎　新　万　衣　然　闪　清　甜　黎　入　晓　声　　　六　起
民　贵　千　坐　明　现　新　睡　明　内　时　寂　　　年　想
　　　　　　　　　　　　　　　　　　　　　　　　　春　到

(In the above poem, it had all of the new ideas and new thoughts of conquering cancer and new therapy in the morning. Time is money and time is life and time is innovation)

自咏

二〇〇六年春

年逾古稀犹自奋

赛因征途不停蹄

躲进小楼研机理

灵思一现靶点明

老骥伏枥志未已

为控转移究歧黄

十栽卓然成夙志

晚霞迷人似晟曦

(The author keeps working hard and persists purse the cancer research and never give up no matter how hard it will be.)

The main topics

A. The outline of conquering cancer

Under the guidance of Xi Jinping's new era of socialism with Chinese characteristics, we should strive to open up a new phase of scientific research in the new era, and the scientific research work to overcome cancer should be advanced. We will strive to follow the path of independent innovation with Chinese characteristics and adhere to the road of independent innovation of Chinese and Western medicine combined with "Chinese-style anti-cancer". China will contribute more to the world's wisdom, China's programs, and China's forces to overcome cancer research, so that the sun of humanity's destiny will shine in the world.

XZ-C proposes to create an environmental protection and cancer prevention research institute and carry out cancer prevention systems engineering and open 21st Century Cancer Research

How to overcome cancer? How to conquer cancer and launch the general attack of cancer?

How to prevent cancer by I see? How to do cancer prevention research by I see?

How to scientifically prevent pollution and treat pollution?

How to scientifically prevent cancer and control cancer?

The purpose of the research work of conquering cancer is to make people's health and to keep away from cancer, and is also a great pioneering work or great initiative for future generations to seek health and welfare.

— *To establish an overall framework for the fight against cancer or for conquering cancer, to create the multidisciplinary of conquering cancer and the science city of the scientific research base of the cancer-related research of conquering cancer, which is the only way to conquering cancer*

— *Proposed the overall design, plan, plan, blueprint and implementation rules of Science City*

---- *Equivalent to designing an overall framework for Chinese characteristics to overcome cancer*

----- *The following is the outline which was proposed by XZ-C of about the implementation of how to overcome cancer:*

The main project to implement the outline of how to overcome cancer is:

The structural work:

Overcoming cancer and launching the general attack of cancer, focusing on prevention, control, and treatment together and at the same attention and at the same level.

Creating multidisciplinary and the scientific research base of cancer-related research---- - Science City

Two-wing project:

A wing - how to overcome cancer? How to prevent cancer?

----- -   to reduce the incidence of cancer

B wing - how to overcome cancer? How to treat cancer?

---- -   to improve cancer cure rate

Aims:

A: *Reduce the incidence of cancer*

B: *Improve cancer cure rate, prolong patient survival, and improve patient quality of life*

If it can be to implement and realize the overall design of cancer, planning blueprints, it is possible to overcome cancer.

How to implement, how to achieve this general guideline, programs, plans, blueprints to overcome cancer?

It should set up the cancer research team to "conquer cancer and launch the general attack of the cancer"

It is to invite famous experts, professors, academic leaders or leading scientists, entrepreneurs, leaders, and volunteers who support "overcome cancer and launch the general attack on cancer" who are invited to work together to make an unprecedented event in human history, "to overcome cancer and to launch the general attack of cancer," and "create a science city that conquers cancer, for the benefit of mankind.

The preparation for setting up:

"The first science city of the scientific research base in the country to overcome cancer"

"The world's first science city of the scientific research base to conquer cancer"

B. The detail of the Table of Contents

Table of Contents

A late scientific research report was 25 years late. The design was put forward during the "Eighth Five-Year Plan" and the plan was completed and the scientific research report was presented after 35 years.

The reason for being late is my acute myocardial infarction, and then there is the resting or recovery time for a long time, then slowly move forward.

A late scientific research report

1. **The source background and experience of scientific research topics**

(1) The source background and the course of completion of scientific research topics (the tortuous course)

(2) Some experiences (Annex 1)

2. Briefly describe the scientific research process of my anti-cancer research

(1) The first stage

(2) The second stage

(3) The third stage

(4) The fourth stage

3. Briefly describe the academic thinking and scientific research thinking of my scientific research process

(1) The first stage (1985-1999)

From the follow-up results it is found:

New findings from animal experiments:

Innovative thinking, changing concepts, and proposing new models and new understandings of cancer treatment

(2) The second stage (after 2001)

Targeting the research goals and the "targets" of cancer treatment to **anti-metastasis**, pointing out that the key to cancer treatment is anti-metastasis

(3) The third stage (after 2006)

The research focuses on the prevention and treatment of the whole process of cancer occurrence and development.

Closely combined with clinical practice, it proposes reform and innovation, research and development in response to the problems and drawbacks of current clinical traditional therapy.

Recognizing that the prevention and treatment strategies for cancer must move forward, the way out for cancer treatment is "three early", and the way out for cancer is prevention.

Put the research focus for the research on prevention and treatment of the whole process of cancer occurrence and development. Closely integrated with clinical practice, in response to the problems and drawbacks of current clinical traditional therapies, it proposes reform and innovation, research and development. Recognizing that the prevention and treatment strategies for cancer must move forward, the way out for cancer treatment is "three early", and the way out for cancer is prevention.

(4) The fourth stage (2011 -)

Now it is the fourth stage of scientific research, which is being carried out and proceeded. The research work is step by step, and the research goal or "target" is positioned to reduce the incidence of cancer, improve the cure rate and prolong the survival period. Professor Xu Ze (XZ-C) proposed an initiative to create the Environmental Protection and Cancer Research Institute and carry out cancer prevention system engineering to reduce the incidence of cancer.

XZ-C proposes to carry out "to overcome conquer and launch the general attack of cancer – cancer prevention, cancer control, cancer treatment at the same attention and at the same level and at the same time"

4. The formation process of the new theory concept of cancer treatment

(1) From the follow-up to the establishment of experimental surgical laboratory

(2) New findings

(3) Animal experimental research on finding new anticancer and anti-metastatic drugs in natural medicine

(4) Clinical verification work

5. The Scientific Research routes and research methods for new theories and new methods of related-cancer treatment

(1) Scientific Research route

(2) Research methods

(3) Academic value and academic status

(4) Dawning or Shuguang scientific research spirit

6.   The tasks, missions, opportunities and challenges of anti-cancer research

(1)   Research on anti-cancer metastasis is a current urgent need

1). It must know the current problems

2). It must know the problems in the current treatment

(2)   Conducting anti-cancer metastasis research is the need for the development of oncology

(3)   What to do and how to do it

7.   The Research of Reform and Development on cancer treatment

8.   What research work have we carried out? What scientific research achievements and scientific and technological innovation series have been made?

Briefly describe scientific research results, scientific thinking, academic thinking, theoretical innovation, and scientific dedication of anti-cancer research.

In the past 30 years, we have made scientific research achievements and scientific technology innovation series in the field of cancer research direction as conquering cancer.

In this series of "Monographs", the following 30 academic arguments are presented for the first time in the world, all of which are original papers, internationally pioneered, and internationally leading, and have reached the forefront of the world.

9.   XZ-C put forward four major scientific contributions, all of which were first proposed internationally, all of which are international leaders.

10. What research work have we carried out?

In order to conquer cancer, a series of scientific research plans, overall design, scheme, projects, blueprints, master plans, overall framework and implementation details or rules are proposed.

"XZ-C proposes a scientific research plan to conquer cancer and launch the general attack of cancer"

(1). It is first proposed at the international level:

"Necessity and Feasibility of Overcoming cancer and launching the General Attack of Cancer"

-- The overall strategic reform of cancer treatment shifts the focus of treatment into prevention and treatment of cancer at the same attention and at the same time and at the same level.

(2) It is first proposed at the international level:

"Preparing for the establishment hospital with cancer prevention and treatment during the whole process of cancer occurrence and development"

—— The global demonstration of the prevention and treatment hospital

(3) It is first proposed at the international level:

"The report of the general attack design for conquering cancer and the basic design and feasibility of building the Science City for conquering cancer"

- It is equivalent to designing an overall framework for conquering cancer design with Chinese characteristics

(4) It is first proposed at the international level:

"The report of the necessity and feasibility which in the construction of a well-off society, it is recommended that "taking a ride to scientific research" to carry out scientific research on cancer prevention and tumors prevention and treatment work"

These four scientific research projects are all proposed for the first time in the world, and are the first in the world. The international leader has opened up a new field of anti-cancer research.

11. How to overcome cancer? How to treat cancer?

XZ-C first proposed in the world: Dawning or Shuguang C-type plan No.1-6

Dawning C-type plan No. 1:

"Conquering cancer and launching the general attack of cancer"

Dawning C-type plan No. 2:

"Creating a full-scale prevention and treatment hospital"

Dawning C-type plan No. 3:

"Building a scientific research base and the science city of conquering cancer"

Dawning or Shuguang C-type plan No. 4:

"Building the multidisciplinary and cancer research group"

Dawning C-type plan No. 5:

"The vaccine is human hope and immunological prevention"

Dawning C-type plan No. 6:

"The prospect of immunomodulatory drugs is gratifying"

12. How to overcome cancer? How to prevent cancer?

The XZ-C first proposed internationally:

Create "Innovative Environmental Protection and Cancer Prevention Research Institute" and carry out cancer prevention system engineering

XZ-C proposes:

Dawning A type cancer prevention plan

Dawning B type cancer prevention plan

Dawning D-type cancer prevention plan

Macro, micro, ultra-micro

13. The scientific research ideas or thinking path of how to fight well and win the three major pollution battles

XZ-C proposes:

How to scientifically prevent pollution and treat pollution?

How to scientifically prevent cancer and control cancer?

How to scientifically design, scheme, plan, scientific thinking, scientific and technological innovation, and win the three major pollution battles by I see (1), (2), (3), (4)

14. The scientific research thought or ideas and words or suggestions of how to fight well or lay a good and win the three major pollution battles

(1) XZ-C proposes:

Advising the World Health Organization:

1). It should promote scientific research ethics, medicine is benevolence, setting up ethics is the first

The scientific Research ethics:

products, achievements, patents, and technologies should have ethical standards

Standard:

the bottom line should not be harmful to human health

Basic ethics:

All products, achievements, patents, technology, goods and people are harmless and do not harm people's health, especially for children, and must not contain carcinogens.

All products, goods, and technology should have ethical standards.

2). It is recommended that all countries, provinces and states should establish anti-cancer research institutes (or institutions) to carry out anti-cancer system projects and carry out anti-cancer projects for their own country, province, state and city (because of various countries, provinces and states) There are a large number of cancer patients in each city)

3). Countries should establish anti-cancer regulations and carry out comprehensively (some should be legislated)

4). implementation of prevention-oriented policy: the way to cure cancer in the "three early", the way out of cancer prevention.

(2) XZ-C proposes:

To the World Health Organization and the United Nations:

1). XZ-C proposes:

It should save the mother river of the world.

2). XZ-C proposal:

"To solve the bell, you need to ring the bell" (all products: airplane, train, car...) should be harmless to human health, no complications, no sequelae, no harm to people's health, especially the three major pollution, can not contain cancer The product should be designed to avoid and remove when designing. When the product leaves the factory, it should be monitored by product ethical standards.

Research ethics:

It should be based on the standard of not damaging human health, especially the carcinogens.

Basic ethics:

All products, achievements, patents, goods and people are harmless and do not harm people's health, especially for children, and must not contain carcinogens.

3). XZ-C proposes an initiative:

The "Innovative Environmental Protection and Cancer Prevention Research Institute" should be established and the cancer prevention system project should be carried out.

—— Open a new era of cancer prevention research and cancer prevention system engineering in the 21st century.

Resolutely fight and win the three major pollution battles, scientific pollution prevention, pollution control, scientific management of smog, scientific cancer prevention, cancer control, this is a great initiative for the benefit of the country and the people, but it is also for the research work of cancer prevention, anti-cancer, and conquering cancer to create good opportunities. Conquering cancer is at the forefront of science and a worldwide problem. Cancer is a human disaster. The whole world and the people all over the world are eager to hope that one day they can overcome cancer and benefit mankind.

15. **Adhere to walk the road of cancer prevention and cancer control innovation in a well-off society with Chinese characteristics**

(1) At the same time as building a well-off society, it is recommended to carry out scientific research of cancer prevention and cancer control and work for cancer prevention and treatment.

(2) Following the scientific development concept and adhering to the innovative road of anti-cancer and anti-metastasis with Chinese characteristics

(3) Energy conservation, emission reduction, pollution prevention, pollution treatment, a well-off society, stay away from cancer

16. **Building a resource-saving and environment-friendly society, which has great correlation with cancer prevention and cancer control.**

17. **The cancer prevention scientific research work cannot walk slowly and it should run ahead, save the wounded**

18. **XZ-C proposed: it should promote scientific research ethics, medicine is benevolence, setting up the ethics it the first**

19. **The past and future of oncology development**

Prospects for cancer treatment, predictive assessment

20. **How to overcome cancer?**

XZ-C proposes that cancer is a disaster for all mankind. It is necessary for the people of the world to work together and China and the United States will jointly tackle the problem.

"Cancer moon shot" (US) and "Dawning C-type plan" (China) - march together and head to the science hall of conquering cancer

Why do you want to move forward together? What are you together? The advantages analysis and complementary advantages for China and the United States itself each

- For the past 100 years, the history record of the "Conquering Cancer" program has been raised or proposed internationally.

- Doing or Be an unprecedented event for the benefit of mankind

- Dawning C plan

- Situation analysis: (1), (2), (3), (4)

Our advantage is:

1. Traditional Chinese medicine, anti-cancer traditional Chinese medicine, immune regulation and control traditional Chinese medicine, activating blood circulation and removing blood stasis anti-cancer thrombus suppository Chinese medicine, Ruanjian Sanjie anti-small nodule Chinese medicine, heat-clearing and detoxifying to improve the micro-environment of cancer cells;

2. Combination of Chinese and Western medicine, combined with innovation

The advantages of the United States are:

Modern medicine, advanced diagnosis and treatment technology, targeted medicine

XZ-C believes that:

We should give full play to China's advantages and potentials. We should increase efforts to develop and explore the advantages of Chinese herbal medicine. Traditional Chinese medicine can improve symptoms, improve physical fitness, increase immunity, and prolong survival. (The lesions generally do not shrink, but they can survive with tumors and live for a long time.) can be used as an adjuvant treatment for surgery.

21. Pathfinding and footprint

- cause

- navigate

- Footprint (scientific footprint)

- Shuguang research spirit

- Thinking in the morning

22. Guide to read

23. Guide to act or to walk

24. Attachment (1——)

Note:

1   XZ-C is Xu Ze-China (Xu Ze - China), because science is borderless, but scientists are national and intellectual property.

2   Cancer is a disaster for all mankind. It must evoke the struggle of the people all over the world. Therefore, 15 of these series are exclusively in English and distributed worldwide.

XZ-C proposes to conquer cancer and to launch the general attack on cancer, and that it must establish the research institute of the environmental protection and cancer prevention and it must carry out cancer prevention system engineering. Open a new era of cancer prevention research and cancer prevention system engineering in the 21st century

While human being is in the search for the cause and condition of cancer, the most prominent thing is that it was found that more than 90% of cancers are caused by or closely related to environmental factors.

The Cancer Prevention Research Institute should conduct cancer prevention research, look for carcinogenic factors, detect damage to humans caused by carcinogens or carcinogenic factors, track the source of carcinogens or carcinogenic factors and study preventive measures of how to reduce or stop these carcinogens.

How to overcome cancer? How to prevent cancer?

XZ-C proposes:

Established the Research Institute of Environmental Protection and Health Prevention Cancer to carry out cancer prevention system engineering and establish a high-level laboratory

XZ-C proposes:

Dawning A type cancer prevention plan

Dawning B type cancer prevention plan

Dawning D-type cancer prevention plan

Because cancer patients cover the whole world, the pollution of industrial and agricultural wastewater, waste residue and waste gas also covers the whole world. Therefore, it is imperative that the global effort be made to conquer cancer and launch the general attack on cancer, or we must globally attack the cancer to attack the general attack, and put cancer prevention, cancer control, cancer treatment at the same level and the same attention and at the same time, especially cancer prevention is the top priority, study these sources of pollution, try to stop at the source, and strive to block the safety risks of cancer in the bud status.

How to fight well and win three major pollution battles?

XZ-C proposed: What is the source of pollution? To solve or to release the bell, you need to ring the bell.

How to <u>scientifically</u> prevent pollution and to treat pollution? How to <u>scientifically</u> prevent cancer and to control cancer?

<u>1.</u>   <u>How to scientifically prevent pollution and to treat pollution?</u>

XZ-C proposes that scientific thinking, scientific research, scientific analysis, and scientific discussion should be conducted:

a. What is the content of pollution? What contents are there? What are the ingredients? What contents are they included in? What are the chemical ingredients?

It should be used for chemical composition detection, analysis, trace element analysis, qualitative and quantitative.

b. Does this ingredient have any effect on human health? What is the damage? Whether is there a carcinogen or not?

c. What is the source of pollution? Why did it happen? Can it be tried to stop at the source? In scientific and research design, how is it avoided?

d. How to stop the pollution at the source?

It is to block at the source of the business.

XZ-C proposed that it is necessary to ring the bell in order to solve the bell, that is, it is to set up a special scientific research team within the enterprise to study and solve it.

Professor Xu Ze proposed to strive to study as much as possible before the product leaves the factory in order not to produce social pollution.

2.   How does it try to stop the pollution at the source? How to prevent it at the source within the company in order to reduce pollution society?

XZ-C proposes:

To solve the bell, it needs to ring the bell.

Industry is the main body of atmospheric pollutant emissions, energy production and consumption are the main sources of air pollutant emissions in China. Special scientific research groups for air pollutants should be established within the enterprise to study the composition analysis of atmospheric pollutants and their emission pathways, and to strive to conduct the research of pollution prevention and pollution control and pollution treatment before the product leaves the factory, and avoid social pollution as much as possible (such as airplanes, trains, cars, thermal power...)

In the route of emission of atmospheric pollutants, it can be purified.

Professor Xu Ze proposed how to overcome cancer and how to prevent cancer by I see

<u>Situation analysis: (1)</u>

- How to prevent cancer? Cancer incidence is rising

<u>Situation analysis: (2)</u>

- Cancer incidence is related to the environment

1). Why does the increase in cancer incidence have a relationship with the environment?

2). The cause of cancer is related to the carcinogenic factors of the external environment and the internal environment.

3). If we have a deeper understanding of the causes of cancer, then we can come up with more valuable suggestions in the future:

How should it prevent cancer-causing factors, how to monitor which carcinogenic factors, and which to eliminate cancer-causing factors, so that we can stay away from cancer and prevent cancer?

<u>Situation analysis: (3)</u>

--- Prevention should be based on improving the carcinogenic factors of external factors (external environment) and internal factors (internal environment)

Professor Xu Ze proposed:

The establishment of an innovative cancer prevention research institute and an innovative cancer prevention system project is an unprecedented and it must be practiced in person to seek health and well-being for mankind.

XZ-C proposed the general design of cancer prevention and cancer prevention system engineering.

Situation analysis: (4)

- **It should set up the Environmental and Cancer Research Group**

It is to monitor environmental pollution-causing factors and data, to research and develop the measures of cancer prevention and cancer control, and to research and develop the method of interventions.

a, from clothing, food, shelter and walking to prevent cancer

b, from the big environment of life to prevent cancer

c, from the small living environment to prevent cancer

d, from life behavior, life hobbies, and living habits to prevent cancer

Under the guidance of Xi Jinping's characteristic socialism in the new era, it strives to open a new situation in scientific research work in the new era, and overcome the scientific research work of cancer, we should make great strides forward, and strives to follow the path of independent innovation with Chinese characteristics and adhere to the road of independent innovation of "Chinese-style anti-cancer" with the combination of Chinese and Western medicine.

Innovation -

It walked out of the road of Immune regulation and control of treatment of cancer with "Chinese-style anti-cancer" of the combination of Chinese and Western medicine while we have accumulated 30 years of the basic and clinical research on anti-cancer and anti-cancer metastasis. We have accumulated clinical application experience more than 12,000 cases in 20 years which can be pushed to the country and can go to the world, can be connected to the "A Belt and A Road" to bring Chinese medicine to the world and to make "Chinese-style anti-cancer" and immune regulation and control of treatment of cancer with the combination of Chinese and Western medicine that not only develops and enriches the content of immunotherapy of cancer, but also brings China's medical modernization into line with international standards and is at the forefront of the world.

One

The Source Background and Experience of the Scientific Research Topics

(1) The source background and the course of the completion of the project (the tortuous path)

My three new monographs are actually the key scientific and technological projects I have undertaken during the" Eighth Five" Plan period-------------------the Project name was:

"The Experimental and Clinical studies of further exploring prevention cancer and anti-cancer Chinese herbal medicine for the prevention and treatment of anti-metastasis on liver cancer, gastric cancer and precancerous lesions with the combination of Chinese and western herbal medicine." The special topic name of Thematic contract of "Eighth Five" National Technology and Science Research plan was :

"Clinical and Experimental Research on Treatment of Gastric Cancer and Precancerous Lesions by Chinese and Western Medicine" was headed or was in charged by the National Science and Technology Commission.

In April 1991, the author submitted an application to the State Science and Technology Commission for key scientific and technological projects during the "Eighth Five Plan" period. The project name is "further explore the experimental and clinical research on the prevention and treatment of anti-cancer and anti-cancer Chinese herbal medicine for the prevention and treatment of precancerous lesions of gastric cancer, liver cancer and gastric cancer." In June, Director of Hubei Provincial Science and Technology Commission Tian organized the three project leaders of the province to apply for the National Science and Technology Commission (1 person from Tongji Medical College, 1 from Hubei Medical College, 1 from Hubei College of Traditional Chinese Medicine) to go to Beijing to report to the Chinese Medicine Administration of the Ministry of Health.

Two months later, Director Tian of the Provincial Science and Technology Commission and three project leaders went to Beijing to report further to the Ministry of Health on design and acceptance of the project. **Two months later, when the project task was**

issued and the "Eighth Five National Science and Technology Research Project Contract" was being signed formally, Professor Xu Ze suddenly developed acute myocardial infarction, anterior wall and high wall myocardial infarction. After rescue and treatment, he was hospitalized for half a year, and he was relieved after a half-year break after leaving the hospital. The National Science and Technology Commission will also be stranded and suspended.

In 1993, Professor Xu Ze's physical condition gradually recovered and also thought about the idea of continuing to study the content of the subject. It was because the author has followed up a lots of the postoperative patients with the radical resection and the results showed that postoperative recurrence and metastasis of cancer were the key factors affecting the long-term outcome after radical resection. The clinical basis and effective methods for preventing postoperative recurrence and metastasis must be studied. It was determined to do some research work that should be done within this capacity. However, there were thoughts but no research funding, so I began to find ways to raise funds for research. In 1993, my wife retired, she applied for a clinic, and her meager income was the starting point for research funding or her meager income started as a research fund. Kunming mice were purchased from the Animal Center of the Medical College for animal experiments, animal cages and related equipment and instruments were prepared, and animal experiments were started. The meager income of the clinic is used to support Professor Xu Ze's animal experiments and scientific research, and to save money in careful calculation or carefully save on applications. Six rooms on the second floor were used for animal experiments. In 1996, Professor Xu Ze was 63 years old and applied for retirement. After that, with the support of this meager income, a series of experimental research and clinical verification work were carried out. After 16 years of hard work and hard work, we finally completed the research project of the State Science and Technology Commission. We collected experimental and clinical research materials, data and summaries, and published three monographs:

1). "New understanding and new model of cancer treatment", Xu Ze, published by Hubei Science and Technology Press, January 2001, Xinhua Bookstore issued;

2). "New Concepts and New Methods for Cancer Metastasis Treatment", Xu Ze, published by the People's Military Medical Press, January 2006, issued by the National Xinhua Bookstore. In April 2007, the General Administration of Press of the People's Republic of China issued the "Three One Hundred" original book certificate.

3). "New Concepts and New Methods of Cancer Treatment" by Xu Ze and Xu Jie, published by Beijing People's Military Medical Press in October 2011. Later, the American medical staff Dr. Bin Wu and others translated into English. The English version was published in Washington, DC on March 26, 2013, and is distributed internationally.

(2) Some experiences

In the past, the author carried out scientific research work in medical colleges, with the guidance of superiors and the help of colleagues, and the laboratory conditions were excellent, undertook the National Natural Science Foundation of China, the National Science and Technology Commission project, provincial science and technology commission project. Two scientific research achievements have been made, one is the domestic advanced level and the other is the international advanced level. He won the second prize of Hubei Province Science and Technology Achievements and won the first prize of Hubei Provincial Health Science and Technology Achievements.

But now it is different. Under such special circumstances, in a clinic or outpatient center, first there is no condition, second there is no equipment, how can we carry out and complete the national task? The author has the following brief experience.

1. Self-reliance and self-raising or self-reliant and self-financing. For the patient service to treat the patient and to work in outpatient and the outpatient income is used as research funding.

2. Keep outpatient medical records and follow up throughout the process.

3. Establish special scientific research collaborations, collaborate and cooperate according to scientific research plans.

4. Establish detailed medical records (including epidemiological data of patients), and analyze in depth the success of each treatment, the failure lessons and the particularity of the condition.

5. Scientific research cooperation strategy of sharing equipment, sharing equipment and sharing results, and not adding large-scale instruments and equipment, and collaborating with the medical college affiliated school, the high-precision equipment inspections are carried out in the medical college affiliated hospital.

6. Selecting scientific frontier topics, failing to apply and to declare the subject (because it has been nearly ancient and rare), and to report the results to the Ministry, the province, and the city.

7. In the private clinic office the old professors can also carry out and complete research projects by fully utilizing the advanced equipment conditions of colleges and universities and combining decades of clinical experience through research and cooperation with universities and colleges, sharing of instruments and equipment, and the strategy of sharing results,

After 20 years of hard work under the heat and cold, I carried out a series of experimental research and clinical verification work, and finally basically completed the "Eighth Five Plan" research project of the National Science and Technology Commission that I applied for. I have compiled experimental and clinical research materials, data, conclusions, and summaries, and have written more than 100 research papers. Since there is no research funding, it is not possible to publish the magazine according to the paper, but it is published according to the new book. Two monographs were published successively. The third book of "New concepts and new methods of cancer treatment" is now published. These three monographs are our difficult moving and the difficult climbing, three different stages with one step and one footprint; is the results from the different levels, three different peaks, which are a series of coherent scientific research steps and scientific research processes.

The above briefly describes the background and ins and outs of my three monographs:

From the discovery of the results of a clinical follow-up to the findings of experimental tumor research; from the review of clinical medical practice cases to the analysis, evaluation and reflection of postoperative adjuvant chemotherapy cases, the drawbacks of traditional chemotherapy were discovered.

Looked for anti-cancer and anti-metastatic new drugs from natural medicines (Chinese medicines):

From performing in vitro and in vivo experiments on cancer-bearing models to the discovery and production of XZ-C series of immunomodulatory Chinese medicines, to go to clinical validation. Now more than 12,000 cases have been clinically validated for more than 16 years.

From the experimental basic research and clinical verification observation moving up to the theoretical understanding, a series of innovative theories are proposed, some are original innovations, and a series of reform measures for traditional therapies are proposed, and the strategies and strategic prospects for conquering cancer are proposed, such as some of the above scientific research contents and scientific research results are the research papers of the original innovative intellectual property that were first reported internationally. All of them are filled in my three monographs and published in the form of books.

Note:

Attachment:

3. Introduction to the Institute of Experimental Surgery, Hubei College of Traditional Chinese Medicine (see page of this book)

4. Science and technology research topics

Two

Briefly describe the scientific research process of anti-cancer research

1. Briefly describe the scientific research process of anti-cancer research

In 1985, I conducted a petition with more than 3,000 patients who were underwent the radical resection of various chest/thoracic surgery and general surgery. The results showed that most patients relapsed and metastasized about 2-3 years after surgery, and some even metastasized within a few months after surgery. I realized that the operation was successful, and the long-term efficacy was unsatisfactory. Postoperative recurrence and metastasis were the key factors affecting the long-term efficacy of the operation.

Therefore, a question is also raised:

Studying prevention and treatment of postoperative recurrence and metastasis is the key to improving postoperative survival.

Therefore, clinical basic research must be carried out, and without breakthroughs in basic research, clinical efficacy is difficult to improve. So we established the Institute of Experimental Surgery and spent 15 years conducting a series of experimental research and clinical validation work from the following three aspects:

1). **Exploring the pathogenesis of cancer, the mechanism of invasion and the mechanism of recurrence and metastasis, and exploring and performing the experimental research on looking for the effective measures to control invasion, recurrence and metastasis.**

My colleagues and I have been conducting experimental tumor research for four years in our laboratory. The selection of research projects is to ask questions from the clinical, to attempt to explain some clinical problems through experimental research, or to solve some clinical problems, all of which are clinical basic research.

2). The experimental research of looking for the new drug of anti-cancer, anti-metastatic, anti-recurrence from natural medicine Chinese herbal medicine.

The existing anticancer drugs not only kill cancer cells but also kill normal cells, and have serious side effects. *Our laboratory uses a tumor suppressor test in cancer-bearing mice to find new drugs that inhibit cancer cells without affecting normal cells from natural Chinese herbal medicines.*

Our lab spent the entire three years, for 200 kinds of Chinese herbal medicines commonly used in traditional anti-cancer prescriptions and anti-cancer prescriptions reported in various places, the anti-tumor or tumor inhibition screening experiments in the cancer-bearing animals were carried out one by one. The result:

It was screened out 48 traditional Chinese medicines that have a good tumor inhibition rate. At the same time, it has a good effect of increasing immune function, and finds the traditional Chinese medicine TG which can inhibit the new micro-vessels.

3). Clinical verification work:

Through the above four years to explore the basic experimental research on the mechanism of recurrence and metastasis, after three or three years of experimental research on natural medicines and Chinese herbal medicines, it was found a batch of XZ-C1-10 anti-cancer immune regulation and control chinese medicine, through the clinical validation of more than 12,000 patients with advanced or postoperative metastatic cancer in 20 years. The application of XZ-C immunomodulation of traditional Chinese medicine has achieved good results, improved quality of life, improved symptoms, and significantly prolonged survival.

Recently, I have reviewed, analyzed, reflected, and experienced the results and findings of my clinical research on clinical practice for more than 60 years, from experiment to clinical, from clinical to experimental, the experimental research and clinical verification data were summarized and collected and organized and published into three monographs:

1)). "New understanding and new model of cancer treatment", published by Hubei Science and Technology Press, Xu Ze, January 2001.

2)). "New Concepts and New Methods for Cancer Metastasis Treatment", Beijing People's Military Medical Press, Xu Ze, January 2006. In April 2007, the

General Administration of the People's Republic of China issued the "Three One Hundred" original book certificate.

3)). "New Concepts and New Methods of Cancer Treatment", published by Beijing People's Military Medical Press, Xu Ze, October 2011. Later, the American medical doctor Dr. BinWu translated into English. The English version was published in Washington, DC on March 26, 2013, and is distributed internationally.

2. Ideological understanding and scientific research thinking of our scientific research journey

The thinking and scientific thinking of our scientific research journey in cancer research for 28 years can be divided into four stages:

1) The first stage 1985-1999

- Identify problems from follow-up results → ask questions → study questions;

- From reviewing, analyzing, reflecting, and discovering the problems of current cancer traditional therapies, further research and improvement are needed;

- Recognize that there are problems, change your mindset, and change your mindset;

- Summarize the materials, collate, collect and publish the first monograph "New Understanding and New Model of Cancer Treatment" published by Hubei Science and Technology Press in January 2001.

2) The second stage After 2001 -

- *Positioning the goals of the study and the "target" of cancer treatment on anti-metastatic, pointing out that the key to cancer treatment is anti-metastatic;*

- Conducted a series of anti-cancer metastasis, recurrence experimental research and clinical basis and clinical validation research, and rose to theoretical innovation, and proposed new ideas and methods for anti-metastasis;

- Summarize the materials, collate, collect and publish the second monograph "New Concepts and New Methods for Cancer Metastasis Treatment" published by People's Military Medical Press in January 2006, issued by Xinhua Bookstore.

In April 2007, he was awarded the "Three One Hundred" Original Book Award by the General Administration of Press and Publication of the People's Republic of China.

3) The third stage After 2006 -

- **Study the goals and priorities of the research on the prevention and treatment of the whole process of cancer occurrence and development;**

- Closely combined with clinical practice, propose reforms and innovations, scientific research and development in response to the problems and shortcomings of current clinical traditional therapies;

- Recognize that the strategy of cancer prevention and treatment must move forward, the way out for anti-cancer treatment is "three early", and the way out for anti-cancer is prevention;

- I have been engaged in oncology surgery for 60 years, more and more patients, the incidence of cancer is rising, and the mortality rate remains high. I deeply understand that cancer should not only pay attention to treatment, but also pay attention to prevention, so as to block it at the source. I conducted a series of related research, did the summary materials and collation and collection and publication of the third monograph "New Concepts and New Methods for Cancer Treatment", published by the People's Military Medical Press in October 2011, and published by Xinhua Bookstore. Later, the American medical professional Dr. Bin Wu translated into English. The English version was published in Washington, DC on March 26, 2013.

4) The fourth stage After 2011 -

- Now is the fourth stage of our research work, which is being developed and carried out; the research work has been to be performed through step by step, positioning the research goal or "target" to reduce the incidence of cancer and to improve the cure rate and to prolong the survival period.

- We have been working on cancer research for 28 years:

The experimental research and clinical research work in the first three stages are mainly to research the new drugs in the treatment aspects and the new methods and new technologies of diagnosis and the new concepts and new methods of treatment.

- But today, in the second decade of the 21st century the cancer is still awkward. The more patients are treated, the higher the incidence rate and the higher the mortality rate.

I am deeply aware that cancer should not only pay attention to treatment, but also pay attention to prevention, in order to stop at the source.

- The current tumor hospital or oncology hospital model is fully focused on treatment, focusing on middle-stage and late-stage patients, the efficacy is poor, it is to exhaust human resource and financial resources, and it failed to reduce the incidence rate. The more the patient is treated, the more the patient comes. The status quo is:

The road that has passed in a century is to attention to or to rectify the treatment with ignoring prevention, or only to treat cancer without prevention at all. For many years we have only been working on cancer treatment. However, work on cancer prevention has been done very little and almost nothing has been done. As a result, the incidence of cancer continues to rise.

Through review, reflection, cliché about cancer prevention and anti-cancer work, what research or work have we done on cancer prevention for a century? What has it been achieved?

The teaching content in the medical school textbook does not pay attention to cancer prevention knowledge;

The setting-up hospital model has not paid attention to the setting up of cancer prevention science;

The scientific research projects in medical schools or hospitals have not paid attention to cancer prevention scientific research projects;

The Journal of Oncology Medicine does not pay attention to cancer prevention work papers.

In short, cancer prevention has not been taken seriously, and prevention has not been taken seriously. The prevention of the old-fashioned talks is mainly based on failure to pay attention.

How to do? How to reduce the incidence of cancer? How to improve the cure rate of cancer? How to reduce cancer mortality? How to prolong the survival period? How to improve the quality of life?

It should launch the general attack of conquering cancer and put the prevention and treatment at the same level and at the same attention and at the same time.

The goal of conquering cancer should be:

To reduce morbidity, improve cure rate, reduce mortality, prolong survival, improve quality of life, and reduce complications.

- At present, the global hospitals and hospitals in China are all devoted to treatment, attention to treatment and light prevention, or only treatment without prevention.

XZ-C believes that this mode of hospitalization or cancer treatment is unlikely to overcome cancer and it is impossible to reduce the incidence.

Global hospitals and hospitals in China must carry out an overall strategic reform of cancer treatment, shifting focusing on treatment into focusing on prevention and treatment at the same level and attention.

- Therefore, we propose to a general plan and design to overcome cancer and launch the total attack. XZ-C (Xu Ze-China) proposed to launch a general attack, which is to carry out the three-stage work of cancer prevention, cancer control and cancer treatment at the same time and the same level.

It is to propose the "Necessity and Feasibility Report for Overcoming cancer and launching the General Attack of Cancer."

It is to propose "XZ-C Scientific Research Plan for Overcoming cancer and launching the General Attack of Cancer"

3. **Why do I study cancer and propose to launch a general attack and to prepare to build a "science city to overcome cancer"?**

It is because:

1). In 1985, I conducted a petition to more than 3,000 patients who had undergone chest and abdominal cancer surgery. I found that most patients relapsed or metastasized within 2-3 years after surgery. Therefore, it is necessary to study methods to prevent postoperative recurrence and metastasis in order to improve the long-term efficacy after surgery.

2). I suddenly had an acute myocardial infarction in 1991. After the treatment was improved and recovered, it was not advisable to go to the operating table again. It was quiet and I went to the small building to concentrate on scientific research.

3). Through experimental research, it was found that thymus atrophy and immune function are low, which is one of the causes and pathogenesis of cancer, and it needs to be further expanded and studied in depth.

4). Through experimental research and clinical validation, after more than 12,000 clinical trials in 28 years, I found this new "Chinese-style anti-cancer" road of the modernization of Chinese medicine with the combination of Chinese and western medicine at the molecular level, which entered into and walked out the new path of the immunomodulation with the combination of the western medicine and the traditional Chinese medicine at the molecular level to prevent thymic atrophy, promote thymic hyperplasia, protect bone marrow hematopoietic function, and improve immune surveillance for conquering cancer, then to stay perversion and to research persistently.

Therefore, it is to propose to overcome cancer and launch the general attack on cancer, prepare to build a "science city" to overcome cancer. **The Attempt is to achieve:**

Reduce the incidence of cancer; improve the cure rate of cancer; prolong the survival of cancer patients; achieve "three early" (early detection, early diagnosis, early treatment), can be cured in the early stage; to achieve prevention, control, and treatment at the same time and at the same level and at the same attention; both prevention and treatment at the same time and level can only overcome cancer and reduce the incidence of cancer.

All basic research must be for the clinical, to improve the patient's efficacy and benefit patients. The criteria for assessing the efficacy of cancer patients should be: The survival period is prolonged, the quality of life is good, and the complications are few.

I came to Wuhan in 1951 and entered the Central South Tongji Medical College. I graduated from Tongji Medical College in 1956 and was assigned to the Affiliated Hospital of Hubei College of Traditional Chinese Medicine. I was the director of surgery and the director of the Institute of Experimental Surgery of Hubei College of Traditional Chinese Medicine.

In 1991, due to sudden acute myocardial infarction, after emergency treatment, I recovered after half a year of hospitalization. It was because he can no longer go to the stage for surgery, I become calm and hide in the small building to conduct basic and clinical research on cancer. Due to the good equipment conditions of my experimental surgical laboratory, a large number of experimental studies on the etiology, pathology, pathogenesis, and cancer metastasis mechanism of cancer were carried out, and the experimental screening of anti-cancer Chinese herbal medicine in the cancer-bearing animal model was conducted.

I was 63 years old in 1996 and applied for retirement. After retiring, I continued my scientific research, and Science will not stop. I have been living in a small building for 20 years, fighting alone (no one cares after retirement, no one knows in the unit and organization, no one asks, no one supports), single-handedly, self-reliant, from the year of the flower to the age of the ancient ; in the year of more than eighty years, I am still persevering and keep perseverance so that a series of experimental studies and clinical validation observations continued. Finally, we have achieved a series of scientific research achievements and technological innovation series.

The experimental and clinical data, information, conclusions, and summaries were collected, and more than 100 scientific research papers were written and published in the new book.

I have published 18 series of monographs that focus on cancer research. Three of them are in Chinese and 15 are in English.

The English version is published in Washington and distributed worldwide.

The book proposes a series of new concepts and new methods to overcome cancer, puts forward the theory of cancer treatment innovation, proposes the road to overcome cancer, and forms the theoretical system of immune regulation and control and treatment, which is the theoretical basis and experimental basis for cancer immunotherapy. It is undergoing clinical application observation and verification, and embarking on the new path to overcome cancer. Why is the English version? It is because cancer is a disaster for all mankind, the people of the world must work together for it. I took my 60 years of medical practice, 30 years of scientific research and clinical verification work of the experimental research of conquering cancer research and the scientific thinking and scientific understanding and skills and lessons and wisdom to contribute to the people, for the benefit of mankind.

I am 87 years old this year. I am the chief designer of the XZ-C research project, "Conquering cancer and launching the General Attack on Cancer and Building Science City for Scientific Research Bases to Conquer Cancer."

I will use my academic, knowledge, wisdom and strength to fully participate in the preparation of the "the Science City of conquering Cancer "practice, to build a "the hospitals for the global demonstration of prevention and treatment ", to prevent and control and treat cancer at the same level, to build a good laboratory and multidisciplinary Cancer Research Group.

It is to change the mode of running a school from paying attention to treatment and ignoring defense into prevention, control, and treatment at the same level and at the same attention and at the same time.

It is to change the treatment mode from paying attention to the treatment for the middle and late stage or severe illness of treatment into focusing on "three early" (early detection, early diagnosis, early treatment) precancerous lesions, early carcinoma in situ. This will benefit mankind and will open up a new era of anti-cancer research, making China's prevention and treatment of cancer and medical care into the forefront of the world.

4. **After 30 years of basic and clinical research on cancer with the direction of research as "to overcome cancer ", we deeply understand that in order to achieve the purpose of cancer prevention and control:**

1). it must launch the general attack.

That is to say, the three stages of cancer prevention, cancer control and cancer treatment at the same time; the three carriages go hand in hand so as to reduce the incidence of cancer, improve cancer cure rate, reduce cancer mortality, and prolong the survival of cancer patients.

If it only is to treat without prevention, or only pays attention to treatment with light prevention, it can never overcome cancer because it can't reduce the incidence, and the patients become more and more because it does not reduce the incidence, the more patients are treated and the more it will have the patients.

How to launch a general attack and implement cancer prevention + cancer control + cancer treatment?

It is necessary to establish a hospital with prevention and treatment of cancer with development and prevention and treatment during the whole process of cancer development and occurrence. It is to change the current hospital mode that can only attention to the treatment without prevention. It is to change the current treatment model which only aims at the middle-stage or late-state cancer.

2). It is necessary for the government to lead and for the experts and scholars to work hard, and for the masses to participate, and thousands of households can participate in it. At present, China is building an innovative country. It is the government-led, mass participation, national mobilization, and the work of thousands of households. This is great timing. If it can carry out medical scientific research to overcome cancer, prevent cancer and control cancer, it will certainly improve the awareness of cancer prevention among the whole people, and achieve the effect of preventing cancer and cancer control. It will receive the effects of significantly reducing the incidence of cancer in China, our province and our city.

3). Why is it to launch a general attack?

It is because the status quo is:

a. The current mode of running a hospital is to pay attention to or to rectify the treatment with light prevention and/ or only have the treatment without prevention ; the more the patient is treated and the more the patients show up.

b. The current treatment mode is mainly in the middle and late stages of cancer, and the effect is very poor.

c. The current radiotherapy and chemotherapy cannot cure, and can only be alleviated. Cancer is still progress during 4 weeks of mitigation period, and the curative effect is very poor. There are still problems and drawbacks.

It is necessary to emphasize early diagnosis, early treatment, and early rehabilitation:

a. It is to change the mode of running a hospital for prevention, control, and treatment at the same attention

b. It is to change the treatment mode into "three early", precancerous lesions.

c. The way out for anti-cancer is prevention, research, and cancer prevention research.

5. **I have been conducting basic research and clinical validation for cancer research for 30 years, both of which are carried out in laboratories and hospitals.** Why is it to think of applying for government support now?

It is because 90% of cancers are related to the environment, the occurrence of cancer is closely related to people's clothing, food, housing, travel and living habits. Therefore, I deeply think that cancer prevention and cancer control work is not only done by medical personnel and experts and scholars which can be done. It must rely on the government's major policy. The current environmental pollution is serious and the ecosystem is degraded, which may be closely related to the rising incidence of cancer.

The treatment of cancer depends on medical personnel and researchers to study new drugs and new treatment techniques.

However, about cancer prevention and control, how to reduce the incidence of cancer, cancer prevention work must rely on the government's major policy, rely on government leadership and mastership and rely on the experts, scholars, and mass participation so as that it can be carried out.

The current status quo is:

1). The more patients are treated, the higher the incidence is, and 90% is related to the environment. We deeply understand that cancer should not only pay attention to treatment, but also pay more attention to prevention, in order to stop it at the source, and it must prevent and treat at the same attention.

2). The current diagnostic method, B-ultrasound, CT, MRI, is currently the most advanced diagnostic means, but once diagnosed, mostly in the middle stage and late-stage, the effect is very poor. Research must be done to find new methods, new reagents, and new technologies for early diagnosis. Early cancer can be cured if it can be diagnosed in early stages and precancerous lesions. Therefore, the way out for cancer treatment is "three early". (early detection, early diagnosis, early treatment).

What should I do next?

Now it is to propose to overcome cancer and launch a general attack. I hope to get support from leaders at all levels. I know that in order to achieve the purpose of cancer prevention, control, and treatment, the government leaders, government masters, experts, and scholars must work hard, and the masses participate and thousands of households participate in.

About 11922 people in China are diagnosed with cancer every day, and 8 people are diagnosed with cancer every minute. Therefore, to study the scientific research work of launching the general attack on cancer, it should not walk slowly, it should run forward and save the wounded.

According to the "2015 China Cancer Statistics" report published by the National Cancer Center, in 2015, the number of new cancer cases in China was about 4.292 million yuan, that is, it should avoid empty talking and should do the hard work, and should always start to walk. No matter how far the road to conquer cancer is, it should always start.

6. **I have been studying in 2013→2014→2015, formulating basic ideas and designs on how to overcome cancer, formulating the theoretical basis and experimental basis for how to overcome cancer, developing the plan and blueprint and the route and the guidelines and the methods for how to overcome cancer. It came up with:**

1). "XZ-C Scientific Research Plan for Overcoming cancer and launching the General Attack of Cancer"

2). "Report on the Necessity of Preparing for the Hospital of Prevention and Treatment of Cancer in the Whole Process"

3). "The report of the necessity and feasibility of at the same time as building a well-off society – it is suggesting "taking a ride to scientific research" - conducting medical scientific research of cancer prevention and treatment and performing the work for cancer prevention and cancer control"

4). "Planning and the overall design of building the Science City for overcoming the cancer and launching the general attack."

These four scientific research projects were first proposed internationally which are opening up thenew areas of anti-cancer research. Professor Xu Ze proposed to the general attack of conquering cancer, which is unprecedented work. As of July 2015, it was formulated as the "Dawning C-type plan". That is, the dawn is morning light, Chaoyang, C type = China, that is, the plan of overcoming cancer with "Chinese model". The "four items" report is generally for "to overcome cancer and to launch a general attack" and for "establish a science city of conquering cancer."

How to implement this plan of conquering cancer in detail?

I have elaborated the overall design, master plan, specific program research team talents, etc. planning and blueprint.

It came up with Total Design • Blueprint of "Science City for Overcoming cancer and launching the General Attack of Cancer"

It was to come up with the overall design and preparation work of Science City

It is to established a trial area for the cancer working group (station)

It is to set up :

1). The Academic Committee of Conquering Cancer

2). The preparation group of the science city (the medical, teaching, research, development science city for conquering cancer and launching the general attack of cancer)

7.   **This work is underway. We have been walking on cancer research of conquering cancer in the 3-4 years, and it is to only slowly moving forward step by step.**

On January 12, 2016, US President Barack Obama proposed the National Cancer Plan in his State of the Union address:

Conquer cancer

The name of the program: "Cancer moon shot"

Goal: Conquer cancer

Nature: National plan to overcome cancer

The person in charge of the plan: Vice President Biden

We have been on the road of conquering cancer for 3-4 years, but only individuals are living in small buildings and fighting alone, step by step, just slowly moving forward.

Now US President Barack Obama announced the National Cancer Plan in his State of the Union address:

Conquer cancer.

It is implemented by the vice president. Vice President Biden is actively implementing it. He goes to the cancer centers in the United States every month to preach: "Cancer moon shot".

On June 29, 2016, the National Cancer Lunar Plan was broadcast to the United States at the White House. Calling on all American scientists to gather wisdom and overcome cancer.

This international scientific research situation is a gratifying situation, and the situation is compelling and inspiring. In this case, the government must be called upon to ask the government to lead and lead the work to support this unprecedented work for the benefit of mankind.

This is a big event. This is an unprecedented event that benefits mankind.

Therefore, XZ-C proposes to move forward together and head to the scientific hall of cancer.

Three

Briefly describe the academic thinking and scientific research thinking of my scientific research process

This is gradually recognized in my scientific research journey in the past 28 years of the research of conquering cancer engaged in. It is our journey of scientific research to complete the application of the "Eighth Five". It is a series of coherent scientific research steps, scientific research stages, scientific research levels, continuous integration, step by step, and different understandings at different stages.

Scientific research is like climbing, and when you reach a mountain peak, you can see a layer of scenery. A mountain is taller than a mountain, and a mountain is better scenery than a mountain scenery.

Following the scientific development concept, the ideological understanding and scientific thinking of my scientific research journey can be divided into three stages:

(1)   The first stage (1985-1999)

New discoveries and new insights :

It was to find out or discover the existing problems – asking questions – innovative thinking, changing ideas.

In 1985, I conducted a petition to more than 3,000 patients who had undergone chest and abdominal cancer surgery. I found that most patients relapsed or metastasized 2-3 years after surgery. Postoperative recurrence and metastasis are the key factors affecting the long-term efficacy of surgery. Clinical basic research to prevent cancer recurrence and metastasis must be carried out. Without breakthroughs in basic research, clinical efficacy is difficult to improve. Since experimental surgery is a key to open the medical exclusion zone, we established a tumor animal laboratory, set up an experimental surgical laboratory, and conducted a series of experimental tumor research:

Performed cancer cell transplantation; Established a cancer animal model; Explored the mechanisms and laws of cancer invasion, metastasis, and recurrence; looked for effective measures to regulate and to control the cancer invasion, recurrence and metastasis.

The new discovery

From experimental tumor research it was found:

1. Removal of the thymus can produce a cancer-bearing animal model. The conclusion of the study:

the occurrence and development of cancer has a positive relationship with the thymus of the host.

2. When we studied the relationship between cancer metastasis and immunity in our laboratory, the experimental results suggest that metastasis is related to immunity.

3. Experimental studies have found that as the cancer progresses, the host's thymus is progressively atrophied.

For further research, the Institute of Experimental Surgery of Hubei College of Traditional Chinese Medicine was established in March 1991 on the basis of the Experimental Surgery Laboratory. Professor Xu Ze is the director, and the academician Qiu fazu was the advisor. The goal and mission of his research is to become "conquer cancer" as the main direction.

In 1994, we established a special outpatient center for oncology clinics. Through the review of clinical medical practice cases and the analysis, evaluation and reflection of postoperative adjuvant chemotherapy, it was found or revealed the existing problems:

1). Some patients with postoperative adjuvant chemotherapy failed to prevent recurrence;

2). Some patients did not prevent metastasis after adjuvant chemotherapy;

3). Some patients have chemotherapy that promotes immune failure.

From the analysis and reflection of clinical practice case, why does the patient's postoperative chemotherapy fail to prevent recurrence and metastasis?

From the analysis of cancer cells in the cancer cell cycle, analysis and reflection from the inhibition of immunity by chemotherapeutic drugs, analysis and reflection from the drug resistance of chemotherapeutic drugs, it was found that there are problems:

1). There are still some important misunderstandings in current chemotherapy;

2). There are still several major contradictions in current chemotherapy, which need further research and improvement.

From the follow-up results, it was found that postoperative recurrence and metastasis is the key to affect the long-term efficacy of surgery. Therefore, we also raised an important question for us:

Clinicians must pay attention to and study the prevention and treatment of postoperative recurrence and metastasis in order to improve the long-term efficacy of postoperative.

From 1985 to 1999, we conducted a series of experimental and clinical research, and reviewed, analyzed and reflected, summed up the positive and negative experiences and lessons of success and failure, and then compiled and published the first monograph "New understanding and new model of cancer treatment", published in January 2001 by Hubei Science and Technology Publishing House, Xinhua Bookstore.

(2) The second stage (after 2001)

The research goals and the "targets" of cancer treatment was positioned on anti-metastatic, it is pointing out that the key to cancer treatment is anti-metastasis.

After 2001, our research work was that **it is in-depth analysis of what the key to the postoperative recurrence and metastasis is**?

Looking back from the 1970s, in view of the recurrence and metastasis rate after cancer surgery, in order to prevent postoperative recurrence and metastasis, a series of adjuvant chemotherapy after surgery was used, and even chemotherapy was started before surgery. But the results are not satisfactory. Recurrence and metastasis still occur soon after surgery. Or there is metastasis while chemotherapy, the more the chemotherapy and the more metastasis. Some cases contribute to immune failure due to intensive chemotherapy. These are all worthy of our clinicians should seriously and objectively think and analyze how cancer treatment work should prevent recurrence and anti-metastasis in order to obtain good long-term therapeutic effects.

Today, the most important problem in cancer treatment is how to resist metastasis. Metastasis is already the bottleneck of cancer treatment.

If the problem of cancer metastasis after radical surgery in patients cannot be solved, cancer treatment can no longer leap forward.

Therefore, the key to current cancer research is anti-metastasis. The core problem of cancer treatment is to resolve metastasis and recurrence.

One of the keys to cancer treatment is anti-cancer metastasis. Metastasis is only a phenomenon. How does it to clearly understand the process, steps and mechanisms of cancer cell metastasis? We should try to understand why cancer cells metastasize? How is it transferred? What are the steps, routes, process shapes and how is the fate of the transfer? What is the molecular mechanism of cancer cell metastasis? Where is the weak link in the process of cancer cell transfer? Which or which link or part is stroke or blocked can achieve the purpose of anti-metastasis?

We spent more than three years experimenting with animal models of cancer metastasis, observing and tracking the regularity of cancer cells on the way to metastasis, looking for ways to interfere with and prevent cancer cells from metastasizing.

Through the review, analysis and evaluation of a large number of cases in clinical practice, we propose:

1. The key to current cancer research is anti-metastasis;

2. Cancer appears in three forms in the human body, and the third form is cancer cells on the way to metastasis;

3. The goal of cancer treatment should be directed to these three forms;

4. "Two-point, one-line theory" cancer treatment in the whole process of cancer development, not only should pay attention to two points, but should also pay attention to cutting off the front line;

5. The specific measures to prevent metastasis should be to carry out the surrounding, chasing, blocking and intercepting of cancer cells during the transfer. It is put forward that in the third field of anti-cancer *metastasis treatment, the "main battlefield" of cancer cells on the way to quenching metastasis is in the blood circulation, and it is important to improve immune regulation and immune monitoring.*

By 2005, we compiled a large amount of data from the above experimental research and clinical verification, summarized, collected and published the second monograph "New Concepts and New Methods for Cancer Metastasis Treatment" published by People's Military Medical Press in January 2006, issued by Xinhua Bookstore. In April 2007, the company won the "Three One Hundred" Original Book Awards issued by the General Administration of Press of the People's Republic of China.

(3) The third stage (after 2006)

The research focuses on the prevention and treatment of the whole process of cancer occurrence and development. It closely combined with clinical practice, it aims at the problems and drawbacks of current clinical traditional therapy, and proposes reform and innovation, research and development. It is recognizing that the strategy of cancer prevention and treatment must move forward, the way out for cancer treatment is "three early", and the way out for cancer is prevention.

The second monograph is moving forward and further based on the first monograph of scientific research, which is positioning **that the "target point" of cancer treatment is anti-metastasis.**

It is pointed out that the key to cancer treatment is anti-metastasis. But metastasis is only the last stage of the whole process of cancer development*, it is only a local problem* in the whole process of cancer, and it cannot reduce the incidence of cancer and **may reduce the mortality rate.**

After 2006, we realized that the goal of cancer treatment is all necessary for the treatment of severely ill patients in the middle and late stages, but the curative effect is very poor. The more new patients are treated, the more the patients we have. Once diagnosed, it is in the middle and late stage, and the effect is not good. In order to overcome cancer, it must be "three early" and must be prevented in order to reduce the incidence of cancer and cancer mortality.

The way out for cancer treatment is "three early", and the study of "three early" must be strengthened.

The occurrence and development of cancer experience the stage of susceptibility - precancerous lesions - the invasive stage. At present, the treatment of cancer in oncology or tumor centers in various cancer hospitals or major hospitals in China, mainly in the middle and late stages, and the treatment effect is poor. If the middle and advanced patients can be operated on, they will be treated surgically. If surgery is not possible, they can only be evaluated. Therefore, the way out for cancer treatment should be "three early", early detection, early diagnosis, early treatment. Early patients generally have better therapeutic effects and improve the therapeutic effect, which inevitably reduces the cancer mortality rate. Therefore, we must pay attention to the study of early diagnosis methods and treatment methods, but also must pay attention to the treatment of precancerous lesions to reduce the middle and late stage patients in the invasion stage.

If we can treat well in precancerous lesions or early stage cancer, the number of patients who progress to invasion and metastasis will decrease, which will also reduce the incidence of cancer. Therefore, we believe that the current local cancer hospitals or oncology departments, mainly in the treatment of middle and late patients, even if the treatment results are good, can only reduce the mortality rate, however it is neglecting the precancerous lesions in the susceptible stage and/or neglecting the early patients, it is unlikely to reduce the incidence of cancer or it is impossible to reduce cancer incidence rate, therefore, we believe that we must pay attention to the occurrence of cancer, the prevention and treatment of the whole process of development, is a strategic overall concept, we must update our thinking and change our mindset.

I have been engaged in oncology surgery for 59 years, and more and more patients, the incidence of cancer is also rising, which makes me deeply understand that cancer should not only pay attention to treatment, but also pay attention to prevention, in order to stop at the source. Therefore, I deeply understand that the cancer treatment is in the "three early days". It is necessary to strengthen the research of "three early" (early detection, early diagnosis, early treatment*). **The way to fight cancer is prevention, and research on preventive measures must be strengthened.***

As mentioned above, the focus of cancer prevention and treatment strategy is shifted forward. Its meaning has two aspects, one is to change lifestyle, to improve environmental pollution and other preventive measures, and the other is to treat precancerous lesions and stop its development to the invasive or mid-late period.

(4) The fourth stage (after 2011)

Putting the focus of cancer prevention and treatment strategies forward and carrying out anti-cancer research to reduce the incidence of cancer, Professor Xu Ze proposed:

the initiative to create an environmental protection and cancer prevention research institute and carry out cancer prevention system engineering and open a new era of cancer prevention research and cancer prevention system engineering in the 21st century.

1. Why did I propose to create an environmental protection and cancer prevention research institute and carry out an cancer prevention system project?

At present, the cancer hospital or oncology department is all to pay heavy attention to treatment with ignoring prevention or only to treat without prevention.

I entered the Central South Tongji Medical College in 1951. It has been 68 years since then, and I have experienced and witnessed the whole process of cancer prevention and control work in China for a century. Looking back at the 20th century, although hospitals in China and around the world are also preventing cancer and anti-cancer work, in fact, the focus is on the treatment of primary cancers that have formed cancerous lesions and the treatment of anti-metastasis, all of which are invasive, middle stage and late stage, and the treatment effect is poor.

So far in the second decade of the 21st century, hospitals all over the world, the oncology departments of the provincial cancer hospitals and the affiliated hospitals of various universities in China, the oncology departments of the top three hospitals are all treatment hospitals, the cancer hospitals are all clinical treatment work, the hospital model is treatment hospitals, and the academic journals of oncology are also clinically diagnosed or clinically based, although there are several journals for cancer prevention and treatment. But there are very few articles on cancer prevention work.

In short, the oncology departments of the cancer hospitals and affiliated hospitals of the 20th century are all attention to treatment with light prevention or only have treatment without prevention.

Looking back, reflecting, old-fashioned cancer prevention and anti-cancer work, what research or work did we do in cancer prevention for a century? What has it been achieved?

The status quo is:

The road that has passed in a century is to pay attention to treatment with light prevention, or only to treatment without prevention. Cancer prevention and anti-cancer are human business and careers and causes, but over the years we have only been working and researching on anti-cancer and cancer treatment. However, work on cancer prevention has been done very little and almost nothing has been done.

There is no emphasis on cancer prevention knowledge in the teaching content of medical school textbooks.

The hospital or the hospital model did not pay attention to the setting up of cancer prevention science.

There is no emphasis on cancer prevention research projects in medical research projects in medical schools or hospitals. The Journal of Oncology Medicine does not pay attention to cancer prevention work papers. In short, cancer prevention has not been taken seriously, and prevention has not been taken seriously.

Old-fashioned cancer prevention and anti-cancer work and that old-fashioned prevention is the main focus did not pay attention to and were implemented.

2. How to launch a general attack to overcome cancer? How can cancer prevention research work be carried out?

XZ-C (Xu Ze-China - China Xu Ze) proposed the general attack, which is that the work for the three stages of cancer prevention and cancer control and cancer treatment should fully developed and synchronized, that is, it is to carry out and to start up cancer prevention research work. And it is the most important and it is the top priority.

As everyone knows:

How to reduce cancer mortality? How to improve the cure rate? How to prolong the survival period?

The way out for cancer treatment is "three early" (early detection, early diagnosis, early treatment), the effect of early cancer treatment is good and works well and it can be fully cured. <u>In particular, cancer lesions are well treated and can be cured.</u>

3. The way out to control cancer is prevention, and research on preventive measures must be strengthened.

Cancer has become the world's largest public health problem, and compared with other chronic diseases, cancer prevention and control will face even greater challenges.

In the past 30 years, the cancer mortality rate in China has shown a clear upward trend, and it has become the first cause of death for urban and rural residents. On average, one out of every four deaths has died of cancer.

Cancer is not only a serious threat to human health, but also an important factor in the rise in medical costs. China's annual direct cost for cancer treatment is nearly 100 billion yuan. The patient and the society as a whole bear a huge economic burden. Many patients have spent tens of thousands or even hundreds of thousands of dollars, and have not achieved corresponding effects. As a result, both human and financial are empty, cancer mortality is still the first, what should I do? It is worthy of our clinician analysis, reflection, and research. How is the research road to go? It is sure to recognize the problems that exist in current treatments.

Although countries have invested heavily in the treatment of cancer patients, the 5-year survival rate of some common cancers has not improved significantly in the past 20 years.

How to do?

The way out of controlling control cancer is prevention. Prevention and intervention are the top priority in the public health field. In recent years, it has been recognized that more than 90% of cancers are caused by environmental factors. Protecting and restoring a good environment is an important part of preventing cancer. One third of cancers are preventable.

The relationship between environment and cancer is extremely close. Environmental pollution can cause various carcinogens to enter the human body or various carcinogenic factors affect the human body. *<u>How to prove the relationship between environmental pollution and cancer has been confirmed by many examples in history.</u>*

<u>Air pollution</u> in environmental pollution can increase the incidence of lung cancer. In industrialized countries, harmful gases such as power generation, steelmaking, automobiles, aircraft, fuel, energy, and large amounts of smoke are emitted into the atmosphere, polluting the air, leading to an increase in the incidence and mortality of lung cancer.

<u>Water pollution in environmental pollution and cancer</u>:

water pollution is mainly caused by industrial and agricultural production and urban sewage. Water pollution can induce or promote cancer.

<u>Chemical carcinogenesis in environmental pollution</u> is also closely related to the incidence of cancer. 80-90% of human cancers are related to environmental factors, among which are mainly chemical factors.

Studying the sources of environmentally-friendly carcinogens and studying how to eliminate such pollution is a very important issue in the prevention of cancer. Prevention of cancer must prevent pollution and control pollution.

I think that energy saving and emission reduction, pollution prevention and pollution control are the first-level prevention of cancer and it is to block the occurrence of cancer at the source. And think this is a good time to help "overcome cancer". I am convinced that building a well-off society will surely achieve the effects of preventing cancer and cancer, and achieving good results, so that the people can be healthy and stay away from cancer.

In order to overcome cancer and conduct cancer prevention and cancer control research, it is necessary to carry out basic and clinical research on anti-cancer metastasis and recurrence, and carry out joint research on multidisciplinary cooperation. It is necessary to establish Wuhan Anticancer Research Association.

With the strong support of the academician Qiu Fazu, Xu Ze, Li Huizhen and other professors applied for preparation. After approval by the higher authorities of Wuhan, the Wuhan Anticancer Research Association was established on June 21, 2009, then it was to establish a professional committee for cancer metastasis treatment and recurrence treatment.

Four

The formation course of new concepts and new methods of cancer treatment

First

From the follow-up to the establishment of experimental surgical research room

Since 1985, the author has conducted a petition to more than 3,000 patients with chest and abdominal cancer after surgery which was performed by my own. It was found that most patients relapsed or metastasized in 2 to 3 years, and some even relapsed, metastasized and died after several months and one year after surgery.

These patients are often not returned to the original surgical surgery center after surgery for review, instead, go to the oncology department or the tumor hospital for chemotherapy and chemotherapy.

- Through large-scale follow-up, the author found an important problem, that is, postoperative recurrence and metastasis are the key factors affecting the long-term efficacy of surgery.

- Therefore, we also recognize that research on the prevention and treatment of postoperative recurrence and metastasis of cancer is the key to improving the long-term efficacy of surgery, which is the key to improve the postoperative survival of patients.

- Therefore, clinicians must conduct clinical basic research to prevent cancer recurrence and metastasis. Without breakthroughs in basic research, clinical efficacy is difficult to improve.

Based on the follow-up results, the next research goals were determined:

1). In order to prevent postoperative recurrence and metastasis so as to improve long-term postoperative efficacy, clinical basic research must be carried out;

2). In order to study prevention of recurrence and metastasis, the experimental tumor models must be established for experimental research.

Therefore, we established an experimental surgical laboratory to conduct experimental tumor research, perform cancer cell transplantation, establish a tumor animal model, and carry out a series of experimental tumor research.

- Explore cancer recurrence, metastasis mechanisms and patterns, and explore the relationship between tumors and immune and immune organs, as well as immune organs and tumors.

- Explore ways to suppress progressive atrophy of immune organs and rebuild immunity when tumor progression.

- Look for effective measures to regulate and to control cancer invasion, recurrence, and metastasis.

- The experimental screening of 200 anti-cancer Chinese herbal medicines commonly used in the literature for the tumor inhibition rate in the cancer-bearing solid tumors animal was performed.

- Search for anti-cancer, anti-metastatic, anti-recurrence new drugs from natural medicines, and use modern science and technology to conduct in-depth research and discovery of cancer prevention and anti-cancer Chinese herbal medicines.

--------- Screening of the anti-cancer Chinese herbal medicines in the traditional understanding of the anti-cancer rate in a strict, scientific and repeated cancer-bearing animal model.

It was to eliminate the effect of no stability, and 48 kinds of XZ-c immunomodulatory anti-tumor Chinese medicines with good curative effect were screened out.

- Based on the success of animal experiments, it has been applied to clinical practice. After 12 years of clinical trials of a large number of clinical cases, the curative effect is remarkable.

Second

The new discoveries

1. Found from the results of follow-up

(1) Postoperative recurrence and metastasis are the key factors affecting the long-term efficacy of surgery. Therefore, we also raised an important issue, that is, clinicians must pay attention to and study the prevention and treatment measures for postoperative recurrence and metastasis, so as to improve long-term postoperative outcomes.

(2) Clinical basic research on recurrence and metastasis must be carried out. Without breakthroughs in basic research, clinical efficacy is difficult to improve.

2. Found from experimental tumor research

(1) Excision of the thymus can produce a model of cancer-bearing animals, and injection of immunosuppressive drugs can also contribute to the establishment of a cancer-bearing animal model.

The conclusions of the study clearly demonstrate that the occurrence and development of cancer has a clear relationship with the immune function of the host's immune organs, thymus and immune organs.

(2) Whether is it immune function decrease first and then easy to get cancer or It is cancer occurrence first and then it causes the low immune function?

Our experimental results are that the immune system is first low and then easy to have cancer. If the immune function is not reduced first, it is not easy to be vaccinated successfully.

The results suggest that improving and maintaining good immune function and protecting the thymus of the immune organs is one of the important measures to prevent cancer.

(3) When studying the relationship between metastasis and immunity of cancer, an animal model of liver metastasis was established, which was divided into two groups, group A and group B. Group A used immunosuppressive drugs, and

group B did not. The result was that the number of intrahepatic metastases in group A was significantly higher than that in group B.

The experimental results suggest that metastasis is associated with immunity, low immune function or the use of immunosuppressive drugs can promote tumor metastasis.

(4) When investigating the effects of tumors on immune organs,

it was found that as the cancer progressed, the thymus showed progressive atrophy. Immediately after inoculation of cancer cells, the thymus of the host showed acute progressive atrophy, cell proliferation was blocked, and the volume was significantly reduced.

The experimental results suggest that the tumor will inhibit the thymus and cause the immune organs to shrink.

(5) It was also found through experiments that some of the experimental mice did not have a successful vaccination or the tumor grew very small, and the thymus did not shrink significantly.

In order to understand the relationship between tumor and thymus atrophy, when transplanted solid cancer in a group of experimental mice grew into the size of the thumb, it was removed. After 1 month of dissection, the thymus did not undergo progressive atrophy.

Therefore, it is speculated that a solid tumor may produce a factor that is not yet known to inhibit the thymus, which is temporarily called "cancer suppressor factor", which needs further study.

(6) The above experimental results prove that the progression of the tumor will cause the thymus to progressively shrink.

Can be there some ways to prevent the host's thymus from shrinking?

Therefore, we began to use immune organ cell transplantation to restore the experimental function of immune organs.

In the study of suppressing/inhibiting the thymus atrophy of the immune organs during the progress of tumors and looking for ways to restore the function of the thymus and rebuild the immune system, the experimental study of transplantation of fetal liver, fetal spleen and fetal thymus cells to restore immune function was performed by using mice.

The results showed that S, T, L three-level or three types cells were transplanted together, and the complete tumor regression rate was 40% in the near future or the short-term, and the long-term tumor complete regression rate was 46.67%. The tumor completely disappeared and survived for a long time.

(7) When investigating the effect of tumor on the spleen of the immune organs of the body, it was found that the spleen had an inhibitory effect on tumor growth in the early stage of the tumor, and in the late stage of the tumor, the spleen also showed progressive atrophy.

The experimental results suggest that the effect of spleen on tumor growth is bidirectional, with some inhibition in the early stage and no inhibition in the late stage. Spleen cell transplantation can enhance the inhibition of tumors.

(8) The results of follow-up suggest that controlling metastasis is the key to cancer treatment. There are many steps and links in the current known cancer cell metastasis. To stop one of the links can prevent their metastasis. In 1986, the author's laboratory carried out microcirculation research work. Microcirculation microscopy was used to observe microvascular formation and flow rate and flow rate of tumor nodules in transplanted mice.

(9) We design looking for anti-tumor angiogenesis drugs from natural medicines. The Olympus microcirculation microscopy system was used to observe the neovascularization process and count the flow rate and flow rate of the arterioles and venules. And the TG of Huang Lateng ethyl acetate extract was found from Chinese herbal medicine to carry out experiments to inhibit blood vessel formation.

It was found that on the first day of vaccination there was no neovascularization; on the second day microscopic neovascularization was observed, and TG reduced the density of neovascularization into and out of the tumor.

(10) From the large number of tumor-bearing animal models in the laboratory, it was also found that the experimental tumors inoculated subcutaneously in some tumor-bearing mice grew larger, the central tissue structure of the transplanted solid tumor is more different from the surrounding cancer cells. The center of

the nodule is mostly sterile necrosis or liquefaction, and the surrounding area is still active cancer cells. Therefore, in the clinical treatment work, measures for treating sterile necrosis can be employed.

According to the results of laboratory experiments, it was found that resection of the thymus can produce a cancer-bearing animal model. *The thymus progressive atrophy was found in cancer, and it was found that immunity is related to the occurrence and development of cancer, and low immunity is related to the metastasis of cancer.*

It was found that excision of the thymus can produce a model of cancer-bearing animals, and it is found that the thymus is progressively atrophied during cancer, and it is found that immunity is related to the occurrence and development of cancer, and low immunity is related to the metastasis of cancer.

The purpose of the next study and treatment determined is to:

1). to prevent thymus atrophy, increase thymus weight, increase immunity, that is, the principle of treatment of protection of Thymus and protection of bone marrow of hematopoiesis or producing the blood.

2). Based on the above experimental findings, data and information, the experimental basis and theoretical basis of new concepts and methods for anticancer and anti-metastasis treatment were established, namely, preventing progressive atrophy of the thymus, protecting the thymus, increasing the weight of the thymus, increasing immunity, and protecting the bone marrow and promoting the production of bone marrow stem cells and immunogenic cells and improving immune surveillance.

3). It was to settle down the experimental basis and theoretical basis of establishing principles, directions, and guidelines for the treatment Established based on new concepts and methods. That is, biological immunotherapy or XZ-C immunomodulation therapy.

How can it be to stop the thymus from shrinking and protecting the thymus?

After three years of basic laboratory research, the thymus progressive atrophy was discovered during cancer; mouse with excision of the thymus can be inoculated with cancer cells to produce a cancer-bearing animal model. Immunization decrease is associated with the occurrence, development and metastasis of tumors. According to the experimental data and information, it is determined that the treatment goal is to try to protect the thymus, increase the weight of the thymus, prevent thymus atrophy, increase immunity, protect Thymus and increase immune function, and protect the marrow from producing blood. ***The theoretical basis for the new concept of anti-cancer and anti-metastatic treatment, the theoretical system of new methods and clinical practice have been established.***

What method can be used to prevent thymus atrophy and protect the thymus?

Through experiments, the author found that when the fetal Thymus, fetal liver and fetal spleen stem cell in the same kind of fetal rat were transplanted, the tumor disappearance rate reached 46.7% and achieved good results. However, the results of this experiment are difficult to be used in clinical practice because human homologous fetal cells cannot be obtained.

So it was to begin to look for drugs that prevent thymus atrophy and protect the thymus from natural medicines.

Third

The experimental research on finding new anticancer and anti-metastatic drugs in natural medicines

The experimental methods of finding new drugs for anti-cancer and anti-metastasis from natural medicines were the followings:

1. In vitro screening experiment

The cancer cells were cultured in vitro to observe the direct damage of the drug to the cancer cells, and the inhibition rate of cell proliferation caused by cytotoxicity was measured.

2. Tumor inhibition rate in tumor-bearing animals

Each batch of experiments consisted of 240 Kunming mice, divided into 8 groups, 30 in each group. Groups 1 to 6 were experimental groups, each group was screened for 1 traditional Chinese medicine, the seventh group was blank control group, and the eighth group was treated with fluorouracil or cyclophosphamide as a control group. The whole group of mice was treated with EA~C or S180 or H22 cancer cells 1×10^7/ml. After 24 hours of inoculation, each rat was orally fed with crude biological powder according to the body weight of 1000mg/kg, 1/d feeding for 4 weeks. It was to observe survival, adverse reactions, calculate prolonged survival, and calculate tumor inhibition rate.

Among the 200 kinds of crude drugs screened by experiments, 48 of them have certain or even good tumor inhibition rate, and the inhibition rate of cancer cells is 70%-90% or more, and the other 152 kinds of traditional Chinese medicines have no inhibition rate for cancer.

After optimized combination, the tumor inhibition rate experiment in the tumor-bearing animal model was carried out to form XZ-C1~XZ-C10 immunoregulatory particles. XZ-C1 can significantly inhibit cancer cells, but does not affect normal cells.

XZ-C4 can protect the Thymus and increase immune function and improve immune function. XZ-C8 can protect the marrow to produce blood, improve the quality of life, increase appetite, enhance physical fitness and prolong survival term.

Fourth

Clinical validation work

1. After 7 years of scientific experiments in the laboratory, it was to screen from natural medicines and to constitute XZ-C immunomodulatory of anti-cancer, anti-metastasis Chinese medicine with the protection of Thymus and increase of immune function, the protection of bone marrow to produce blood, promoting the blood circulation and dissolving the blood stasis, and the clinical validation work is carried out on the basis of the success of the animal experiment or on the basis of the success of animal experiments, clinical validation work was carried out.

2. Since 1985, one side of the tumor-bearing mouse tumor-bearing animal experiment, clinical efficacy in the outpatient clinic.

2. Since 1985, on the one hand, the tumor-bearing mice were tested in the tumor-bearing mice, and on the other hand, the efficacy was verified in the outpatient clinic. However, there are few patients, and there is no medical record in the outpatient clinic (the medical records are all issued to patients), and it is impossible to accumulate scientific research materials. It must take the road of scientific research and cooperation.

3. Set up an anti-cancer research collaboration group, take the road of scientific research and cooperation, and jointly set up the research road, and set up the Dawn or Shuguang Oncology Clinic.

4. Resume outpatient medical records, fill in complete and detailed outpatient medical records, obtain complete information of clinical verification, facilitate analysis and statistics, and be conducive to outpatient clinical research to improve medical quality.

5. The outpatient cases were kept, and they were followed up regularly. The experience and lessons of the diagnosis and treatment of this case were analyzed briefly to observe the long-term effects.

6. The oncology clinic outpatient medical records are designed in a tabular format, which contains all relevant medical information and relevant epidemiological data to facilitate statistical analysis of possible pathogenic factors.

7. After more than one year of follow-up, outpatient medical records, the medical records are summarized, and the large table analysis is carried out. The contents of the large table include the contents of the outpatient medical record form, which are concise and detailed, and detailed.

The Twilight Oncology Clinic has been verified for 14 years, and the large table has accumulated more than 10,000 outpatient clinical data for outpatient clinical research.

7. The cases and Outpatient medical records which follow up more than 1 year are all written into medical records summary and add on the big table analysis, each item in the large form contains the contents of the outpatient medical record form. That is to be concise and detailed, and that has both the detailed and throughout. Dawning or Twilight Oncology Clinic has been verified for 14 years. The large table has accumulated nearly 10,000 outpatient clinical data for outpatient clinical research.

8. From experimental research to clinical research, from clinical to experimental, the collaborative group has experimental research bases and clinical application verification bases. The former is in the medical school laboratory, and the latter is in the Twilight Oncology Clinic. From experiment to clinical, that is, based on the success of experimental research, it is applied to the clinic, and new problems are found in the clinical application process. Further basic research is carried out, and new experimental results are applied to clinical verification.

For example, outpatients with liver cancer with portal vein tumor thrombus, renal cancer patients with inferior vena cava tumor thrombus. Some are CT reports, and some are pathological sections of surgically removed specimens. **In fact, the cancer plug is the cancer cell group on the way to transfer, is the third manifestation of cancer in the human body. After we found** a cancer thrombus problem, we began the experimental study of cancer thrombus formation. It was to look for new ways to fight against cancerous plugs and dissolve cancerous plugs. As a result, we found four kinds of traditional Chinese medicines that help to dissolve cancerous plugs and found out their active ingredients.

Such experiments → clinical → re-experiment → re-clinical, continuous cyclical rise, after 12 years of clinical practice experience, awareness continues to rise, it was to sum up practice; after conducting analysis and reflection and evaluation, it has risen to the theory and proposes new understanding, new thinking, and new treatment ideas.

9. In the past 12 years, through a large number of outpatient consultations after analysis, evaluation, reflection, a series of clinical problems was found, further research and improvement is needed.

10. From the review, analysis and reflection of a large number of outpatient medical records, it is recognized that postoperative adjuvant chemotherapy in many patients fails to prevent recurrence and even promotes immune failure. This indicates that chemotherapy needs further research and improvement.

11. From the review, analysis and reflection of a large number of outpatient medical records, it is recognized that many patients have recurrence and metastasis soon after surgery. The design of "radical surgery" needs further research and improvement. *How to do the intraoperative tumor-free technology to prevent and treat the shedding and planting of cancer cells in the thoracic cavity or abdominal cavity or surgical field cancer cells is an important measure to prevent postoperative recurrence and metastasis.*

12. Through the collaborative group to focus on a large number of cases of treatment practice, evaluation, analysis, reflection, and experience the following points:

(1) Current postoperative adjuvant chemotherapy:

Many patients fail to prevent cancer recurrence and metastasis.

(2) The focus of anti-cancer should be anti-metastasis and recurrence, which is the key to improve the long-term efficacy of postoperative patients.

(3) The "threshold" of anti-cancer should be "three early".

(4) Anti-cancer recurrence must start from the surgery:

From the data of outpatients, some radical hospitals underwent radical surgery without rules and regulation, therefore, the recurrence is early and the abdominal cavity is widely metastasized or there were recurrence early and extensive intra-abdominal metastasis. The education and learning of standardized and regulated cancer surgery should be strengthened.

(5) Some patients with postoperative cancer have weak constitution and it is 4 cycles of chemotherapy or 6 cycles of chemotherapy, which promotes the decline of immune function and even exhaustion. Why do you want 4 cycles or 6 cycles, and what is the theoretical basis or experimental data?

The theoretical basis of laboratory experimental research with 4 courses of chemotherapy or 6 courses of treatment has not been found in domestic and foreign literatures.

13.

Through review, analyze, reflect, evaluate from 14 years of access to a large number of outpatients, the diagnosis of current cancer mainly relies on pathological sections. However, pathological sections must be obtained after surgery, intraoperative or endoscopic biopsy or puncture, which is in the middle and late stages. *Therefore, we should try to study new methods of early diagnosis and new tumor markers.*

14. Looking back or Judging from the positive performance of CT, MRI, and color Doppler examinations in a large number of outpatients, once CT, MRI, color Doppler, etc. see the place, most of the patients are mostly in the advanced stage, and some have lost the opportunity for surgery. Therefore, we should try to study and find new new technologies, new markers and new diagnostic methods that can be discovered early.

15. Clinical efficacy observation:

On the basis of experimental research, since 1994 the medications have been applied to clinically various types of cancer, which mostly patients are with stage III or IV.

That is, advanced cancer that cannot be removed by exploration; recent or long-term metastasis or recurrence after various cancer operations; liver metastasis, lung metastasis, brain metastasis, bone metastasis or cancerous pleural effusion and cancerous ascites in various advanced or late-stage cancers; various cancer palliative resection, exploration can only do gastric thoracic anastomosis or colostomy can not be removed; patients who are not suitable for surgery, radiotherapy or chemotherapy.

XZ-C immunomodulation anticancer Chinese medicine has been clinically applied for 14 years, and systematic observation has achieved obvious curative effect. No adverse reactions were observed after long-term use. Clinical observations have proven that XZ-C immunomodulatory Chinese medicine can comprehensively improve the quality of life of patients with advanced cancer, improve the body's immunity, control cancer cell proliferation, consolidate and enhance the long-term efficacy after surgery or chemotherapy or radiotherapy.

16. **Oral administration and external application of XZ-C drug have a good effect on softening and reducing body surface metastasis.** Combined with intervention or intubation pump treatment, it can protect the liver, kidney, bone marrow hematopoietic system and immune organs, and improve immunity.

In the Dawning or Twilight Oncology Clinic, 4,698 patients with stage III, IV or metastatic recurrent cancer were treated for long-term follow-up or follow-up.

17. **The evaluation of the quality of life of patients with advanced cancer with taking XZ-C immunomodulatory Chinese medicine :**

The patients were all middle-advanced patients. After taking the drug, the improvement of symptoms was 93.2%, the mental improvement was 95.2%, the appetite was improved by 93%, and the physical strength was increased by 57.3%. The overall quality of life of patients with advanced cancer was improved.

The 42nd Annual Meeting of the American Society of Clinical Oncology (ASCO) proposed that comprehensive assessment of the quality of life of loyalists is one of the main treatment goals. A total of 223 articles in the 2006 ASCO conference papers were related to the quality of life of patients, accounting for 5.8 of the total number of papers. %, quality of life has become an important factor that people must consider when choosing a treatment strategy.

For understanding the purpose of anti-tumor treatment, as people continue to improve the quality of life of cancer loyalists as one of the main purposes of treatment, a large number of studies have begun to take the impact of treatment on quality of life as the main evaluation indicators.

A total of 223 articles in the ASCO conference papers in 2006 were related to the quality of life of patients, accounting for 5.8% of the total number of papers. Quality of life has become an important factor that must be considered when people choose treatment strategies. The understanding of the purpose of anti-tumor treatment has made people increasingly improve the quality of life of cancer patients as one of the main purposes of treatment. A large number of studies have begun to take the impact of treatment on quality of life as the main evaluation index.

18. XZ-C anti-cancer analgesic effect:

Pain is a more obvious and painful symptom in patients with advanced cancer. General analgesics have little effect on cancer pain, and narcotic analgesics are addictive and analgesic. XZ-C anti-cancer analgesic cream has strong analgesic effect and lasts for a long time. After 298 cases of clinical verification, the effective rate was 78.0%, and the total effective rate was 95.3%. Repeated use did not show obvious adverse reactions, no addiction, and the analgesic effect was stable. It is an effective treatment for cancer patients to relieve pain and improve their quality of life.

19. Efficacy evaluation:

Paying attention to the short-term efficacy and imaging indicators, and paying more attention to the long-term efficacy of survival, quality of life and immune indicators. The goal is to have a long life and good quality of life. During the course of medication, it is necessary to pay attention to changes in self-conscious symptoms and improvement of self-conscious symptoms for more than one month, otherwise it is invalid. It is effective to pay attention to the spirit, good appetite, and quality of life (Carson's score) for more than one month, otherwise it will be invalid. The evaluation criteria for solid tumor mass were classified into 4 grades according to the size of the tumor, that is, the grade 1 mass disappeared, the grade II mass was reduced by 1/2, the grade III mass became soft, and the grade IV mass did not change or increase.

In this book, Xu Ze published the basic research and clinical research of the new concept and new method of cancer metastasis treatment. The new findings of a series of experimental research and the theoretical innovation of clinical research are original innovations: Xu Ze first discovered and proposed the following five clinically applied oncology theoretical innovations in the world: theoretical innovation content:

1. Three manifestations of cancer in the human body; theoretical innovations;

2. The "two points and one line" theory of the whole process of cancer development; theoretical innovation content;

3. cancer transfer treatment "three steps"; theoretical innovation content;

4. Open up the third field of human anti-cancer metastasis treatment; theoretical innovation;

5. The new concept, new model of XU ZE cancer therapy.

Printed in the United States
By Bookmasters